The Human Body

in Health and Disease

Fifth Edition

Ruth Lundeen Memmler, M.D.

*Professor Emeritus, Life Sciences;
formerly Coordinator, Health, Life Sciences, and
Nursing,
East Los Angeles College, Los Angeles,
California*

Dena Lin Wood, R.N., B.S., P.H.N.

*Staff Nurse, Memorial Hospital of Glendale,
Glendale, California*

Illustrated by Anthony Ravielli

J. B. Lippincott Company

Philadelphia
London   Mexico City   New York   St. Louis
São Paulo   Sydney

Sponsoring Editor: Bernice Heller
Manuscript Editor: Helen Ewan
Indexer: Gene Heller
Art Director: Tracy Baldwin
Cover Photograph: Steve Allen—Peter Arnold, Inc.
Designer: William Boehm
Production Supervisor: N. Carol Kerr
Production Coordinator: Charles W. Field
Compositor: Kingsport Press
Printer/Binder: Kingsport Press

Fifth Edition

Library of Congress Cataloging in Publication Data

Memmler, Ruth Lundeen.
    The human body in health and disease.

    Bibliography: p.
    Includes index.
    1. Human physiology. 2. Physiology,
Pathological. 3. Anatomy, Human. I. Wood, Dena
Lin. II. Title.
QP34.5.M48   1983   612   82–12743
ISBN 0–397–54385–9
ISBN 0–397–54386–7 (pbk.)

To our students and to our families

Preface

In this, the fifth edition of *The Human Body in Health and Disease,* we have taken note of many important recent developments and concepts related to human physiology. At the same time, we have tried to avoid complicating the material for beginning students—the audience to which this book is addressed. As has been true of previous editions, the primary aim is to describe and explain the fundamental facts and principles of human structure (anatomy) and function (physiology), and abnormalities of structure and function (pathology). We have included discussions of those disorders that the health worker is most likely to encounter in the community or in the hospital. Rare diseases that are managed mainly in intensive or special care facilities are not covered.

In response to instructors' requests and suggestions, the physiology content has been expanded throughout the book. For example, material on cell development and function has been both simplified and expanded, to give the student a complete picture of this essential topic.

Former Chapter 9, Bones, Joints, and Muscles, has been divided into two chapters, Chapter 9, Bones and Joints, and Chapter 10, The Muscular System. This separation has allowed us to provide better coverage of each of the topics, and to pay proper attention to principles of muscle physiology, which is essential to understanding the whole of human physiology.

Chapter 7, Disease and Disease-Producing Organisms, and Chapter 13, The Blood, are additional examples of the greater emphasis on physiology and on providing the total picture.

Placing the content on body fluids and electrolytes in a separate chapter has enabled us to give broader and more accurate coverage of this topic.

Instructors who have used earlier editions of the book will notice a few changes in chapter sequence. We believe that both they and their students will find the new sequence more logical and easier to follow than was the case with previous editions. Nevertheless, the book retains the unique quality of being readily adaptable to class needs. For example, some instructors have told us that they begin with the chapter on digestion because of the importance of diet and of the health worker's role in teaching patients, while other instructors prefer to begin with the chapter on the brain, the spinal cord, and the nerves, because the nervous system controls the all-important processes of circulation and respiration. This flexibility appears to be desirable in an introductory textbook.

As before, our goal has been to explain every topic clearly and simply, so that students having their initial exposure to human anatomy and physiology can immediately feel at ease with the material. It is our hope that this introduction will serve to motivate students to study further.

Ruth L. Memmler, M.D.
Dena L. Wood, R.N., B.S., P.H.N.

Acknowledgments

We thank the many readers who have taken the time to make suggestions about changes to improve the book. Particularly do we thank Lea Tupper Davidson, Professor of Medical Record Science, Department of Health Sciences, East Los Angeles College, who has used *The Human Body in Health and Disease* over a period of years and who has made useful recommendations to us. We express our appreciation and indebtedness to the staff of the J. B. Lippincott Company, especially Bernice Heller, Development Editor for Basic Sciences, and David T. Miller, Vice President.

Contents

22

Heredity and Hereditary Diseases *321*

23

Immunity, Vaccines, and Serums *329*

Glossary Guide

To the Student:
To aid you in your study of this text, a complete list of glossary terms is provided below. For convenience, the chapter number in which each term is introduced is also listed.

Chapter 1

The General Plan of the Human Body

1

Glossary

Anterior, ventral   Near the belly surface or front of the body

Caudal   Inferior; away from the head

Cell membrane   Outer covering of the cell

Cranial   Near the head

Cytoplasm   The cell protoplasm outside the nucleus

Diaphragm   Any partition that separates one area from another, especially the dome-shaped musculomembranous partition between the thoracic and abdominal cavities

Distal   Farthest from a point of reference

Dorsal, posterior   Near the back of the body

Lateral   Toward the side of a body or structure

Medial   Near the midline of a body or structure

Nucleolus   A tiny globule located within the nucleus of a cell

Organ   Groups of tissues that together perform a single function

Organelle   A specific particle of living material present in most cells and serving a specific function in the cell

Protoplasm   The living building material of all organisms, plants, and animals; the only matter in which life is manifested

Proximal   Nearest to a point of reference

Superior   Above; in a higher position

System   Groups of organs that together perform certain functions

Tissue   Groups of cells having a specialized function

What Are Living Things Made Of?

According to a nursery rhyme, children are made of sugar and spice, or perhaps of puppy dogs' tails, depending on which sex we are discussing. More accurately, the "stuff" of which all living things are made is called *protoplasm* (pro'to-plazm). This word is made up of two Greek words: *proto,* meaning "original," and *plasm,* meaning "substance." Chemically, protoplasm is composed of quite ordinary elements, such as carbon, oxygen, hydrogen, sulfur, nitrogen, and phosphorus. There is nothing extraordinary, either, in the appearance of protoplasm; it looks very much like the white of an egg. Yet, nobody has been able to explain why protoplasm has that characteristic which we call life. We shall learn more about this intricate substance in later chapters.

The building material of all living things, both plants and animals, is protoplasm, and the building blocks made of this material are called *cells* (see Fig. 1-1). Cells vary a great deal in size. Something as small as a worm may be composed of millions of cells, yet we all are familiar with at least one of the larger kinds of cells, of which an egg is a perfectly good example. In fact, if we keep the egg in mind, the construction of the cell will be quite easy to visualize. Let us work our way from the outside to the center.

First comes the outer covering, called the *cell membrane.* Next is the main substance of the cell, the *cytoplasm* (si'to-plazm), which might be likened to the white of the egg. The cytoplasm contains water, food particles, pigment, and other special-ized materials. In the center of the cell, comparable with the egg yolk, is a globule called the *nucleus* (nu'kle-us), containing the chromatin (kro'mah-tin) network. The nucleus controls some of the activities of the cell, including its reproduction. Within the nucleus is still another tiny globule of matter called the *nucleolus* (nu-kle'o-lus), the function of which is related to reproduction. The unique ability of a cell to reproduce, as well as the structure and function of organized particles within the cytoplasm, called organelles (or''gan-els'), are discussed in Chapter 2.

The scientific study of cells began with the invention by Anton van Leeuwenhoek of the microscope some 350 years ago. In time, his single-lens microscope was replaced by the modern compound microscope which has two sets of lenses. This is the type in use in most laboratories. In recent years, a great boon to microbiologists has been the development of the electron microscope, which by a

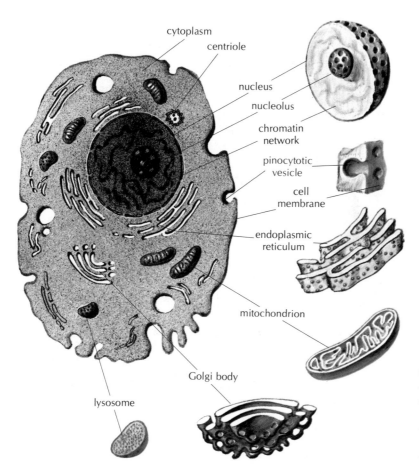

cytoplasm
centriole
nucleus
nucleolus
chromatin network
pinocytotic vesicle
cell membrane
endoplasmic reticulum
mitochondrion
Golgi body
lysosome

Fig. 1-1 A typical cell. The nucleus is the control center. The organelles—the endoplasmic reticulum, the mitochondrion, the Golgi body, and the lysosomes—perform specialized tasks.

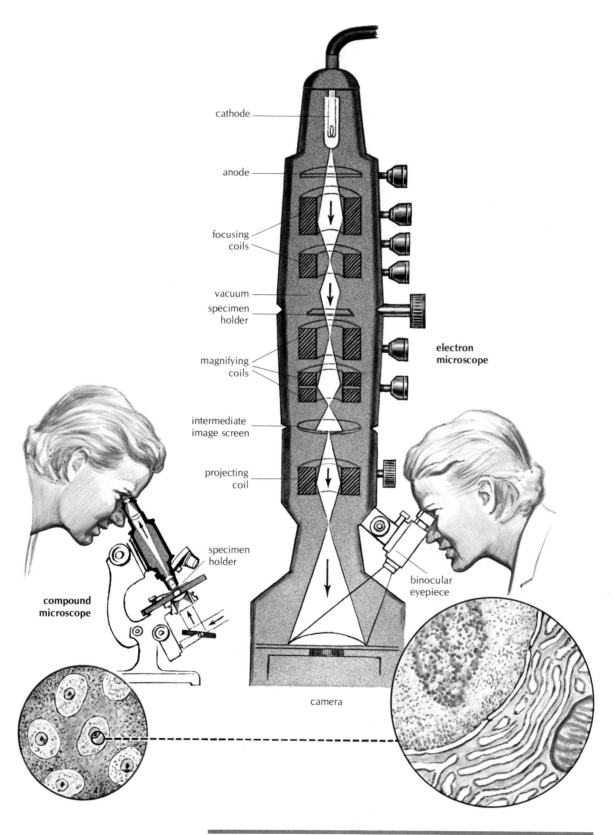

cathode

anode

focusing
coils

vacuum

specimen
holder

magnifying
coils

intermediate
image screen

projecting
coil

**electron
microscope**

**compound
microscope**

specimen
holder

binocular
eyepiece

camera

Fig. 1-2 *A simplified comparison of an optical microscope and
an electron microscope.*

combination of magnification and enlargement of the resulting image affords magnification to one million times or more (Fig. 1-2).

The cell, then, is the basic unit of all life. When you study the causes of disease, you will encounter a number of primitive living things that are composed of but one cell. However, for the moment we shall confine our discussion to the human body, which is made up of many millions of cells. The body is composed of specialized groups of cells, the first of which are called *tissues.* Various tissues that together perform a single function form *organs,* and several organs and parts grouped together for certain functions form *systems.* The heart is an organ composed of muscle tissue, connective tissue, and nerve tissue, all working together to pump blood. The heart and the blood vessels constitute the circulatory system.

Body Systems

The body systems have been variously stated to be nine, ten, or eleven in number, depending on how much detail one wishes to include.
Here is one list of systems:

1 The **skeletal system.** The basic framework of the body is a system of over 200 bones with their joints, collectively known as the skeleton.
2 The **muscular system.** Body movements result from the action of the muscles which are attached to the bones. Other types of muscles are present in the walls of such organs as the intestine and the heart.
3 The **circulatory system.** The heart and blood vessels make up the system whereby blood is pumped to all the body tissues, bringing with it food, oxygen, and other substances, and carrying away waste materials. Lymph vessels and nodes play an important supporting role.
4 The **digestive system.** This system comprises all organs that have to do with taking in food and converting the useful parts of it into substances that the body cells can use. Examples of these organs are the mouth, the teeth, the alimentary canal (esophagus, stomach, and intestine), the liver, and the pancreas.
5 The **respiratory system.** This includes the lungs and the passages leading to them. The purpose of this system is to take in air and from it extract oxygen which is then dissolved into the blood and conveyed to all the tissues. A waste product of the cells, carbon dioxide, is taken by the blood to the lungs, whence it is expelled to the outside air.
6 The **integumentary** (in-teg-u-men′tar-e) **system.** The word integument (in-teg′u-ment) means skin. The skin is considered by some authorities to be a separate body system. It includes the skin and its appendages, the nails and sweat and oil glands.
7 The **urinary system.** This is also called the excretory system. Its main components are the kidneys, the ureters, the bladder, and the urethra. Its chief purpose is to rid the body of certain waste products and excess water. (Note that other waste products are removed by the digestive and the respiratory systems.)
8 The **nervous system.** The brain, the spinal cord, and the nerves make up this very complex system by which most parts of the body are controlled and coordinated. The organs of special sense (such as the eyes, ears, taste buds, and organs of smell), sometimes classed as a separate *sensory system,* together with the sense of touch, receive stimuli from the outside world. These stimuli are converted into impulses that are transmitted to the brain. The brain determines to a great extent the body's responses to messages from without and within, and in it occur such higher functions as memory and reasoning.
9 The **endocrine system.** A few scattered organs known as endocrine glands produce special substances called hormones, which regulate such body functions as growth, food utilization within the cells, and reproduction. Examples of endocrine glands are the thyroid and the pituitary glands.
10 The **reproductive system.** This system includes the external sex organs and all related inner structures that are concerned with the production of new individuals.

Directions in the Body

Because it would be awkward and incorrect to speak of bandaging the "southwest part" of the chest, a number of terms have been devised to

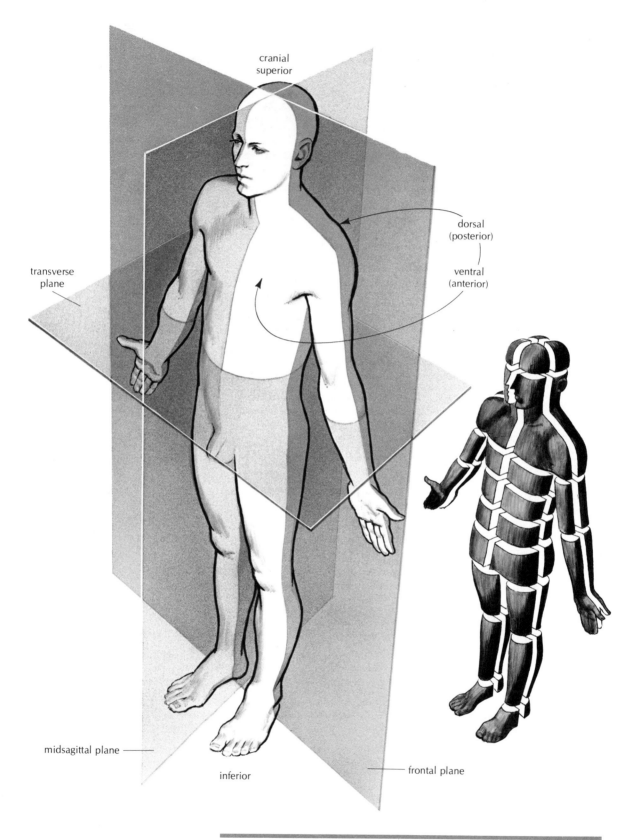

cranial
superior

transverse
plane

dorsal
(posterior)

ventral
(anterior)

midsagittal plane

inferior

frontal plane

Fig. 1-3 Body planes and directions.

designate specific regions and directions in the body. Some of the more important of these are listed as follows (note that they refer to the body in the *anatomic position*—upright with palms facing forward):

1 **Superior** is a relative term meaning above or in a higher position. Its opposite, **inferior,** means below or lower. The heart, for example, is superior to the intestine.
2 **Ventral** and **anterior** mean the same thing in humans: located near the belly surface or front of the body. Their corresponding opposites, **dorsal** and **posterior,** refer to locations nearer the back.
3 **Cranial** means near the head; **caudal,** near the sacral region of the spinal column (*i.e.,* where the tail is located in lower animals).
4 **Medial** means near an imaginary plane that passes through the midline of the body, dividing it into left and right portions. **Lateral,** its opposite, means farther away from the midline, toward the side.
5 **Proximal** means nearest the origin of a structure; **distal,** farthest from that point. For example, the part of your thumb where it joins your hand is its proximal region. The tip of the thumb is its distal region.

For convenience in visualizing the spatial relationships of various body structures to each other, anatomists have divided the body by means of three imaginary planes. Think of a body plane as a huge cleaver (Fig. 1-3).

1 The **midsagittal** (mid-saj′i-tal) **plane.** If the cleaver were to cut the body in two down the middle in a fore-and-aft direction, separating it into right and left portions, the sections you would see would be midsagittal.
2 The **frontal plane.** If, instead of the above operation, the cleaver were held in line with the ears and then were brought down the middle of the body, creating a front and a rear portion, you would see a front (anterior or ventral) section and a rear (posterior or dorsal) section.
3 The **transverse plane.** If the cleaver blade were swung horizontally, it would divide the body into an upper (superior) part and a lower (infe-

rior) portion. There could be many such cross sections, each of which is on a transverse plane.

Body Cavities

The body contains a few large internal spaces or *cavities* within which various organs are located. There are two groups of cavities: *dorsal* and *ventral* (Fig. 1-4).

Dorsal Cavities

There are two dorsal cavities: the *cranial cavity,* containing the brain, and the *spinal canal,* enclosing the spinal cord. Both of these cavities join, hence they are a continuous space.

Ventral Cavities

The ventral cavities are much larger than the dorsal ones. There are two ventral cavities: the *thoracic* (tho-ras′ik) *cavity,* containing mainly the heart, the lungs, and the large blood vessels, and the *abdominal cavity.* This latter space is subdivided into two portions, one containing the stomach, most of the intestine, the kidneys, the liver, the gallbladder, the pancreas, and the spleen, and a lower one called the *pelvis,* or pelvic cavity, in which are located the urinary bladder, the rectum, and the internal parts of the reproductive system.

Unlike the dorsal cavities, the ventral cavities are not continuous. They are separated by a muscular partition, the *diaphragm* (di′ah-fram), the function of which is discussed in Chapter 17.

Regions in the Abdominal Cavity

Because the abdominal cavity is so large, it is helpful to divide it into nine regions. These are shown in Fig. 1-5. The three central regions are the *epigastrium* (ep-i-gas′tre-um), located just below the breastbone; the *umbilical* (um-bil′i-kal) *region* about the umbilicus (um-bil′i-kus), commonly called the navel; and the *hypogastric* (hi-po-gas′trik) *region,* the lowest of all of the midline regions. At each side are the right and left *hypochondriac* (hi-po-kon′dre-ak) regions, just below the ribs; then the right and left *lumbar* regions; and, finally, the right and left *iliac,* or *inguinal* (in′gwi-nal), regions. A much simpler division into four

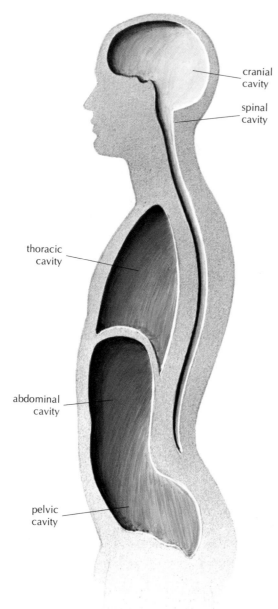

cranial
cavity

spinal
cavity

thoracic
cavity

abdominal
cavity

pelvic
cavity

▓ **ventral body cavity**

░ **dorsal body cavities**

Fig. 1-4 *Side view of body cavities.*

quadrants (right upper, left upper, right lower, left lower) is now less frequently used.

The Metric System

Now that we have set the stage for further study of the body and its structure and processes, a look at the metric system would be in order since it is rapidly replacing the present system of measurement in the United States. The drug industry and the health-care industry already have converted to the metric system, so anyone who plans a career in health should be acquainted with metrics.

To use the metric system easily and correctly may require a bit of effort as is often the case with

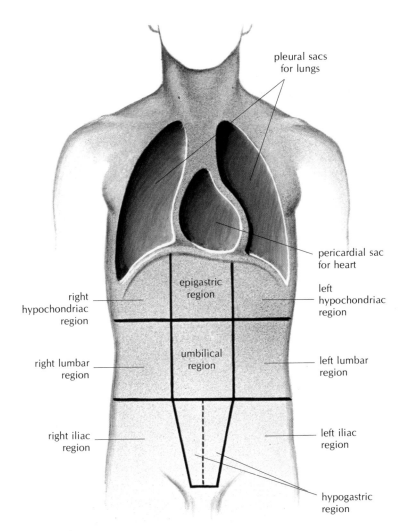

pleural sacs
for lungs

pericardial sac
for heart

right
hypochondriac
region

epigastric
region

left
hypochondriac
region

right lumbar
region

umbilical
region

left lumbar
region

right iliac
region

left iliac
region

hypogastric
region

Fig. 1-5 *Front view of body cavities and the regions of the abdomen.*

any new idea. Actually, you already know something about the metric system because our monetary system is similar to it in that both are decimal systems. One hundred cents equals one dollar; one hundred centimeters equals one meter. The first step is to learn the meanings of the following prefixes:

Centi (1/100)—100 centimeters (cm) = 1 meter (m)

Milli (1/1000)—1000 millimeters (mm) = 1 meter (m)

Kilo (1,000)—1000 meters = 1 kilometer (kil′o-me-ter) (km)

The metric system includes other measurements, but these are the ones used most frequently. Millimeters, centimeters, meters, and kilometers are linear measurements that correspond to inches,

feet, yards, and miles, respectively. In this text, we have included the metric equivalents for inches, feet, and so on to indicate the size of an organ or part (Fig. 1-6). Some equivalents that may help you to appreciate the size of various body parts are as follows:

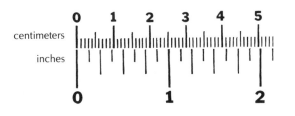

Fig. 1-6 *Comparison of centimeters and inches.*

1 mm = 0.04 in, or 1 in = 25 mm
1 cm = 0.4 in, or 1 in = 2.5 cm
1 m = 3.3 ft, or 1 ft = 30 cm

The same prefixes are used as for the linear measurements. The meter is the standard for length, and the gram, for weights. Thirty grams is approximately equal to one ounce, and one kilogram to two and two tenths pounds. Drug dosages are usually stated in grams or milligrams. One thousand milligrams equals one gram; a 500-milligram (mg) dose would be the equivalent of 0.5 gram (g), and 250 mg is equal to 0.25 g.

The dosages of liquid medications are indicated as volume. The standard metric measurement for volume is the liter (le'ter). There are 1000 milliliters (ml) in a liter (l). A liter is slightly greater than a quart, a liter being equal to 1.06 quarts. For smaller quantities, the milliliter (ml) is used most of the time. There are 5 ml in a teaspoon and 15 ml in a tablespoon. A fluid ounce contains 30 ml.

The Celsius (centigrade) temperature scale, now in use by most other countries as well as by scientists in this country, is discussed in Chapter 6.

Summary

1 Living matter.
  A Basic substance—protoplasm.
  B Structural unit—cell.
  C Principal parts of cell—cell membrane, cytoplasm, nucleus, nucleolus.
  D Organization of body cells—tissues, organs, systems.
2 Body systems—skeletal, muscular, circulatory, digestive, respiratory, integumentary, urinary, nervous (and sensory), endocrine, reproductive.
3 Body directions.
  A Superior, near head; inferior, away from head.
  B Ventral (anterior), near belly; dorsal (posterior), near back.
  C Cranial, near head; caudal, near end of spinal column.
  D Medial, near midsagittal plane; lateral, toward side.
  E Proximal, near origin; distal, distant from origin.

  F Body division by planes.
    (1) Midsagittal—left and right portions.
    (2) Frontal—front and rear portions.
    (3) Transverse—top and bottom portions.
4 Body cavities.
  A Dorsal.
    (1) Cranial.
    (2) Spinal.
  B Ventral.
    (1) Thoracic.
    (2) Abdominal.
      (a) 9 regions include epigastric, umbilical, hypogastric, right and left hypochondriac, right and left lumbar, and right and left iliac, or inguinal.
      (b) 4 quadrants (no longer extensively used).
  C Dorsal cavities continuous, abdominal cavities separated by diaphragm.
5 The metric system.
A logical decimal system.

Questions and Problems

1 Of what substance is living matter composed?
2 Define a cell. Name 4 main components of a typical cell.
3 Define tissue, organ, body, system.
4 List the body systems, including a brief description of each with respect to its function.
5 List the opposite term for each of the following body directions: superior, ventral, anterior, cranial, medial, proximal. Define each item in the complete list.
6 What are the 3 main body planes? Explain the division of each.
7 Make a rough sketch of the 2 principal groups of body cavities, indicating the 9 divisions of the largest cavity.
8 Why should you learn the metric system? What are its advantages?

Chapter 2

Cells, Tissues, and Tumors

2

Glossary

Adipose Fat; containing fat, as adipose tissue.

Anabolism The building-up phase of metabolism, in which the cell uses simple substances such as amino acids to assemble more complex substances.

Axon The nerve fiber that carries impulses away from the nerve cell body.

CAT, CT Computerized axial tomography, performed with a special scanner that produces cross-sectional views of body parts, for detection of tumors.

Catabolism The degradation, or breaking-down, phase of metabolism in which the cell nutrients are changed from complex to simple forms.

Chromosomes Small rod-shaped bodies that stain deeply and appear in the nucleus at the time of cell division (mitosis). They contain the hereditary factors, the genes.

Collagen A protein that serves as the "glue" that provides for structure in cells and connective tissue throughout the body.

Dendrite A nerve fiber that conducts impulses to the cell body.

Deoxyribonucleic acid, DNA The nucleic acid primarily found in the nucleus of cells; the hereditary material of each cell.

Diffusion The process of becoming spread out, as any gaseous substance that spreads throughout a room; the movement of molecules from any area of high concentration to one of lower concentration.

Enzyme A specialized protein that speeds up the chemical reactions within the body; enzymes help the organelles in the vital process of metabolism, energy conversion, reproduction, and elimination of waste products.

Epithelium The tissue that forms the outer part (epidermis) of the skin; it lines blood vessels, hollow organs, and passages that lead to the outside of the body, and makes up the active part of many glands.

Extracellular Outside a cell or cells.

Filtration The passage of a liquid through a filter or a membrane that acts as a filter.

Immunotherapy A type of passive immunization in which antibodies are administered to increase the body defenses against cancer.

Intracellular   Within the cell.

Laser   *L*ight *a*mplification by *s*timulated *e*mission of *r*adiation. A device that produces a very highly concentrated and intense beam of light.

Metabolism   The physical and chemical changes or processes by which living substance is maintained and by which energy is produced.

Metastasis   The process of spread of tumor cells from their original location.

Myelin   The fatlike substance that forms a covering for many nerve fibers; these are called myelinated nerve fibers.

Neoplasm   Any new, abnormal growth of cells.

Neurilemma   A very thin membrane wrapping the nerve fibers of the peripheral nervous system.

Neuroglia   The special connective tissue of the central nervous system.

Neuron   The nerve cell body plus its processes; the structural unit of nerve tissue.

Nevus (pl. nevi)   A small skin tumor, usually congenital in origin, which may be vascular or nonvascular. It is sometimes called a mole.

Osmosis   The passage of a pure solvent, such as water, from a solution of lesser concentration to one of greater concentration through a semipermeable membrane.

Ribonucleic acid, RNA   The substance that carries DNA, the blueprint for all cells, to all parts of the body.

More About Cells

In Chapter 1, we learned that the cell is the fundamental building block of all life, no matter whether the living thing is made of one cell or many millions of them. A cell may live alone or may be only one unit of a complex structure. Wherever it exists, the cell, during its life cycle, performs those activities characteristic of living matter. The life functions are carried out by the specialized *organelles* within each cell. In order that cells may undergo chemical changes vital to sustaining life, without using large amounts of energy, specialized proteins called *enzymes* are present to assist the organelles

in metabolizing nutrients, in eliminating waste products, in converting stored nutrients to energy, and in reproducing.

Protein Synthesis

Since protein molecules play an indispensable part in the body's activities, we need to identify the cellular substances that direct the production of protein. In the cytoplasm and in the nucleus are chemicals called *nucleic* (nu-kle′-ik) *acids*. The two nucleic acids important in protein production are *ribonucleic* (ri-bo-nu-kle′-ik) *acid,* abbreviated *RNA,* and *deoxyribonucleic* (de-ok-se-ri-bo-nu-kle′-ik) *acid,* or *DNA.* DNA molecules are found in the cell nucleus, arranged in a double spiral (Fig. 2-1). The strands of the spiral are held together by hydrogen bonds. In the nucleus, which is the control center of the cell, DNA exists in this spiral form on the *chromosomes* (kro′-mo-soms). Chromosomes are spindle-shaped rods made up primarily of DNA; they contain the genes, which are the hereditary factors of each cell. It is the genes that carry the messages for the development of particular inherited characteristics, such as brown eyes or long noses. Thus, the nucleus is considered the cell's control center and DNA, the master blueprint.

A blueprint is only a map. The directions it illustrates must be translated into appropriate actions. RNA carries the DNA message and transmits it to the organelles responsible for protein synthesis, the ribosomes ("protein factories") on the endoplasmic reticulum. DNA sends the code by breaking its hydrogen bonds and uncoiling into single spirals. The sequence of molecules on the single strand of DNA contains the map for the production of a particular protein. RNA is a substance with a structure similar to that of single-stranded DNA. When the DNA uncoils and reveals its sequence of molecules, RNA copies the message and carries it to the ribosomes on the endoplasmic reticulum. Here the message is decoded to produce chains of amino acids, the building blocks of protein.

Cell Division

To ensure that every cell in the body has similar genetic information, cell reproduction occurs by

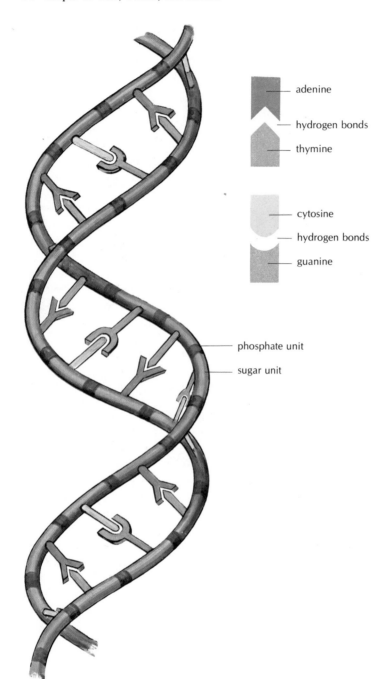

adenine

hydrogen bonds

thymine

cytosine

hydrogen bonds

guanine

phosphate unit

sugar unit

Fig. 2-1 *Schematic representation of the basic structure of a DNA molecule. Each structural unit consists of a phosphate group and a sugar group to which is attached a nitrogen base (adenine or thymine, cytosine or guanine). Adenine, thymine, cytosine, and guanine are enzymes that "spell out" all the genetic instructions that control all activities of the cell.*

a dividing process called mitosis. The original parent cell divides to form two identical daughter cells.

During every cell division spectacular changes occur in the nucleus. DNA uncoils from its double-stranded spiral form and each strand duplicates itself. The strands return to their spiral organization. Now, two spiral structures of DNA exist to supply identical genetic information to each of the future daughter cells. The chromatin material, DNA and other protein molecules, found in the nucleus during times between active division, compacts to become rod-shaped bodies—the chromosomes—which contain the genes. Remember, there are two sets of chromosomes.

Meanwhile, in the cytoplasm, one pair of centrioles moves to the opposite side of the cell, trailing threadlike substances which form a structure resembling a spindle stretched across the cell. Then, the chromosomes line up in the nuclear area along the threadlike spindles, and one of each of the duplicated chromosomes begins to move toward opposite sides of the cell. As mitosis continues, the nuclear area becomes pinched in the middle until two nuclear regions have formed. A similar change occurs in the cell membrane and proceeds until the cell resembles a dumbbell. Now, each pair of centrioles replicates (is repeated). The midsection between the two halves of the dumbbell becomes smaller and smaller until, finally, the cell splits in two. There are now two identical daughter cells, which are themselves identical to, but smaller than, the parent cell (Fig. 2-2).

So far, so good; we have two new cells identical to the parent cell, but smaller and less mature. Therefore, the new cells need to grow and mature in order to carry out the life functions.

Cell Nourishment

In order to grow, cells require food and must have a method to receive this nourishment. This would seem to be a problem, since we learned that most cells are surrounded by a protective membrane. However, if the cell is bathed in a liquid containing dissolved food materials, an interesting thing happens: the liquid with the dissolved food particles passes through the cell membrane. Not only do the dissolved nutrient molecules pass in, but waste products pass out of the cell in the opposite direction, enabling the cell to perform the function of elimination. The membrane also keeps valuable protein and other substances from leaving the cell and prevents the admission of undesirable substances. For this reason, the cell membrane is classified as a *semipermeable* (sem-e-per′me-ah-b'l) membrane, being very selective in what it allows to enter and to leave the cell. It is permeable or passable to some molecules but is impassable to others.

Water, a tiny molecule, is always able to penetrate the membrane; whereas certain sugars, such as sucrose, cannot pass through because the molecules are too large, even though readily soluble. So, by the processes of metabolism, sucrose is converted to glucose, which can diffuse through the membrane because its molecule is smaller.

A combination of various physical processes is responsible for the phenomenon of exchanges through the cell membrane or through the tissue membranes that are made up of a combination of many cells. Some of these processes are as follows:

1 **Diffusion,** the constant movement of molecules from a region of relatively higher concentration

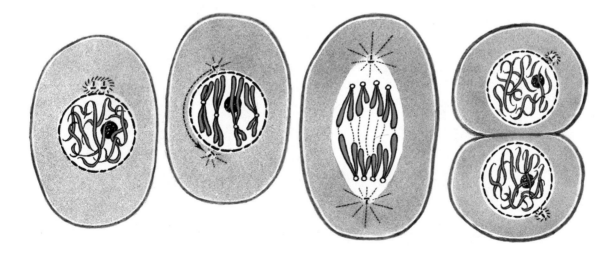

Fig. 2-2 *Mitosis. One pair of centrioles migrate, the chromatin material of the nucleus changes into rod-shaped chromosomes, and two daughter cells form within the cell membrane.*

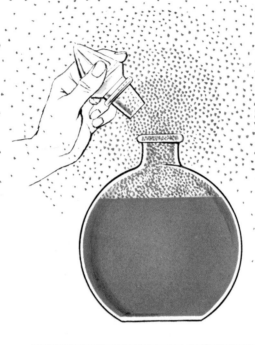

Fig. 2-3 Diffusion of gaseous molecules throughout a given space. The bottle could contain perfume, a spray of some kind, a chlorine bleach, etc. In any case, there is a tendency for the molecules to spread throughout the area.

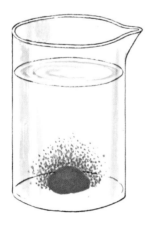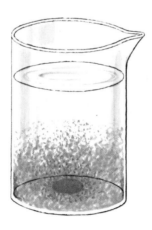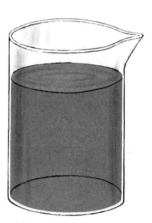

Fig. 2-4 Diffusion of a solid and a liquid. The solid diffuses into the water; the water diffuses into the solid; the molecules of solid tend to spread throughout the water.

to one of lower concentration. Molecules, especially those in solution, tend to spread throughout an area until they tend to become equally concentrated in all parts of the container (Figs. 2-3 and 2-4).

2 **Osmosis,** the diffusion of water through a semipermeable membrane, with the water molecules going from the less concentrated solution to the one that is more concentrated. The dissolved molecules in the more concentrated solution "pull" the water molecules from the less concentrated solution across the semipermeable membrane. In addition, both the size of the molecules of the dissolved substance and the nature or type of membrane are factors that determine the osmotic ("pulling") ability of the concentrated solution (Fig. 2-5).

3 **Filtration,** the passage of water containing dissolved materials through a membrane as a result of a greater mechanical ("pushing") force on one side (Fig. 2-6). Normally, large particles cannot pass through an intact membrane (Fig.

2-7). An example of filtration in the human body is the formation of urine in the microscopic functional units of the kidney as described in Chapter 19.

It is important to recognize that our bodies are composed of large amounts of fluids. Certain kinds of fluids bathe the cells, carry nutrient substances to and from cells, and transport the nutrients in and out of the cells. This group of fluids is called *extracellular fluid* because it includes all body fluids outside of the cells. A second type of fluid is that contained within the cells, called *intracellular fluid.* Extracellular and intracellular fluids account for approximately 65% of an adult's weight. Each type of fluid consists of electrolytes, such as sodium, chloride, and potassium ions, and nutrient substances, such as protein and carbohydrate substances, dissolved or suspended in water. Chemical reactions that are necessary for proper body functioning are carried on much more readily in a watery solution. Substances that do not go into

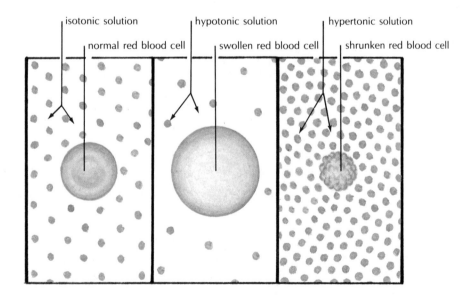

Fig. 2-5 *Osmosis. Water molecules moving through a cell membrane into a solution of salts in high concentration. The normal saline solution has a concentration nearly the same as that inside the cell; the dilute solution causes the cell to swell and eventually hemolyze because of the large number of water molecules moving into the cell; the concentrated solution causes the water molecules to move out of the cell, leaving it shrunken.*

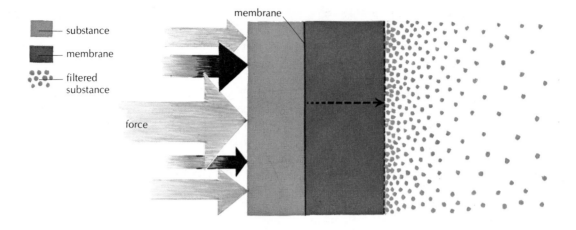

Fig. 2-6   *Filtration. A mechanical force pushes a substance through a membrane.*

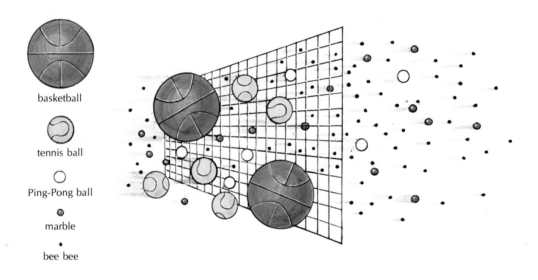

Fig. 2-7   *Filtration. Large objects (basketballs and tennis balls) cannot pass through the net. In the human body, large particles (proteins and blood cells) do not pass through intact membranes.*

solution may be suspended in the various liquids of the body, many of which circulate; and, thus, they may be moved from place to place. Water is indispensable for cell life, and lack of water causes death more rapidly than the lack of any other dietary constituent.

The solution of water and other materials in which the tissues are bathed is slightly salty, owing to the presence of electrolytes, an interesting reminder of the first living cells which originated in the sea.

The distribution of ions in intracellular and extracellular fluids differs in an important way. There is relatively more sodium in extracellular fluid than in intracellular fluid. Likewise, there is more potassium in intracellular than in extracellular fluid. One consequence of this ionic distribution is described by the saying, "Where salt is, water follows." When the body retains salt, large amounts of water may also be retained. The largest amount of this water will remain in the extracellular fluid spaces. This condition is called *edema*. If the body excretes large amounts of salt, water will also be lost. This process may lead to a condition called *dehydration*.

The Cellular Factory

A cell is very much like a tiny factory, complete with its own power plant, the mitochondria. All the chemical reactions by which food is transformed for use by the cells is given the broad general name of *metabolism*. The cell consumes nutrients and breaks them down to simpler forms. This breaking-down phase of metabolism is called *catabolism*. Catabolism releases energy from the complex nutrients. This energy is trapped in the high-energy bonds of the compound *adenosine* (ahden′-o-sēn) *triphosphate* (ATP) and made available for the process of anabolism. *Anabolism* is the building-up phase of metabolism. The cells use ATP to assemble simple structures, such as amino acids, into complex structures needed by the cell to build and repair its cytoplasm and organelles. As after any fire, waste products are left over. These are removed from the cell, to be carried away by blood and other fluids and eliminated from the body.

Some kinds of cells reproduce more readily than others; certain types, if they die, are not replaced at all. On the other hand, many thousands of new cells are formed daily in the skin and other tissues to replace those destroyed by injury, disease or certain natural processes. As a person ages, characteristic changes in the overall activity of his body cells take place. One example of these is the slowing down of repair processes. The fracture of a bone, for example, takes considerably longer to heal in an aged person than in a young one.

At this point, we are ready to proceed from the individual cell to the specialized groups of cells of which our bodies are made. Such groups are known as *tissues*.

On Tissues in General

Although the basic structure of cells, as well as certain behavior patterns, remains constant regardless of the type of cell under discussion, cells themselves vary enormously with respect to shape, size, color and specialty. Many cells, for example, are transparent; some of these form the "window" of the eye. Other cells may have extensions in the form of thin fibers over a yard long, as in the case of some nerve cells. Some produce secretions; others transmit electrical impulses.

Tissues are groups of cells similar in structure and substance and arranged in a characteristic pattern, and specialized for the performances of a specific task. In some ways, the tissues in our bodies might be compared with the different materials which we use to clothe ourselves. Think for a moment of the great variety of materials employed in covering the body according to the degree of protection needed, the time of year, and so forth—wool, cotton, silk, rayon, leather, and even straw. All of these have different properties; so do tissues.

Tissue Classification

The four main groups of tissue are the following:

1 **Epithelium** forms glands, covers surfaces, and lines cavities.
2 **Connective tissue** holds all parts of the body in place.
3 **Nerve tissue** conducts nerve impulses.
4 **Muscle tissue** is designed for power-producing contractions.

Blood is considered a tissue, since it contains cells and performs many of the functions of tissues. However, the blood has so many other unique characteristics and purposes that an entire chapter is devoted to it.

Epithelium

Epithelium (ep-e-the′le-um) forms a protective covering for the body and all its organs; in fact, it is the main tissue of the outer layer of the skin. It forms the lining of the intestinal tract, the respiratory and urinary passages, the blood vessels, the uterus, and other body cavities.

Epithelium has many forms and many purposes, and the cells of which it is composed vary accordingly (Fig. 2-8). For instance, the cells of some kinds of epithelium produce secretions, such as *mucus* (mu′kus) (a clear, sticky fluid), digestive juices, perspiration and other substances. The digestive tract is lined with a special kind of epithelium whose cells not only produce secretions but are

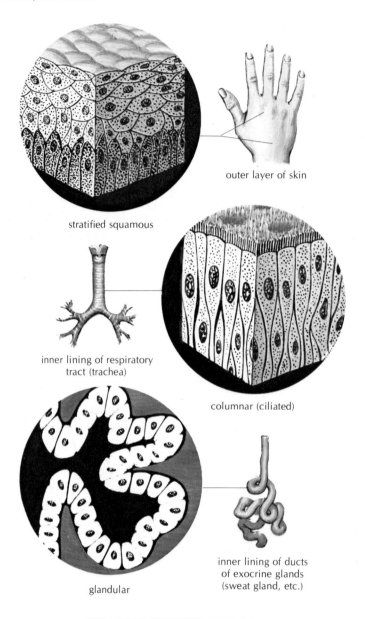

outer layer of skin

stratified squamous

inner lining of respiratory
tract (trachea)

columnar (ciliated)

glandular

inner lining of ducts
of exocrine glands
(sweat gland, etc.)

Fig. 2-8   Three types of epithelium.

also designed to absorb digested foods. The air that we breathe passes over yet another form of epithelium that lines the respiratory tract. This lining secretes mucus and is also provided with tiny hairlike projections called *cilia* (sil′e-ah). Together, the mucus and the cilia help to trap bits of dust and other foreign particles which could otherwise reach the lungs and damage them. Some organs, such as the urinary bladder, must vary a great deal in size during the course of their work;

and for this purpose there is a special wrinkled, crepelike type of tissue, called transitional epithelium, which is capable of great expansion, yet will return to its original form once the tension is relaxed—as when, in this case, the bladder is emptied. Certain areas of the epithelium that forms the outer layer of the skin are capable of modifying themselves for greater strength whenever they are subjected to unusual wear and tear; the growth of calluses is a good example of this.

Epithelium will repair itself very quickly if it is injured. If, for example, there is a cut, the cells near and around the wound immediately form daughter cells which grow until the cut is closed. Epithelial tissue reproduces frequently in areas of the body subject to normal wear and tear, such as the skin, the inside of the mouth, and the lining of the intestinal tract.

Connective Tissue

The supporting fabric of the organs and other parts of the body is connective tissue (Fig. 2-9). If we were able to dissolve all the tissues except connective tissue, we would still be able to recognize the contour of the parts and the organs of the entire body. There are three distinct kinds of connective tissue, which are classified quite simply:

1 **Soft** connective tissues
2 **Hard** connective tissues
3 **Blood** and **lymph**

Soft Connective Tissues

This group of connective tissues serves a number of different purposes. One type, called *adipose*

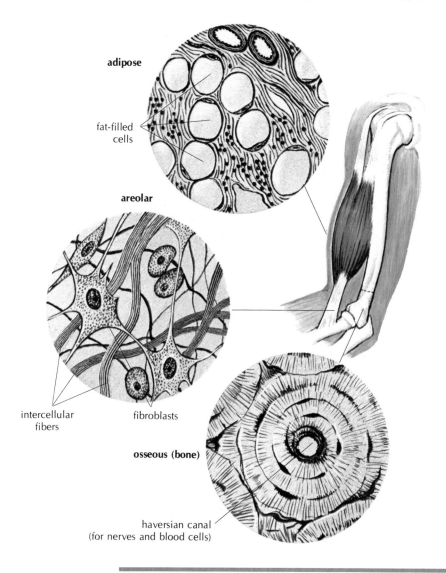

Fig. 2-9 Connective tissue.

(ad′e-pose) tissue, stores up fat for use by the body as a reserve food, as a heat insulator, and as padding for various structures. Another kind of soft connective tissue serves as a binding between organs, as well as a framework for some organs which are otherwise made of epithelium. There is yet another form of this tissue which is particularly strong, being built up of fibers much like the strands of a cable. And, like a cable, this form of tissue serves to support certain organs which are subjected to powerful strains. A good example is a tendon, a cordlike band of tissue that connects muscles to bones.

There is another interesting function of soft connective tissue, and this is its use by nature to repair muscle and nerve tissue as well as to repair connective tissue itself. Like epithelial tissue, soft connective tissue can repair itself easily. A large, gaping wound will require a correspondingly large growth of this new connective tissue; the new growth is called scar tissue. The process of repair includes stages in which new blood vessels are formed in the wound, followed by the growth of the scar tissue. An excessive development of the blood vessels in the early stages of repair may lead to the formation of so-called proud flesh. Normally, however, the blood vessels are gradually replaced by white fibrous connective tissue which forms the scar. Suturing (sewing) the edges of a clean wound together, as is done in the case of operative wounds, decreases the amount of scar tissue needed and hence reduces the size of the resulting scar. Such scar tissue may be stronger than the original tissue.

Hard Connective Tissues

The hard connective tissues, which, as the name suggests, are more solid than the other group, include cartilage and bone. Cartilage, popularly called gristle, is a tough, elastic, and translucent material which is found in such places as between the segments of the spine and at the ends of the long bones. In these positions, cartilage acts as a shock absorber as well as a bearing surface which reduces the friction between moving parts. Cartilage is found in other structures also, such as the nose, the ear, and parts of the larynx, or "voice box."

The tissue of which bones are made, called *osseous* (os′e-us) tissue (see Fig. 2-9), is very much like cartilage in its cellular structure. In fact, the bones of the unborn baby, in the early stages of development, are (except for some of the skull bones) nothing but cartilage. However, gradually this tissue becomes impregnated with calcium salts; and since calcium is another word for lime, we see that a mineral deposit is going on which finally leaves the bones in their characteristically hard and stony state. Within the bones are nerves, blood vessels, bone-forming cells, and a special form of tissue, bone marrow, in which certain ingredients of the blood are manufactured.

In soft and hard connective tissue, the major extracellular protein is *collagen* (kol′-ah-jen). Since it is a protein, the major function of collagen is to provide for structure in cells and connective tissue throughout the body. Therefore, when a person suffers from a connective tissue, or collagen, disease, such as lupus erythematosus or rheumatoid arthritis, collagen fibers in many body parts may be affected. Blood and lymph connective tissue are discussed in Chapters 14 and 15, respectively.

Nerve Tissue

The human body is made up of countless structures both large and small, each of which contributes something to the action of the whole organism. This aggregation of structures might be considered as an army, all of whose members must work together. In order that they may do so, there must be a central coordinating and order-giving agency somewhere; otherwise chaos would ensue. In the body this central agency is the brain. Each structure of the body is in direct communication with the brain by means of its own set of telephone wires, called nerves. The nerves from even the most remote parts of the body all come together and form a great trunk cable called the spinal cord, which in turn leads directly into the central switchboard of the brain. Here, messages come in and orders go out 24 hours a day. This entire communication system, brain and all, is made of nerve tissue.

The basic structural unit of nerve tissue is the *neuron* (nu′-ron) (Fig. 2-10). A neuron consists of a nerve cell body plus small branches like those of a tree. These are called fibers. One group of these fibers, the *dendrites,* carries nerve impulses or messages to the nerve cell body. A single fiber, the *axon,* carries impulses away from the nerve

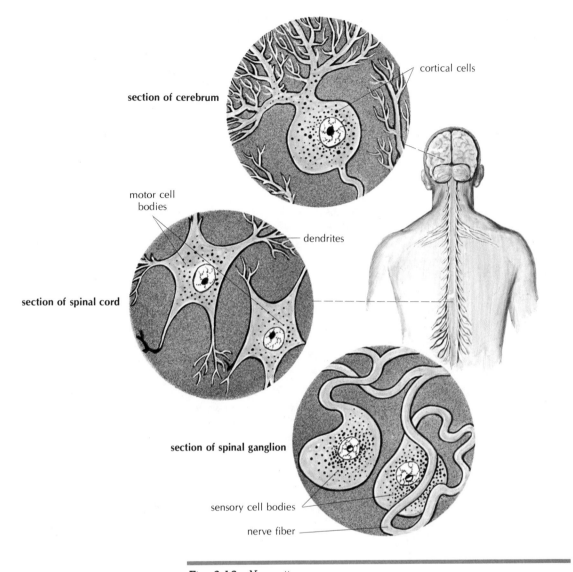

section of cerebrum

cortical cells

motor cell bodies

dendrites

section of spinal cord

section of spinal ganglion

sensory cell bodies

nerve fiber

Fig. 2-10   Nerve tissue.

cell body. Neurons may be quite long, since their fibers can extend for several feet.

Nerve tissue (clusters of neurons) is supported by ordinary connective tissue everywhere except in the brain and spinal cord. Here, the supporting tissue is *neuroglia,* which has a protective function as well.

All the nerves outside the brain and the spinal cord, called the *peripheral* (peh-rif′er-al) nerves, have a thin coating known as *neurilemma* (nu-re-lem′mah). Neurilemma is a part of the mechanism by which the peripheral nerves repair themselves when damaged. The brain and the spinal cord, on the other hand, have no neurilemma; if they are injured, the injury is permanent. However, even in the peripheral nerves, repair is a slow and uncertain process.

Telephone wires are insulated to keep them from being short-circuited, and so are nerve fibers, which actually do transmit something very much like an electric current. The insulating material of nerve fibers is called *myelin* (mi′el-in), and groups of these fibers form "white matter," so-called because of the color of the covering; it is very much like fat in appearance and consistency. Not all nerves have myelin, however; some of the nerves of the system that controls the action of the glands, the smooth muscles, and the heart do not have myelin. The cell bodies of all nerve cells also are unmyelinated (without a myelin cover). Since all nerve cells are gray to begin with, and large collections of cell bodies are found in the brain, the great mass of brain tissue is popularly termed "gray matter." A more detailed discussion of nerve tissue is taken up in Chapter 11.

Muscle Tissue

Muscle tissue is designed to produce power by a forcible contraction. The cells of muscle tissue are threadlike, and so are called muscle fibers. If a piece of well-cooked meat is pulled apart, small groups of these muscle fibers can be observed. Muscle tissue is usually classified as follows (Fig. 2-11):

1　**Skeletal muscle,** which combines with connective tissue structures, such as tendons (discussed later along with the skeleton), to provide for movement of the body. This type of tissue is also known as *voluntary* muscle, since it can be made to contract by those nerve impulses from the brain that originate from an act of will. In other words, in theory at least, any of your skeletal muscles can be made to contract as you want them to.

　　The next two groups of muscle tissue are

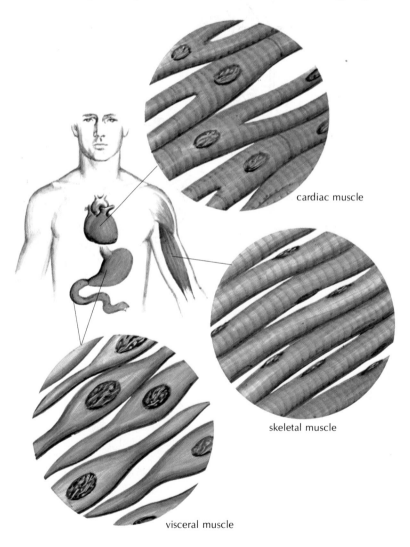

cardiac muscle

skeletal muscle

visceral muscle

Fig. 2-11　Muscle tissue.

known as *involuntary* muscle, since they typically contract independently of the will. In fact, most of the time we do not think of their actions at all. These are

2 **Cardiac muscle,** which forms the bulk of the heart wall and is known also as *myocardium* (mi-o-kar′de-um). This is the muscle that produces the regular contractions known as heartbeats.

3 **Visceral muscle,** known also as *smooth* muscle, which forms the walls of the *viscera* (vis′er-ah), meaning the organs of the ventral body cavities (with the exception of the heart). Some examples of visceral muscles are those that move the food and waste materials along the digestive tract. Visceral muscles are found in other kinds of structures as well. Many tubular structures contain them, such as the blood vessels and the tubes that carry urine from the kidneys. Even certain structures at the bases of body hair have this type of muscle. When they contract, there results the skin condition that we call gooseflesh. Other types of visceral muscles are taken up under the various body systems.

There is a general disorder of the muscles which might be mentioned here. It is called a *spasm* and is a sudden and involuntary contraction of a muscle. A spasm is always painful. A spasm of the visceral muscles is called *colic,* and a good example of colic is the spasm of the intestinal muscles often referred to as bellyache. Spasms may occur also in the skeletal muscles; if the spasms occur in a series, the condition may be called a *seizure* or *convulsion.* Specific diseases of which these abnormal muscle contractions are symptomatic are discussed later.

Muscle tissue, like nerve tissue, repairs itself only with difficulty or not at all, once an injury has been sustained. These tissues, when injured, are replaced frequently with connective tissue.

Tumors, Benign and Malignant

In the study of cells and tissues we gain some insight into the laws of growth. For reasons that still remain obscure, cells develop various forms, and those that are of the same kind congregate to form one of the basic tissues. These tissues become, in turn, the specialized organs. In the early stage of the body's development, the cells multiply rapidly, and hence the body with all its structures grows in size until a point of maximum growth has been reached. From here on, cell division is not so rapid; it continues, however, at a rate sufficient to replace cells which for one reason or another have become used up and discarded. This complete picture of growth is neat and logical: the tissues are maintained, and every cell and formation of cells has its purpose.

It may happen, however, that the normal pattern of growth is broken by an upstart formation of cells having no purpose whatsoever in the body. Any abnormal growth of cells is called a *tumor,* or *neoplasm.* If the tumor is confined to a local area and does not spread, it is called a *benign* (be-nine′) tumor. If the tumor spreads to neighboring tissues or to distant parts of the body, it is called a *malignant* (mah-lig′-nant) tumor. The general term for any type of malignant tumor is *cancer.* The process of tumor cell spread is called *metastasis* (ma-tas′-ta-sis).

Tumors are found in all kinds of tissue, but they occur most frequently in those tissues which repair themselves most quickly: namely, epithelium and connective tissue, in that order.

Benign Tumors

Benign tumors, theoretically at least, are not dangerous in themselves; that is, they do not spread. Their cells adhere together; and, often, they are encapsulated, that is, surrounded by a containing membrane. Benign tumors grow as a single mass within a tissue, lending themselves neatly to complete surgical removal. Of course, some benign tumors can be quite harmful in their effect; they may grow within an organ, increase in size, and cause considerable mechanical damage. A benign tumor of the brain, for example, can kill a person just as a malignant one can, since the tumor grows in an enclosed area and compresses vital brain tissue. Some examples of benign tumors (note that most of the names end in -oma, which means tumor) include:

1 **Papilloma** (pap-i-lo′mah). These grow in epithelium as projecting masses. One example is a wart.
2 **Adenoma** (ad-e-no′mah). These are epithelial,

growing in and about the glands (aden- means gland).

3 **Lipoma** (lip-o′mah). These are connective tissue tumors, originating in fatty (adipose) tissue.

4 **Osteoma** (os-te-o′mah). These are also connective tissue tumors, but originate in the bones.

5 **Myoma** (mi-o′mah). These are tumors of muscle tissue. Rare in voluntary muscle, they are common in some types of involuntary muscle, particularly the uterus (womb). When found in this organ, however, they are ordinarily called *fibroids*.

6 **Angioma** (an-je-o′mah). This tumor usually is one composed of small blood or lymph vessels; an example is the birthmark.

7 **Nevus** (ne′vus). These are small skin tumors of various tissues. Some are better known as moles. Some are angiomas. Ordinarily, they are harmless but can become malignant.

Malignant Tumors

Malignant tumors, unlike benign tumors, can cause death no matter where they occur. The word cancer means "crab," and this is descriptive: a cancer sends out clawlike extensions into neighboring tissue. Not only does this happen, but also a cancer literally spreads its own "seeds" which plant themselves in other parts of the body. These seeds are, of course, cancer cells, and they are transported everywhere by either the blood or the lymph (a fluid related to the blood). When the cancer cells reach their destination, they immediately form new (secondary) growths (*metastases*). Malignant tumors, moreover, grow much more rapidly than benign ones.

Malignant tumors generally are classified in two categories according to the type of tissue in which they originate:

1 **Carcinoma** (kar-si-no′mah). These are cancers originating in epithelium and are by far the most common type of cancer. Common sites of carcinoma are the skin, the mouth, the lung, the breast, the stomach, the colon, and the uterus. These are usually spread by the lymphatic system (see Chap. 15).

2 **Sarcoma** (sar-ko′mah). These are cancers of connective tissue of all kinds and hence may be found anywhere in the body. Their cells are usually spread by the blood stream, and they often form secondary growths in the lungs.

There are other types of malignant tumors: for example, those that originate in birthmarks or in moles, called *melanomas* (mel″ah-no′mahs), and tumors that originate in the connective tissue of the brain and spinal cord, called *gliomas* (gli-o′mahs).

The Symptoms of Cancer

Everyone should be familiar with certain signs that may be indicative of early cancer, so that they can be reported immediately before the condition can spread. It is unfortunate that early cancer is painless; otherwise, cancer would not be the problem that it is. Early symptoms may include unaccountable loss of weight, any unusual bleeding or discharge, persistent indigestion, chronic hoarseness or cough, changes in color or size of moles, any kind of sore that does not heal in a reasonable time, the presence of any unusual lump, and the presence of white patches inside the mouth or white spots on the tongue.

Detection and Treatment of Cancer

Cancer diagnosis is becoming increasingly specific, leading to more precise methods of treatment. High-frequency sound waves (ultrasound) and the CT (computed tomography) scanner which uses x-rays to produce a cross-sectional picture of parts of the body, such as the brain, are methods to provide a better indication of the size and location of the tumor. This, along with the study of the cells themselves, leads to a process called staging. This determination leads to an orderly use of the various available treatment methods.

While benign tumors can be removed completely by surgery, malignant tumors cannot be treated so easily, for a number of reasons. If cancerous tissue is removed surgically, there is always the probability that a few hidden cells will be left behind, to grow anew. If the cells have spread to distant parts of the body, there is little that anyone can do. Sometimes surgery is preceded by or followed by radiation. Radiation therapy is administered by x-ray machines or by the placement of radioactive seeds within the involved organ. Radiation destroys the more rapidly dividing cancer cells while causing less damage to the more slowly dividing normal cells. Methods are being developed that will permit focusing the beam of radiation more accurately and thus reduce the damage to normal body structures.

Drugs used for the treatment of cancer include those that act selectively on tumor cells. They are known as *antineoplastic* (an″ti-ne″o-plas′-tik) agents and are most effective when used in combination. This is because each drug exerts its specific effects; when several drugs are used together, they exert very powerful effects on the cancer cells. The treatment of cancer with antineoplastic agents is one form of chemotherapy (keem-oh-ther′-a-py) (see Chap. 7). Certain types of leukemia and various cancers of the lymphatic system are often effec-

tively treated by this means. Research continues to develop new drugs and more effective drug combinations.

A newer technique is the use of immunotherapy (i-mu″-no-ther′-ah-pe) agents. Immunotherapy involves giving the patient a special type of inoculation to strengthen his own body defenses and thus prevent the spread of the cancer cells.

The *laser* (la′zer), a device that produces a very highly concentrated and intense beam of light, may sometimes successfully destroy the tumor, or may be employed as a cutting device for removing the growth. Important advantages of the laser are its ability to coagulate blood so that bleeding is largely prevented and the capacity to direct a narrow beam of light accurately to attack harmful cells and avoid normal ones.

Summary

Characteristics of cells.
A The building block of living things.
B Organelles are responsible for various life functions within the cell.
C Enzymes assist cells in functioning.
D Protein synthesis.
E The cell reproduces by mitosis.
F Physical and biologic processes bring materials through the semipermeable cell membrane.
  (1) Diffusion, osmosis, filtration.
  (2) Extracellular fluid, intracellular fluid.
  (3) Distribution of sodium and potassium, edema; dehydration.
G Chemical action within the cell is called metabolism; catabolism, anabolism.
2 Tissues.
A Tissues made of specialized cells.
B Tissue compares with cloth; properties vary with function.
3 Tissue classification.
A Epithelium.
B Connective tissue.
C Nerve tissue.
D Muscle tissue.
4 Epithelium.
A Forms protective covering of the body and its organs.
B Forms lining of the intestinal tract, respira-

tory and urinary passages, blood vessels, uterus and other body cavities.
C May produce secretions.
D May have cilia or other special characteristics.
E Some types are wrinkled.
F Repairs itself quickly and easily.
5 Connective tissue.
A Supports organs and other body structures; collagen is major extracellular protein.
B Divided into types.
  (1) Soft. Stores fat, binds organs, forms organ framework, supports organs with heavy strains, forms scar tissue.
  (2) Hard. Bones and cartilage.
C Repairs itself easily.
D Blood and lymph are two special connective tissue types.
6 Nerve tissue.
A Basic structure is neuron; neuroglia is supporting tissue.
B Composes coordinating and communication systems of the body.
C Neurons vary greatly in length; have fibers, axon, and dendrites.
D Neurilemma helps nerves to repair themselves. Peripheral nerves have neurilemma, brain and spinal cord do not, so are incapable of repair.

E Repair of nerves even with neurilemma is slow and uncertain.

F Myelin insulates some nerves.

7 Muscle tissue.

A Primary purpose is to provide forcible contractions.

B Fiber-like cells.

C Three kinds.

(1) Skeletal. Forms the body muscles proper, also called voluntary muscle.

(2) Cardiac. Contracts regularly to produce heartbeat. An involuntary muscle.

(3) Visceral. Known also as smooth muscle. Forms the walls of internal organs (heart excepted) including tubular structures.

D Muscle disorders: spasm, colic, seizure.

E Repairs itself with difficulty or not at all. Injured tissue may be replaced with scar tissue.

8 Tumors, or neoplasms.

A Characteristics.

(1) Abnormal cell growths.

(2) Found mainly in epithelium and connective tissue.

B Kinds of tumors.

(1) Benign.

(2) Malignant.

C Benign tumors.

(1) Do not spread.

(2) Completely removable by surgery.

(3) Examples—papilloma, adenoma, lipoma, osteoma, myoma, angioma, nevus.

D Malignant tumors.

(1) Send out appendages into neighboring tissue.

(2) Cells spread to other parts of the body and cause secondary growths.

(3) Cells grow more rapidly than those of benign tumors.

(4) Can kill victim no matter where they grow.

(5) Categories of malignant tumors (cancer).

(a) Carcinoma. Epithelial, usually spread by lymphatic system. Most common.

(b) Sarcoma. Connective tissue cancer. Usually spread by blood stream.

E Cancer symptoms—unaccountable weight loss, cough, persistent indigestion, unusual lumps, bleeding, discharge, nonhealing sores, change in color or size of moles, white patches inside the mouth or on the tongue.

F Treatment of tumors—surgery, radiation, drugs, laser.

Questions and Problems

1 Define each of the following: organelle, mitochondria, enzyme, semipermeable membrane, DNA.

2 Why is protein synthesis vital to cell division?

3 Outline the various stages of cell division. What is the name of this process?

4 What are some examples of processes that are responsible for the exchange of materials through membranes?

5 What goes on inside the cell once it receives these materials? Give the name for this process.

6 Define anabolism and catabolism.

7 Define a tissue. Give a few general characteristics of tissues.

8 Define epithelium and give 2 examples. How easily does it repair itself?

9 Define connective tissue. Name the main kinds of connective tissue and give an example of each. How easily does it repair itself?

10 What is the main purpose of nerve tissue? What is its basic structural unit called?

11 Define neurilemma. Where is it present or absent?

12 Define myelin. Where is it found?

13 How easily does nervous tissue repair itself?

14 Name the 3 kinds of muscle tissue and give an example of each.

15 What is the difference between voluntary and involuntary muscle?

16 Name a general disorder of muscle tissue. Name 2 different variations of this and define them.

17 How easily does muscle tissue repair itself?

18 What is a tumor? In what kinds of tissue are they most commonly found?

19 Name the 2 general categories of tumors.

20 Name 4 examples of benign tumors and tell where each is found.

21 What is the difference between a benign and a malignant tumor?

22 Name the 2 categories of malignant tumors. In what kind of tissue are they found? Which is the most common?

23 In what ways is cancer treated?

24 Name some early symptoms of cancer.

Chapter 3

Membranes

3

Glossary

Capsule A structure that encloses a body part or organ.

Fascia A layer or band of connective tissue, especially that which holds the skin to the surface muscles, or any of the sheets enclosing muscles or other organs.

Membrane A thin layer of tissue that covers a surface, lines a cavity, or divides a space or an organ.

Meninges The 3 membranes that cover the brain and spinal cord.

Mesothelium A layer of epithelium that covers the serous membranes.

Mucosa A lining membrane that produces mucus and is found in spaces connected with the outside, such as the alimentary and respiratory tracts; mucous membrane.

Parietal Relating to the walls of a space or cavity.

Pericardium The serous membrane that lines the sac enclosing the heart, plus the reflection that attaches itself to the heart itself.

Perichondrium A membrane that covers the surface of cartilage.

Periosteum The special fibrous connective tissue membrane covering the bones of the body; the surface tissue which plays an important part in the repair of bone fractures and other injuries.

Peritoneum The large serous membrane that lines the abdominal cavity and is reflected over the organs within.

Pleura (pl. pleurae, pleuras) A membrane that covers the lung and lines the thoracic cavity.

Serosa A serous membrane; one that is found lining the body cavities, such as the pleural and peritoneal cavities.

Synovial Relating to a thick fluid found in joints, bursae and tendon sheaths.

Viscera (sing. viscus) The organs in the 3 large body cavities, such as the stomach and the liver in the abdominal cavity.

Now that we have discussed the fundamental cell groupings—the tissues—we are ready to proceed to the next step and see in what ways the tissues are combined to form the body structures. The simplest of these tissue combinations are called *membranes*.

In our discussion of cells, we encountered the

word "membrane" for the first time and noted that a membrane is the wall of a cell through which various materials in solution (oxygen, food materials) can enter and through which other substances (waste materials, secretions) can leave. This wall is called the *plasma membrane.*

In this chapter, however, we consider only those membranes that are made up of a multitude of cells—that is, tissues. These are known as *tissue membranes,* but, for the sake of convenience, they shall henceforth be referred to simply as membranes.

Membranes are thin sheets of tissue. Their properties vary: some are fragile, and others are tough. Some are transparent while others are opaque, that is, they cannot be seen through. Membranes may serve as dividing partitions, or may line hollow organs and body cavities. They may cover a surface, may serve as dividing partitions, or may line hollow organs and body cavities. Other membranes serve to anchor various organs. They may contain secreting cells that produce lubricants that ease the movement of organs such as the heart and the movement of the joints.

Kinds of Membranes

There are two broad categories of membranes. The first of these are the *epithelial membranes,* so-called because their outer surfaces are faced with epithelium. Their deep surfaces, however, have a layer of connective tissue, which strengthens the membrane. Epithelial membranes are in turn divided into two subgroups:

Mucous (mu'kus) **membranes** line tubes and other spaces that open to the outside of the body.
Serous (se'rus) **membranes** line the external walls of body cavities and are folded back onto the surface of exposed organs, forming the outermost layer of many of them.

The second category of membranes is known as *fibrous connective tissue membranes.* Unlike epithelial membranes, those of this group are composed entirely of connective tissue. This category of membranes also can be divided into two subgroups:

1 **Fascial** (fash'e-al) **membranes** serve to anchor and support the organs.
2 **Skeletal membranes** cover bone and cartilage.

Epithelial Membranes

Epithelial membranes are made of closely crowded active cells which manufacture lubricants and protect the deeper tissues from invasion by microorganisms. Mucous membranes produce a rather thick and sticky substance called mucus, while serous membranes secrete a much thinner lubricant. (Note that the adjective in each case contains an "o," while the nouns naming the secretion do not.)

In referring to the mucous membrane of a particular part, the noun *mucosa* (mu-ko'sah) may be used, while the special serous membrane lining a closed cavity or covering an organ is called the *serosa* se-ro'sah).

Mucous Membranes

Mucous membranes form extensive continuous linings in the digestive, the respiratory, the urinary, and the reproductive systems, all of which are connected with the outside of the body. They vary somewhat both in structure and function. The cells that line the nasal cavities and most parts of the respiratory tract are supplied with tiny hairlike extensions of the protoplasm, called cilia, which have been mentioned previously. The microscopic cilia move in a wavelike manner that forces the secretions outward away from the deeper parts of the lungs. In this way foreign particles such as bacteria and dust become trapped in the sticky mucus and are prevented from causing harm. Ciliated epithelium is also found in certain tubes of both the male and the female reproductive systems.

The mucous membranes that line the digestive tract have their own special functions. For example, the mucous membrane of the stomach serves to protect the deeper tissues from the action of certain powerful digestive juices. If for some reason a portion of this membrane were injured, these juices would begin to digest a part of the stomach itself—which, incidentally, is exactly what happens in the case of peptic ulcers. Mucous membranes located farther along in this system are designed to absorb food materials which are then transported to all the cells of the body. But we are getting too far ahead in our story; other mucous membranes are discussed as we encounter them.

Serous Membranes

Serous membranes, unlike mucous membranes, do not usually communicate with the outside of the body. This group lines the closed ventral body cavities. There are three serous membranes:

1 The two **pleurae** (ploor′e) or pleuras (ploor′ ahs), form two separate sacs, one for each lung in the thoracic cavity.
2 The **pericardium** (per-e-kar′de-um) is a sac that covers the heart. It fits into a space in the chest between the two lungs.
3 The **peritoneum** (per-i-to-ne′um) is the largest serous membrane, and it lines the abdominal cavity. This cavity is closed in the male, but it is connected with the outside by the reproductive system in the female (Fig. 3-1).

The epithelium covering serous membranes is of a special kind called *mesothelium* (mes-o-the′ le-um), which is smooth and glistening, and is lubricated so that movements of the organs can take place with a minimum of friction.

Serous membranes are so arranged that one portion forms the lining of the closed sac, while another part of the membrane covers the surface of the organs. Since the word *parietal* (pah-ri′e-tal) refers to a wall, the serous membrane attached to the wall of a cavity or sac is known as the parietal layer. There is, for example, parietal pleura lining the chest wall, and parietal pericardium lining the sac that encloses the heart. Because organs are called *viscera,* the membrane attached to the organs is the *visceral* layer. On the surface of the heart is visceral pericardium, while each lung surface is made up of visceral pleura.

Connective Tissue Membranes

Compared with epithelium membranes, connective tissue membranes are static, serving chiefly as retaining and supporting structures. These membranes, as has been mentioned, are divided into two subgroups, fascial and skeletal membranes.

Fascial Membranes

The word fascia means band; hence fascial membranes are bands or sheets the purpose of which is to support the organs and hold them in place. An example of a fascial membrane is the continuous sheet of tissue which underlies the skin. This contains fat (adipose tissue or ''padding'') and is called the *superficial fascia.* Superficial refers to a surface; so the superficial fascia is closer than any other kind to the surface of the body.

As we penetrate more deeply into the body, we find examples of the *deep fascia,* which contains no fat and has many different purposes. Fascial membranes enclose the glands and the viscera; these envelopes are called *capsules.* Deep fascia covers and protects the muscle tissue, and these coverings are known as *muscle sheaths.* The blood vessels and the nerves also are sheathed with fascia; the brain and the spinal cord are encased in a multilayered covering called the *meninges* (me-nin′jez). In addition, fascia serves to anchor muscle tissue to structures such as the bones.

Skeletal Membranes

Skeletal membranes cover bones and cartilage. The membrane that covers the bones is known as *periosteum* (per-e-os′te-um), and that which covers cartilage is called *perichondrium* (per-e-kon′dre-um).

The cavities of the joints are lined with connective tissue membranes called *synovial* (si-no′ve-al) membranes, and their particular purpose is to secrete a lubricating fluid that reduces the friction between the ends of bones, thus permitting free movement of the joints.

With this we conclude our brief introduction to membranes. As we study each system in turn, other membranes will be encountered. They may have unfamiliar names, but they will be either epithelial or connective tissue membranes, and we shall also become familiar with their general locations. In short, they will be easy to recognize and remember.

Membranes and Disease

We are all familiar with a number of diseases that directly affect membranes. These range all the way

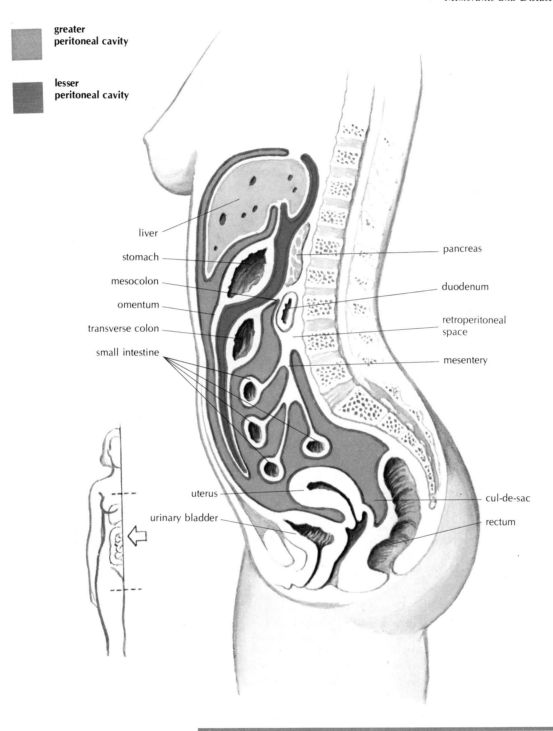

greater
peritoneal cavity

lesser
peritoneal cavity

liver

stomach

mesocolon

omentum

transverse colon

small intestine

uterus

urinary bladder

pancreas

duodenum

retroperitoneal
space

mesentery

cul-de-sac

rectum

Fig. 3-1 Abdominal cavity showing peritoneum.

from the common cold, which is an inflammation of the mucosa of the nasal passages, to the sometimes fatal condition known as peritonitis, an infection of the peritoneum, which can follow the rupture of the appendix. More of these diseases of membranes will be covered in due course.

Membranes can act as pathways along which disease may spread. In general, epithelial membranes seem to have more resistance to infections than do those layers made of connective tissue. However, lowered resistance may allow the transmission of infection along any membrane. For example, infections may travel along the lining of the tubes of the reproductive system into the urinary system, in either sex. In addition to this, in the female, an infection may travel up the tubes and spaces of the reproductive system into the peritoneal cavity.

Sometimes connective tissue membranes form planes of division extending in such a way that infection in one area is prevented from reaching another space. In other cases a vertical plane which separates two areas may seem to encourage the travel of bacteria either upward or downward. An infection of the tonsils, for example, may travel down to the chest.

Certain diseases considered to be metabolic disorders may also attack membranes. In *lupus erythematosus* (er″i-them′-ah-to-sus) serous membranes such as the pleura, pericardium, and peritoneum are often involved. In rheumatoid arthritis, the synovial membrane is inflamed and may be replaced by fibrous connective tissue.

Summary

1 Characteristics of membranes.
   A Simplest combinations of tissue.
   B Thin, skinlike layers of tissue.
   C Secrete substances, line cavities, support organs.
2 Kinds of Membranes.
   A Epithelial—outer surface is epithelium; deep surface is connective tissue.
   B Connective tissue—composed entirely of connective tissue.
3 Epithelial membranes.
   A Mucous membranes—secrete mucus, line passages that communicate with the outside of the body.
   B Serous membranes.
      (1) Characteristics—are covered with mesothelium, line body cavities, are lubricated thinly, have parietal and visceral layers.
      (2) 3 serous membranes—pleurae (lung cavities), pericardium (heart sac), peritoneum (abdominal cavity).

4 Connective tissue membranes.
   A Characteristics—static, retaining and supporting structures.
   B Kinds.
      (1) Fascial membranes; superficial fascia has fat, is below dermis of skin; deep fascia forms capsules, muscle sheaths; sheaths for nerves and blood vessels; anchors muscle fibers to bones.
      (2) Skeletal membranes—cover bones and cartilage. Periosteum (bone covering); perichondrium (cartilage covering). Synovial membranes line joint cavities and secrete joint lubricant.
5 Membranes and disease.
   A Membrane inflammations—common cold, peritonitis.
   B Can be pathways along which disease spreads. Can also block off spaces from infection.
   C Lupus erythematosus and arthritis may involve membranes.

Questions and Problems

1 What does the word membrane mean, generally speaking?
2 What is the general name for the membranes with which this chapter deals?
3 Name some general characteristics of membranes.
4 What are the 2 broad categories of membranes?

5 What are some general characteristics of epithelial membranes?
6 Name the 2 subgroups of epithelial membranes.
7 Give some characteristics of mucous membranes and name 2 examples of them.
8 Name some characteristics of serous membranes.

9 Name the three serous membranes and locate each.

10 What is the name for the kind of epithelium that covers serous membranes?

11 Name the 2 layers of serous membranes and tell what each means.

12 Give some general characteristics of connective tissue membranes.

13 Name the 2 subgroups of connective tissue membranes.

14 What are the main purposes of fascial membranes?

15 Name 2 kinds of fascia.

16 Give 3 examples of deep fascia.

17 What are the main purposes of skeletal membranes?

18 Name 3 examples of skeletal membranes.

19 Name 2 diseases of membranes.

20 How do membranes figure in the penetration and progress of disease organisms within the body?

Chapter 4

Chemistry, Matter, and Life

4

Glossary

Acid   A substance that can donate a proton to another substance.

Anion   An ion having a negative charge.

Atom   Any one of the ultimate units of an element that can exist and still have the properties of the element; the particles that together form a molecule in a compound.

Base   A substance that can accept a proton from another substance.

Cation   An ion having a positive charge.

Compound   A substance made of 2 or more elements.

Electrolyte   A solution that conducts electricity by means of ions that are positively or negatively charged.

Electron   The unit of negative electricity.

Element   In chemistry, a simple substance that cannot be decomposed into simpler substances by chemical means.

Homeostasis   A consistency and uniformity of the internal body environment which maintains normal body function; stability of body fluids and their constituents.

Ion   An atom having a positive or a negative charge.

Isotope   A chemical element that has the same atomic number as another but a different atomic weight.

Mixture   A combination of two or more substances that are not bound to each other.

Molecule   A minute mass of matter; a combination of atoms that form a given chemical substance or compound; the smallest particle in a chemical compound that can exist in a free state.

Neutron   A noncharged particle within the cell nucleus.

Proton   A positively charged particle within the cell nucleus.

What Is Chemistry?

Great strides toward understanding living organisms, including the human being, have come to us through *chemistry,* the science that deals with the composition of matter. Knowledge of chemistry and chemical changes helps us in the understanding of the normal and the abnormal functioning of the body and its parts. The digestion of food in the intestinal tract, the production of urine by the kidneys, the regularity of breathing—all body processes—are based on chemical principles. Chemistry also is important in *microbiology* (the study of microscopic plants and animals) and *pharmacology* (the study of drugs). The various solutions that are used to cleanse the skin before a surgical operation are chemicals, as are aspirin, penicillin, and all other drugs used in treating disease. In order to have some understanding of the importance of chemistry in the health field, this chapter briefly describes *atoms* and *molecules, elements, compounds,* and *mixtures,* which are the fundamental units of matter.

A Look at Atoms

Atoms are small particles that form the building blocks of matter, the smallest complete units of which all matter is made. To visualize the size of an atom, one can think of placing millions of them on the sharpened end of a pencil and still having room for many more. Everything about us, everything we can see and touch, is made of atoms—the food we eat, the atmosphere, the water in the oceans, the smoke coming out of the chimney.

Despite the fact that the atom is such a tiny particle, it has been carefully studied and has been found to have a definite structure. An atom is made up of a nucleus which contains positively charged electric particles called *protons* and noncharged particles called *neutrons.* Rotating around the nucleus in regions called orbitals are negatively charged particles called *electrons* (Fig. 4-1).

The protons and electrons usually are equal in number in any atom. Collectively, they are responsible for all of the atom's characteristics; individually, they play a role in the atom's function. The neutrons and protons are tightly bound in the nucleus, contributing nearly all of the atom's weight and mass. The positively charged protons keep the negatively charged electrons in the orbital

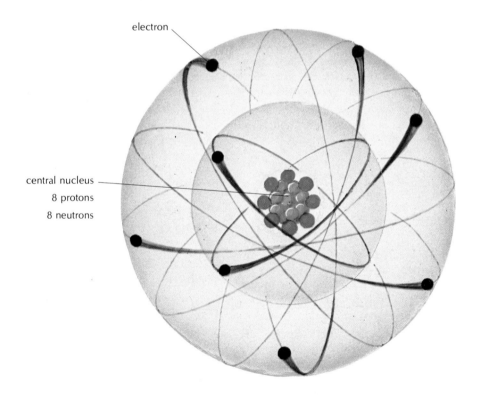

electron

central nucleus
8 protons
8 neutrons

Fig. 4-1 *Representation of oxygen atom. Eight protons and eight neutrons are tightly bound in the central nucleus, around which the eight electrons revolve.*

area around the nucleus because of the opposite charge that each particle possesses. Positively (+) charged protons attract negatively (−) charged electrons. The electrons contribute important chemical characteristics of the specific atom.

Most atoms have several orbitals of electrons. However, each orbital can hold only two electrons. The orbitals are arranged into energy shells. Energy shells are identified by their distance from the nucleus of the atom. The first energy shell, the one closest to the nucleus, is composed of one orbital. The second shell, the next in distance away from the nucleus, can have four orbitals. Since each orbital can contain only two electrons, the second shell has the capacity to hold eight electrons. The electrons farthest away from the nucleus are the particles that give the atom its chemical characteristics.

If the outermost shell has more than four electrons, but less than its capacity of eight, the atom normally tends to complete this shell by gaining electrons. Such atoms are called nonmetals. The oxygen atom illustrated in Figure 4-1 has six electrons in its second, or outermost, shell. When oxygen enters into chemical reactions, its chemical behavior is to gain two electrons in order to fill up the second or outermost shell. The oxygen atom, then, would have two more electrons than protons. If the outermost shell has less than four electrons, that atom normally tends to lose those electrons to attain a complete outer shell. Such atoms are called metals.

Molecules, Elements, Compounds, and Mixtures

When two or more atoms unite, a *molecule* is formed. It can be made of *like* atoms, as in the case of the oxygen molecule which is made of two identical atoms; such substances are called *elements*. An element cannot be decomposed—that is, changed into something else—by physical means (e.g., by the use of heat, pressure, electricity). Examples of elements include various gases, such as hydrogen, oxygen, and nitrogen; liquids, such as the mercury used in thermometers and blood pressure instruments; and many solids, such as iron, aluminum, gold, silver, and carbon. Graphite (the

so-called lead in a pencil), coal, charcoal, and the diamond are examples of the element carbon. The entire universe is made up of about 105 elements.

Elements can be identified by their names, their symbols, or their atomic numbers. Chemists use symbols as shorthand methods to name elements. The atomic number of an element is equal to the number of protons that are present in the nucleus. Since the number of protons is equal to the number of electrons in an element, the atomic number also identifies the number of electrons whirling about the nucleus. Table 4-1 lists some elements found in the human body.

Usually, we think of molecules as including two or more different atoms. For example, a molecule of sodium chloride (NaCl), or common table salt, includes one atom of sodium (Na) and one of chlorine (Cl). Those substances that contain molecules formed by the union of two or more different atoms are called *compounds*. Compounds may be made of a few elements in a simple combination or they may be very complex; some, such as proteins, have thousands of atoms. The simplest compound would have molecules each of which contains one atom of each of the two elements that unite to form the compound. An example of such a compound is the gas carbon monoxide (CO), which contains one atom of carbon (C) and one atom of oxygen (O). Some compounds are called organic because they were first found only in living organisms. They are usually complex compounds and contain the element carbon as an im-

Table 4-1 Common chemical elements.

Name	Symbol	Atomic Number
Hydrogen	H	1
Carbon	C	6
Nitrogen	N	7
Oxygen	O	8
Sodium	Na	11
Phosphorus	P	15
Sulfur	S	16
Chlorine	Cl	17
Potassium	K	19
Iron	Fe	26

portant constituent. The starch found in potatoes, the fatty layer of tissue under the skin, and many drugs are organic compounds.

It is interesting to observe how different a compound is from any of its constituents. For example, two atoms of hydrogen (2H), which we know as a gas, unite with one atom of oxygen (O), also a gas, to form a molecule of a liquid, water (H_2O) (Fig. 4-2). Water is remarkably different in its appearance and its properties from its component gases. Another example is a sugar, glucose ($C_6H_{12}O_6$), a thick syrupy liquid. Its constituents include twelve atoms of the gas hydrogen, six atoms of the gas oxygen, and six atoms of the solid element carbon. In this case, the component gases and the solid carbon do not in any way resemble the glucose.

It is fortunate that not all elements or compounds combine chemically when brought together. If such were the case we would be unable to keep intact the hundred or so different compounds in blood plasma while it is dried or frozen. Dried (powdered) plasma may be sent long distances easily and inexpensively. It may then be reconstituted by adding sterile water as it is needed in a war zone or at the scene of a major disaster. The many valuable compounds in the plasma remain separate entities with their own properties. Such combinations are called *mixtures*—blends of two or more substances. Salt water is a mixture, both the salt and the water remaining separate compounds. The substances in a mixture can be present in any proportion, while in a compound the elements combine in definite proportions. You can stir any amount of salt into a given amount of water and still have a mixture. However, if one more atom of oxygen (O) were added to a water molecule (H_2O), you would have an entirely new compound called hydrogen peroxide (H_2O_2) not water. Air is a mixture of gases. Seawater is a mixture of water and dissolved solids; the amount of each will vary in different places, the water being less salty near the mouths of rivers. The compounds in a mixture can usually be separated by mechanical means, such as dissolving or boiling. If salt water is boiled, the compound water will eventually escape as steam or vapor, which, if collected in a bottle and cooled, regains its water state. The compound salt will remain in the pan, appearing as the original white granules.

To better understand the relationship of mix-

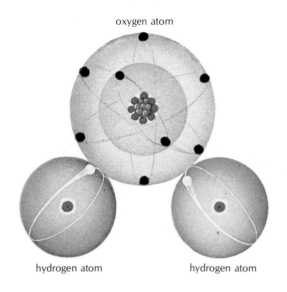

oxygen atom

hydrogen atom   hydrogen atom

Fig. 4-2 Molecule of water.

tures, compounds, elements, molecules, and atoms, we can follow the changes that occur in the transfer of a mixture to the individual atom. As was previously mentioned, salt and water in a saltwater mixture regain their original properties by simply boiling. If we were able to take one gram of salt and cut it into halves, cut one section in half again, and continue doing so, it would still have the same properties as salt. The smallest particle obtainable that would still have the properties of salt is the salt molecule, which is made up of one atom of the element sodium and one atom of the element chlorine. Thus, we have regressed from the mixture to the atom. To summarize, we can say that salt water, a mixture, is made up of two compounds, NaCl and H_2O. The components of salt are atoms of the element sodium and atoms of the element chlorine. The water, of course, can be broken down in like manner to its atoms of hydrogen and oxygen.

Ions and Electrolytes

When discussing the structure of the atom, we mentioned the positively charged (+) protons that are located in the nucleus, with the corresponding number of negatively charged (−) electrons rotating in the surrounding space and neutralizing the protons. If we can imagine removing a single electron from the sodium atom, it would leave one proton not neutralized, and the atom would have a positive charge (Na^+). This can actually happen—the freely whirling electron can leap out of its orbital. Likewise, atoms can gain electrons so that there are more electrons than protons. Chlorine, which has seven electrons in its outermost shell, tends to gain one electron to fill the shell to its capacity. Such an atom of chlorine is negatively charged (Cl^-). (Fig. 4-3). An atom with a positive or negative charge is called an *ion.* An ion that is positively charged is a *cation,* while a negatively charged ion is an *anion.*

When an atom loses an electron, it searches for another electron and will attach itself to an anion that has an extra one. The anion, in turn, is eager to give up its extra one to the cation. Let us imagine a sodium atom coming in contact with a chlorine atom. The chlorine atom gains an electron from the sodium atom, and the two newly formed ions (Na^+ and Cl^-), because of their opposite charges which attract each other, will cling together and produce the compound sodium chloride. As was previously mentioned, this is ordinary table salt. A vast number of chemical compounds are made by this method of electron transfer (Fig. 4-4).

In the fluids and in the cells of the body, ions make it possible for materials to be altered, broken down, and recombined to form new substances. Calcium ions (Ca^{++}) are necessary for the clotting of blood, the normal relaxation of muscle, and the health of bone tissue. Bicarbonate ions (HCO_3^-) are required for the regulation of acidity and alkalinity of the tissues. The stable condition of the normal organism, called *homeostasis* (ho-me-o-sta′-sis), is influenced by ions (see Chap. 6).

Compounds that form ions whenever they are in solution are called *electrolytes* (e-lek′tro-lites).

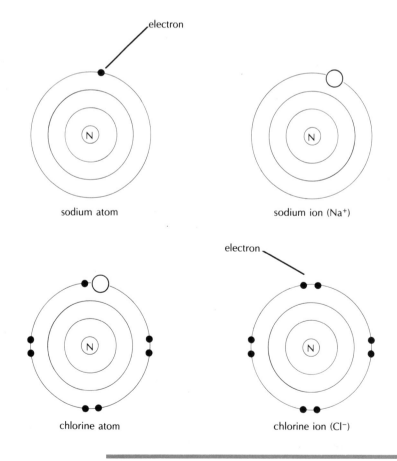

Fig. 4-3 *Formation of Na⁺ cation and Cl⁻ anion.*

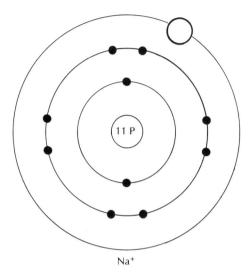
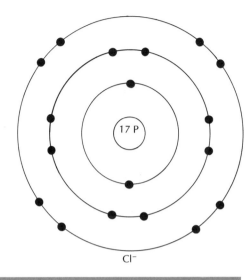

Fig. 4-4 *Sodium ion with 11 protons in nucleus and 10 electrons in orbitals is attracted to chlorine ion with 17 protons in nucleus and 18 electrons in orbitals to form compound sodium chloride.*

Electrolytes are responsible for the acidity and the alkalinity of solutions. They also include a variety of mineral salts, such as sodium and potassium chloride. Electrolytes must be present in exactly the right quantities in the fluid within the cell (intracellular) and outside the cell (extracellular) or there will be very damaging effects on the cells in the body, preventing them from functioning properly.

Since ions are charged particles, electrolytes can conduct an electric current. Records of electric currents in tissues are valuable indications of the functioning or malfunctioning of tissues and organs. The *electrocardiogram* (e-lek-tro-kar′de-o-gram) and the *electroencephalogram* (e-lek-tro-en-sef′ah-lo-gram) are graphic tracings (recorded by special instruments) of the electric currents generated by the heart muscle and the brain, respectively (see Chap. 11 and 14).

Acids and Bases

A delicate balance exists in the acidity or alkalinity of body fluids. If a person is to remain healthy, these chemical characteristics must remain within narrow limits. The substances responsible for the balanced chemical state are acids, bases, and buffers. *Buffers* form a chemical system that prevents changes in hydrogen ion concentration and thus maintains a relatively constant pH.

Acids are chemical substances capable of donating a proton, or H^+, to another substance. A *base* is a chemical substance that can accept a proton. For example, when hydrochloric acid is in a solution of water, the HCl acts as an acid, giving a proton to the base, H_2O.

$$HCl + H_2O \rightarrow H_3O^+ + Cl^-$$

You can see that the water has received a hydrogen ion from the hydrochloric acid. The greater the concentration of hydrogen ions (H^+) in a solution, the greater is the acid strength of that solution. Acidity is indicated by pH units, pH is the symbol for hydrogen ion concentration (Fig. 4-5).

A pH of 7 is neutral, having an equal number of cations and anions. Each degree on the scale represents a tenfold increase in the number of ions present. A solution registering 9 on the scale would have 10 times the number of anions as one that registers 8. A solution registering 5 would have 10 times the cations as one registering 6. Therefore, the lower the pH rating, the greater the acidity, and the higher the pH, the greater the alkalinity. Blood is only slightly alkaline, with a pH range of 7.35 to 7.45, or nearly neutral.

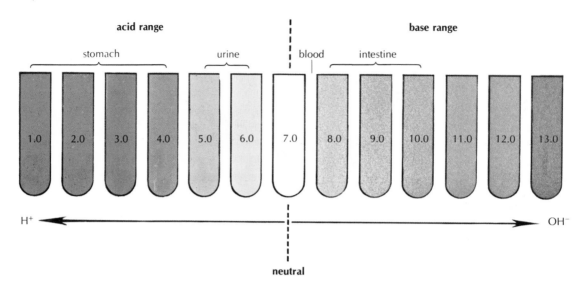

Fig. 4-5   *The pH scale measures degree of acidity or alkalinity.*

Radioactivity

No discussion of atoms is complete without reference to the part some play in the diagnosis and treatment of disease. Atoms of an element may exist in several forms called *isotopes*. These forms are alike in their chemical reactions but differ in weight. For example, heavy oxygen is much like regular oxygen except for its weight. This greater weight is due to the presence of one or more extra neutrons in the nucleus of the heavier isotope. Isotopes may be stable and maintain a constant character; others disintegrate (fall apart) as they give off small particles and rays, and these are said to be *radioactive.* Radioactive elements may occur naturally, as is the case with such very heavy isotopes as radium and uranium. Others may be produced artificially from nonradioactive elements such as iodine and gold by bombarding (smashing) the atoms in special machines.

The rays given off by some radioactive elements have the ability to penetrate and destroy tissues and so are used in the treatment of cancer. Radiation therapy is often given by means of special machines (such as linear accelerators) that are able to release particles to destroy tumors. The sensitivity of the younger and the dividing cells in a growing cancer allows selective destruction of the abnormal cells with a minimum of damage to normal tissues. Modern radiation instruments produce tremendous amounts of energy (in the multimillion electron-volt range) and yet can destroy deep-seated cancers without causing serious skin reactions.

Radioactive isotopes, such as cobalt 60, in the form of pellets, may be sealed in stainless-steel cylinders. These cylinders are mounted on arms or cranes that permit the proper alignment for directing the beams through a porthole to the area to be treated.

In the form of needles, seeds, or tubes, implants containing radioactive isotopes are widely used in the treatment of many types of cancer.

In addition to its therapeutic values, radiation is extensively used in diagnosis. X-rays penetrate the tissues and produce an impression of their interior on a photographic plate. Radioactive iodine and other "tracers" taken orally or injected into the bloodstream are used to diagnose abnormalities of several body organs. Rigid precautions must be followed by hospital personnel to protect themselves and the patient when using radiation in diagnosis or therapy because the rays can destroy healthy as well as diseased tissues.

The Chemistry of Living Matter

Perhaps the most interesting and baffling of all substances is protoplasm, the component of all living cells and tissues. Living matter is made up of atoms and molecules that are readily identifiable. Nevertheless, scientists have tried in vain over the years to produce protoplasm in the laboratory. Of the 100 or more elements that have been found in nature, only a relatively few, and those the lighter ones, are important components of protoplasm. Hydrogen, oxygen, carbon, and nitrogen are the elements that make up about 99% of protoplasm. Calcium, sodium, potassium, phosphorus, sulfur, chlorine, and magnesium are the seven elements that make up most of the remaining 1% of the tissue elements. There are a number of others that are present in trace amounts, such as iron, copper, iodine, and fluorine.

From these elements, the compounds that are formed and are most important in the human organism include the proteins, carbohydrates, and lipids (fatlike substances). The carbohydrates and lipids contain carbon, hydrogen, and oxygen as their chief and usually only elements. A group of complex lipids, important in living material, contains phosphorus, in addition to carbon, hydrogen, and oxygen. These compounds are called *phospholipids* (fos″fo-lip′ids). *Proteins* are carbon, hydrogen, and oxygen compounds that contain nitrogen and, in some cases, sulfur. These compounds are present in nutrients. Nutrients, which are necessary for normal body functions, are supplied by foods and include carbohydrates, proteins, lipids, mineral salts, and vitamins. These will be discussed in Chapter 18.

As previously mentioned, in appearance, protoplasm resembles the white of an egg.

Protoplasm is not of a uniform composition but includes a variety of substances, intricately organized. Dissolved in the water of protoplasm are mineral (inorganic) salts, simple sugars, and other substances. In addition to this complex solution, there is a variety of protein and fat molecules which seem to change from a fluid or *sol* state to a semisolid condition, known as the *gel* state. If we think of gelatin, we may remember that changes in temperature can cause it to become liquid with warmer conditions or solid in colder states. Such factors as the concentration of salts, pressure, and agitation (shaking), as well as temperature variations cause changes back and forth between the sol state and the gel state within the protoplasm.

Summary

1 Chemistry.
  A Deals with composition of matter.
  B Includes study of atoms, elements, molecules, compounds, and mixtures.
2 A look at atoms.
  A Atoms are the smallest building blocks of all matter.
  B The atomic nucleus consists of protons and neutrons.
  C Electrons rotate around the nucleus.
3 Molecules, elements, compounds, and mixtures.
  A Union of 2 or more atoms is called molecule.
  B Molecule may be made of like atoms (*e.g.,* oxygen molecule); when made of 2 different atoms, is a compound (*e.g.,* protein).
  C Elements made of 1 type of atom.
  D Elements cannot be subdivided chemically.
  E Compounds contain 2 or more elements.
  F Complex molecular structure in many organic compounds.
  G Substances in a mixture are not combined chemically.
  H Mixtures are made of substances in any proportions.
4 Ions and electrolytes.
  A Atoms with electronic charges are ions.
  B Many chemical compounds are made by electron transfer.
  C Electrolytes are compounds that ionize when in solution.
5 Acids and bases.
  A Cation is positive ion. Anion is negative ion.
  B Acid is cationic solution; base is anionic solution.

C pH is symbol for hydrogen ion concentration—indicates acidity or alkalinity of the solution.
6 Radioactivity important in medicine and industry.
7 The chemistry of living matter.

A Hydrogen, oxygen, carbon, and nitrogen are elements in largest quantity in protoplasm.
B Proteins, carbohydrates, and lipids are compounds in protoplasm.

Questions and Problems

1 Define chemistry and tell something about what is included in this study.
2 What are atoms and what is known of their structure?
3 Define molecule, element, compound and mixture.
4 What is an element and what are some examples of elements?
5 What are organic compounds and what element is found in all of them?
6 How does a mixture differ from a compound?
7 What are ions and how are they related to electrolytes? What are some examples of ions and of what importance are they in the body?
8 What would "pH 11.5" indicate?
9 What is meant by radioactivity and what are some of its practical uses?
10 What elements are found in the largest amounts in protoplasm?

Chapter 5

Body Fluids

5

- Importance of body water
- Homeostasis
- Function of electrolytes
- Intake and output
- Imbalances of body fluids

Glossary

Ascites Abnormal collection of serous fluid in the peritoneal cavity.

Dehydration An extreme deficit of body fluids.

Edema Abnormal accumulation of fluid in the body's intercellular spaces.

Effusion Escape of fluid into a part, such as pleural effusion, the accumulation of fluid in the space between the lung membrane and the membrane lining the thoracic cavity.

The most abundant compound in the protoplasm is water. No plant or animal, including the human, can live very long without it. Water is of critical importance in all physiologic processes that go on in body tissues. Water carries substances to and from the cells and makes possible the essential processes of absorption, exchange, secretion, and excretion. The percentage of water in the human varies from 50% in an obese person to 75% in a lean person. (Adipose tissue has a very low water content which accounts for the lower percentage of water in an obese person.) The average adult is approximately 60% water. All of which serves to remind us of our heritage from the sea.

Water molecules are relatively small and far apart. This attribute gives water its remarkable property as a solvent. Water is often referred to as the universal solvent because of this ability to dissolve a vast array of substances.

However, of what importance is water—that colorless, tasteless, odorless liquid that contains no calories—in the study of health and disease? If you keep in mind that you are mostly water, you can appreciate that any time the volume or chemical makeup of the body fluids deviates even slightly from the safe bounds of the normal, disease will result.

How the Body Fluids Maintain Homeostasis

Every one of the body's cells depends on homeostasis, the constancy of the body's internal environment. The body fluids are the chief regulators that ensure homeostasis. Their regulatory functions include the following:

1 Activation of the thirst mechanism maintains the volume of water at a constant level. Any time there is an increase in concentration of body fluids, it is sensed by the hypothalamus, which sends out the "thirst" message and causes the person to drink water or another fluid containing liberal amounts of water.
2 The kidneys regulate retention and excretion of water, thereby maintaining the proper concentration of minerals in the plasma.
3 The quantities of the mineral salts (such as sodium and potassium) that are excreted by the kidneys are regulated by hormones, notably the hormone aldosterone, which is secreted by the adrenal cortex.
4 The pH, or acid–base balance, is kept constant by the body fluid buffers (see Chap. 2), the lungs, and the kidneys.
5 Water or water-containing liquids in the diet stimulate the flow of digestive juices.

Electrolytes and Their Functions

Remember that water occupies three locations, or compartments, in the body. The greatest volume of water is found inside the cells—the intracellular water. The water outside the cells—the extracellular water—is located in two compartments: one is the microscopic spaces between cells (where it is called interstitial fluid) and the other is the blood (where it is called plasma) (Fig. 5-1).

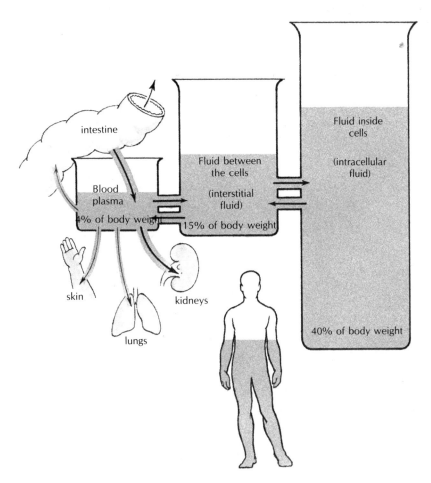

Fig. 5-1 *Diagram to show absorption, circulation, and excretion of body fluids.*

Most of the substances dissolved in the body water are electrolytes (see Chap. 4). In normal health, the distribution of electrolytes in the body fluid is exactly right, both intracellularly and extracellulary. The electrolytes, you recall, dissociate or break down into cations or anions, and the cations and anions have vital roles to play in the health of the body. A few of the most important roles are described below:

1 **Sodium,** a cation, is chiefly responsible for maintaining osmotic balance and body fluid volume. With the cells, sodium is required for vital chemical reactions. It stimulates nerve action and is essential in maintenance of acid–base balance.
2 **Potassium,** a cation, is primarily involved in cellular enzyme activities, and it helps regulate the chemical reactions by which carbohydrate is converted to energy and amino acids are converted to protein.
3 **Calcium,** a cation, is required for bone formation, the maintenance of muscle excitability, and blood clotting.
4 **Phosphate,** an anion, is probably the single most important mineral constituent needed by cells. It is essential in the metabolism of carbohydrates, bone formation, and acid–base balance.
5 **Chloride,** an anion, is essential for formation of the hydrochloric acid of the gastric juice.

Intake and Output of Water

The quantity of water consumed in a day varies considerably. The average adult in a comfortable environment takes in about 2500 ml of water daily. About half of this quantity comes from drinking water and other beverages, and about half comes from foods—fruits, vegetables, soups, milk.

In a person whose health state is normal, the quantity taken in (intake) is approximately equal to the quantity lost (output). In many disorders, it is important for the health-care team to know whether the patient's intake and output are approximately equal, and a 24-hour intake–output record

will be kept. The intake record includes *all* the liquid the patient has consumed, in the form of water, beverages, and food, as well as the quantity and kinds of foods that have been eaten in each 24-hour period. The output record includes the quantity of urine excreted in the 24-hour period, as well as an estimation of fluid losses due to fever, vomiting, diarrhea, bleeding, wound discharge, or other causes.

Disorders Involving Body Fluids

1 **Edema** is the accumulation of excessive fluid in the intercellular spaces. In some kinds of edema, salt is retained, and "where salt is, water follows." Edema of the hands and the feet will cause these organs to swell and to have a boggy appearance. Among the underlying causes of edema are kidney failure, congestive heart failure, and too much dietary salt. Protein loss and too little dietary protein over an extended period of time are also important causes of edema. Some women experience premenstrual edema.
2 **Water intoxication** is a drastic dilution of body fluids in both the intracellular and extracellular compartments. The resulting extreme imbalance can cause convulsions leading to death. Some underlying causes are the administration of very high quantities of intravenous fluids and inappropriate (abnormal) secretion of the antidiuretic hormone.
3 **Dehydration** (de″hi-dra′shun) is a severe deficit of body fluids which will result in death if prolonged. The causes include vomiting, diarrhea, drainage from burns or wounds, excessive perspiration, and too-little fluid intake.
4 **Effusion** (e-fu′shun) is the collection of fluid in a part or a space. An example is pleural effusion, fluid within the pleural sacs; the fluid compresses the lung so that normal breathing is not possible. Tuberculosis, cancer, and some infections may give rise to effusion.
5 **Ascites** (ah-si′tez) is effusion with accumulation of fluid within the abdominal cavity. It may occur in disorders of the liver, the kidneys, and the heart, and in cancers and infection.

Summary

1 Water essential to human life, processes of absorption, exchange, secretion, and excretion.
2 Homeostasis: dependent on water balance.
3 Electrolytes in body water—essential to normal function.
4 Normal fluid losses: through lungs, intestine, skin, and urinary tract.
5 Intake should equal output. Intake–output record: valuable information about certain disorders.
6 Disorders—water intoxication, edema, dehydration, effusion, ascites.

Questions and Problems

1 Describe the main functions of water.
2 What is the significance of the statement that water is the universal solvent?
3 State 3 or more ways in which the body fluid maintains homeostasis.
4 In a healthy person, what is the ratio of fluid intake to output?
5 What is the importance of an intake–output record?
6 Describe 4 or more disorders involving body fluids.

Chapter 6

Body Temperature and Its Regulation

6

- Homeostasis
- Heat production and loss
- The "thermostat" of the body
- Normal and abnormal temperature
- Effects of heat and cold

Glossary

Conduction The transfer of heat, electricity, or sound waves.

Convection Transmission of heat in a liquid or a gas by circulation carried on by the heated particles.

Crisis A turning point, especially a sudden change in the course of a disease.

Evaporation Conversion of a liquid or a solid to vapor.

Hypothermia An extremely low body temperature.

Lysis The gradual lessening of symptoms of a disease.

Pyrogen A substance that produces fever.

Radiation Transmission of heat from its source in the form of heat waves or rays.

Body Temperature and Homeostasis

Heat is an important by-product of the many chemical activities constantly going on in the tissues all over the body. Simultaneously, heat is always being lost through a variety of outlets. Yet, by virtue of a number of regulatory devices the body temperature remains constant within quite narrow limits under normal conditions. The maintenance of a constant temperature in spite of both internal and external influences is one phase of the concept of homeostasis, the tendency of the body processes to maintain a normal state despite forces that tend to alter them. Other examples of the maintenance of homeostasis are the heart rate, respiratory rate and blood pressure, which all tend to remain within their normal limits. In addition to these more obvious types of homeostasis, there are many other examples that involve the composition of body fluids.

Heat Production

Heat is produced when oxygen combines with food products in the cells. Thus heat is a by-product of the reactions in all cells as they produce energy. Oxygen enters the cell and there it is used to break down the carbohydrates, proteins, and fats that occur in foodstuffs. The end products of these reactions are energy, water, and carbon dioxide. Energy liberated from food is seen as external work (muscle movement), energy storage (as energy-rich compounds for future work), and heat. The amount of heat produced by a given organ varies with the kind of tissue and with its activity. While at rest, muscles may produce as little as 25% of the total body heat, but when numbers of muscles contract, the heat production may be multiplied hundreds of times owing to the increased metabolic rate needed for energy production. Under basal conditions (rest), the abdominal organs, particularly the liver, produce about one half of the body heat; but during vigorous muscular activity, this ratio is greatly changed. While the body is at rest, the brain may produce 15% of the body heat, but an increase in activity in nerve tissue produces very little increase in heat production. The largest amount of heat, therefore, is produced in the muscles and the glands. It would seem from this description that some parts of the body would tend to become much warmer than others. The circulating blood, however, distributes heat fairly evenly throughout the entire body.

The rate at which heat is produced is affected by a number of factors which may include activity level, hormone production, food intake, and age. When the body is at complete rest (basal condition), the glandular organs such as the liver continue to add some heat constantly with but slight variations. But the amount of heat produced in muscles during activity is hundreds of times as great as during rest. In addition to these causes of variation, certain hormones, such as thyroxine from the thyroid gland and epinephrine (adrenaline) from the medulla of the adrenal gland, may increase the rate of heat production. The intake of food also is accompanied by increased heat production. The reasons are not entirely clear. More fuel is poured into the blood and is therefore more readily available for cellular "combustion." The glandular structures and the muscles of the digestive system generate additional heat as they set to work. This does not account for all the increase, however, nor does it account for the much greater increase in metabolism following a meal containing large amounts of protein. Whatever the reasons, the intake of food definitely increases the chemical activities that go on in the body and thus adds to heat production.

Heat Loss

More than 80% of heat loss occurs through the skin. The remaining 15% to 20% is dissipated by the respiratory system and with the urine and feces. Networks of blood vessels in the deeper part (corium, or dermis) of the skin are capable of bringing considerable quantities of blood near the surface so that heat can be dissipated to the outside. This can occur in several ways. Heat can be transferred to the surrounding air (*conduction*). Heat also travels from its source in the form of heat waves or rays (*radiation*). If the air is moving so that the layer of heated air next to the body is constantly being carried away and replaced with cooler air (as by an electric fan), the process is known as *convection*. Finally, heat loss may be produced by *evaporation*. Any liquid uses heat during the process of changing to the vapor state. Rub some alcohol on your arm; it evaporates rapidly, and in so doing uses so much heat, taking it from the skin, that your arm feels cold. Perspiration does the same thing, though not as quickly. The rate of heat loss through evaporation depends upon the humidity of the surrounding air. When this exceeds 60% or so, perspiration will not evaporate so readily, and one feels generally miserable unless some other means such as convection (by a fan) can be resorted to.

If the temperature of the surrounding air is lower than that of the body, excessive heat loss is prevented by both natural and artificial means. Clothing checks heat loss by trapping "dead air" both in its material and its layers. This noncirculating air is a good insulator. An effective natural insulation against cold is the layer of fat under the skin. Even though the skin temperature may be low, this fatty tissue prevents the deeper tissues from losing too much heat. This layer is, on the average, slightly thicker in the female than in the male. Naturally there are individual variations, but as a rule the degree of insulation depends on the thickness of this layer of subcutaneous fat.

Other factors that play a part in heat loss include the volume of tissue compared with the amount of skin surface. A child loses heat more rapidly than an adult. Such parts as the fingers and the toes are affected more by exposure to cold, because in each case there is a greater amount of skin compared with total tissue volume.

Temperature Regulation

Since the body temperature remains almost constant in spite of the wide variations in the rate of heat production or loss, obviously there must be a temperature regulator. Actually, many areas of the body take part in this process, but the most important heat-regulating center is an area inside the brain, located just above the pituitary gland, called the *hypothalamus* (hi-po-thal'ah-mus). Some of the cells in the hypothalamus control the production of heat in the body tissues, while another group of cells controls heat loss. This control comes about in response to the heat brought to the brain by the blood as well as to nerve impulses from the temperature receptors in the skin. If these two factors indicate that too much heat is being lost, impulses are sent quickly from the hypothalamus to the autonomic (involuntary) nervous system which, in turn, causes constriction of the skin blood vessels in order to reduce heat loss. Other impulses are sent to the muscles to cause shivering, a rhythmic contraction of many body muscles, which results in increased heat production. The output of epinephrine may be increased, also, if conditions call for it. Epinephrine increases cell metabolism for a short period of time, and this, in turn, increases heat production. Also, the smooth muscle around the hair roots contracts, forming "gooseflesh," a reaction that conserves little heat in humans.

If, on the other hand, there is danger of overheating, the hypothalamus will transmit impulses that stimulate the sweat glands to increased activity and also dilate the blood vessels in the skin so that there is increased blood flow with a correspondingly greater loss of heat. The hypothalamus also may encourage relaxation of muscles and thus minimize the production of heat in these organs.

Muscles are especially important in temperature regulation because variations in the amount of activity of these large masses of tissue can readily increase or decrease the total amounts of heat produced according to the needs of the body. Since muscles form roughly one third of the bulk of the body, either an involuntary or a purposeful increase in the activity of this big group of organs can form enough heat to offset considerable decrease in the temperature of the environment.

Very young and very old persons are limited in their ability to regulate body temperature when exposed to extremes in environment. The newborn infant will have lowering of body temperature if exposed to a cool environment for a long period of time. The elderly also are not able to produce enough heat to maintain body temperature in a cool environment. Heat loss mechanisms of the newborn are not fully developed; the elderly do not lose as much heat from their skin. Both groups should be protected from extreme temperatures.

Normal Body Temperature

The normal temperature range obtained by either glass or electronic thermometers may extend from 97°F to 100°F (36.2°C to 37.6°C). Temperature of the body varies with the time of day. Usually it is lower in the early morning, since the muscles have been relaxed and no food has been taken in for several hours. Temperature tends to be higher in the late afternoon and evening because of physical activity and consumption of food.

Normal temperature also varies with the part of the body. Skin temperature as obtained in the *axilla* is lower than mouth temperature, and mouth temperature is a degree or so lower than rectal temperature. If it were possible to place a thermometer inside the liver, it is believed that it would register a degree or more higher than the rectal temperature. The temperature within a muscle might be even higher during its activity.

Although the Fahrenheit scale is used in the United States, in most parts of the world temperature is measured using the *Celsius* (sel'se-us) thermometer. The ice point is at 0°, and the normal boiling point of water is at 100°, the interval between these two points being divided into 100 equal units. The Celsius scale is also called the centigrade scale (think of 100 cents).

On the Fahrenheit thermometer, there are 180 divisions; one Fahrenheit division equals 5/9 Celsius division, and one Celsius division equals 9/5 Fahrenheit divisions. It is a simple matter to convert one to the other: C = (F − 32) × 5/9; F = (C × 9/5) + 32.

1 0°C = 32°F = The freezing point of water.
2 10°C = 50°F = Cool, mild weather.
3 20°C = 60°F = Comfortable weather temperature.
4 30°C = 86°F = Warm weather.
5 37°C = 98.6°F = Normal body temperature.
6 40°C = 104°F = Hot weather.
7 100°C = 212°F = Boiling temperature of water.

Abnormal Body Temperature
Fever

Fever is a condition in which the body temperature is higher than normal. Usually the presence of fever is due to an infection, though there can be many other causes such as malignancies, brain injuries, toxic reactions, reactions to vaccines, and diseases involving the central nervous system. Sometimes emotional upsets can bring on a fever. Whatever the cause, the effect is to reset the body's thermostat in the hypothalamus.

Curiously enough, fever usually is preceded by a chill—that is, a violent attack of shivering and a sensation of cold that such measures as blankets and hot water bottles seem unable to relieve. Owing to these reactions heat is being generated and stored in the body; and when the chill subsides, the body temperature is elevated.

The old adage that a fever should be starved is completely wrong. During a fever there is an increase in metabolism that is usually proportional to the amount of fever. In addition to the use of available sugar and fat there is an increase in the use of protein, and during the first week or so of a fever there is definite evidence of destruction of body protein. A high calorie diet with plenty of protein is therefore desirable.

When a fever ends, sometimes the drop in temperature to normal occurs very rapidly. This sudden fall in temperature is called the *crisis,* and is usually accompanied by symptoms indicating rapid heat loss: profuse perspiration, muscular relaxation, and dilated blood vessels in the skin. A gradual drop in temperature, on the other hand, is known as *lysis.*

The mechanism of fever production is not completely understood, but we might think of the hypothalamus as a thermostat which is set higher at this time. This change in the heat-regulating mechanism often follows the injection of a foreign protein or the entrance into the blood stream of bacteria or their toxins. Those substances that produce fever are called *pyrogens* (pi'ro-jens). Up to a point, fever may be beneficial because it steps up *phagocytosis,* the process by which white blood cells surround, engulf, and digest bacteria and other foreign bodies, inhibits the growth of certain organisms, and increases cellular metabolism, which may be helpful in recovering from disease.

It is extremely important that the health worker keep accurate daily temperature records of patients, since a knowledge of the temperature level and its fluctuations is invaluable in aiding diagnosis and monitoring response to treatment. The temperature chart is a "picture" which tells a lot to the practiced eye.

Effects of Extreme Outside Temperatures

The body's heat-regulating devices are efficient, but there is a limit to what they can accomplish. High outside temperature may overcome the body's heat-loss mechanisms. Body temperature will rise. Cellular metabolism and accompanying heat production will increase. When the body temperature goes up, the individual is apt to suffer from a series of disorders, beginning with heat cramps, then heat exhaustion, and finally, if untreated, heat stroke.

In *heat cramps,* there is localized muscle cramping of the extremities and, occasionally, of the abdomen. This will respond to rest in a cool environment and adequate fluids.

With further heat retention and more fluid loss, *heat exhaustion* follows. Symptoms of this disorder include headache, tiredness, vomiting, and a rapid pulse. There may be a decrease in circulating blood volume and lowered blood pressure. Heat exhaustion also responds to rest and fluid replacement.

Heat stroke (also called sunstroke) is a final stage and a medical emergency. Heat stroke can be recognized by a body temperature of up to 41°C (105°F), hot, dry skin, and central nervous system symptoms including confusion, dizziness, and loss of consciousness. The body has responded to the loss of fluid from the circulation by reducing blood flow to the skin and sweat glands. The most important treatment is to lower body temperature immediately, by removing the individual's clothing, placing him in a cool environment, and cooling him with cold water or ice. The individual must have treatment with appropriate fluids containing the vital electrolytes including sodium, potassium, calcium, and chloride. Supportive medical care is necessary, since heat stroke can cause fatal complications.

The body is no more capable of coping with prolonged exposure to cold than to heat. If, for example, the body is immersed in cold water for a time, the water (a better heat conductor than air) removes more heat from the body than can be replaced, and the body temperature falls. This can happen too, of course, in cold air—particularly when clothing is inadequate. An excessively low body temperature is termed *hypothermia* (hi-po-ther′me-ah), and its main effects are uncontrolled shivering, lack of coordination, and decreased heart and respiratory rate. Speech becomes slurred, and there is overpowering sleepiness with possible coma and death. Outdoor activities in cool, not necessarily cold, weather cause many unrecognized cases of hypothermia. Wind, fatigue, and depletion of water and energy stores all play a part. Once cooled below a certain point, cellular metabolism is slowed and heat production is inadequate for maintaining a normal body temperature. The person must be warmed by heat from an outside source. The best first-aid measure is to put the individual in a warmed sleeping bag with an unclothed companion until shivering stops. Administering hot, sweetened fluids also helps.

Exposure to cold, particularly to moist cold, can cause permanent local tissue damage. The areas most likely to be affected by cold are the face, the ears, and the extremities. The causes include ice crystal formation resulting in tissue damage and the reduction of the blood supply to the area. This condition causes interference with cell nutrition and metabolism, and necrosis of the tissues with gangrene can result. Examples of cold damage are *chilblains* (localized itching and painful red areas on the skin), *frostbite,* and immersion foot or trench foot. Immersion or trench foot resembles frostbite, but results from prolonged exposure to water, rather than cold air. The very young, the very old, and those who suffer from disease of the circulatory system are particularly susceptible to cold injuries.

A frostbitten area should *never* be rubbed, but should be rapidly thawed by immersion in warm water or by contact with warm bare skin. The affected area should be treated very gently; if the feet are frostbitten, the individual should not be permitted to walk. Persons with cold-damaged extremities frequently have some lowering of body temperature. Warming of the whole person should not be neglected during the warming of the affected part.

Hypothermia is employed in certain types of surgery. In such cases the hypothalamus is depressed by drugs and the body temperature may be reduced to 25°C (77°F) before the operation is begun. Then, in the case of heart surgery, further cooling down to 20°C (68°F), is accomplished as the blood goes through the heart-lung machine. This has been successful even with tiny infants suffering from congenital heart abnormalities.

Summary

1 Body temperature and homeostasis.
  A Homeostasis—tendency of body processes to maintain normal state.
  B Body temperature regulation a phase of homeostasis.
2 Heat production.
  A Produced constantly in metabolic processes.
  B Muscles and glands produce most heat.
  C Heat distributed through body by blood.
  D Heat production rate determined by muscle and glandular activity, food intake, age.

3 Heat loss.
  A Outlets—chiefly skin; also respiratory system, urine, feces.
  B Heat loss from skin—conduction, radiation, convection, evaporation.
  C Excess heat loss prevented by artificial means (clothing), natural means (subcutaneous fat).
4 Temperature regulation.
  A Chief center is hypothalamus.
  B Information reaches it by blood and also nerves from temperature receptors.

C Hypothalamus causes either increased heat production (blood vessel constriction in skin, shivering, "gooseflesh," increased epinephrine) or increased heat loss (activation of sweat glands, blood vessel dilation, muscular relaxation).

5 Normal body temperature.
  A Normal range 97°F–100°F (36.2°C–37.6°C).
  B Varies with time of day, part of body.
  C On Celsius, or centigrade, scale, water freezes at 0° and boils at 100°; on Fahrenheit scale water freezes at 32° and boils at 212°.

6 Abnormal body temperature.
  A Fever.
    (1) Abnormally high body temperature, usually caused by infection.
    (2) Preceded by chill; terminates in crisis or lysis.
    (3) Causes destruction of some body protein; increases phagocytosis and possibly antibody production.
  B Extremes in outside temperature.
    (1) Heat—can cause heat exhaustion or sunstroke.
    (2) Cold—can cause hypothermia (sometimes but rarely of pathologic origin); cold injuries (chilblains, frostbite, immersion foot, trench foot).

Questions and Problems

1 What is homeostasis? Name 4 aspects of it.
2 How is heat produced in the body? What structures produce the most heat during increased activity?
3 Name 4 factors affecting heat production.
4 By what channels is heat lost from the body?
5 Name 4 ways in which heat escapes to the environment.
6 In what ways is heat kept in the body?
7 Name the main temperature regulator and describe what it does when the body is too hot and when it is too cold. What part do muscles play?
8 What is the normal body temperature range? How does it vary with respect to the time of day and the part of the body?
9 Define fever, name some aspects of its course, and list some of its beneficial and detrimental effects.
10 Name and describe 2 consequences of excessive outside heat. Why do these conditions occur?
11 What is the prime emergency measure for sunstroke?
12 What is hypothermia? Under what circumstances does it usually occur? List some of its effects. In what types of surgery is hypothermia induced?
13 Name and describe 2 common injuries resulting from cold. What happens in the body to bring these conditions about?

Chapter 7

Disease and Disease-Producing Organisms

7

Glossary

Ameba A single-celled protozoon, a minute irregular mass of protoplasm which propels itself by extending a branch, or "false foot," and then flowing over it.

Antisepsis The process of rendering pathogens incapable of multiplying.

Ascaris (pl. ascarides) An intestinal parasitic worm; a roundworm.

Bacilli (sing. bacillus) Bacteria having straight, slender shapes. Bacilli cause diphtheria and tuberculosis.

Bacteriology The study of the plantlike organisms called bacteria.

Bacteriostasis A condition in which bacteria are inhibited in their growth, but not killed.

Chemotherapy The treatment of disorders by chemicals, especially those that harm the disease organisms without harming the patient.

Ciliate A group of protozoa covered with cilia (tiny hairs) which propel the organism by producing a wave motion.

Cocci (sing. coccus) Spherical bacterial cells that resemble dots.

Disinfection The process of killing all pathogens on an object.

Etiology The study of causes of disease, including theories of origin and organisms that may be involved in causation.

Flagella (sing. flagellum) Microscopic whiplike processes or threadlike appendages that enable certain bacteria to move rapidly.

Helminthology Systematic study of worms and wormlike parasites.

Microbiology The science dealing with microscopic plants and animals, including bacteria, fungi, viruses, and protozoa.

Microorganism A tiny living organism (sometimes called a microbe or a germ) that cannot be seen with the naked eye.

Parasitology The study of those organisms that live in or on another at the latter's expense.

Pathogen Any disease-producing organism.

Chlamydias A group of microorganisms that can exist only within living cells. They cause trachoma and some respiratory diseases.

Protozoology Systematic study of single-celled animals.

Rickettsias Microscopic oval to rod-shaped organisms classified as bacteria although they are much smaller and can grow only in living matter.

Spirochetes   A group of bacteria capable of wavelike and twisting motions.

Sterilization   The process of killing all living microorganisms on an object.

Virus   The smallest known agent capable of causing infection.

What Is Disease?

Disease may be defined as the abnormal state in which part or all of the body is not properly adjusted or is not capable of carrying on all its required functions. There are marked variations in the extent of the disease and in its effect on the person. Disease can have a number of direct causes such as the following:

1 **Disease-producing organisms.** Some of these are discussed in this chapter. These are believed to play a part in at least one half of human illnesses.

2 **Malnutrition.** This means a lack of essential vitamins, minerals, proteins, or other substances required for normal life processes to take place.

3 **Physical agents.** These include excessive heat or cold, or injuries that cause cuts, fractures, or crushing damage to tissues.

4 **Chemicals.** Some may be poisonous or otherwise injurious if present in excess, such as lead compounds (in paints), carbolic acid (in certain antiseptic solutions), certain laundry aids, and other products.

5 **Birth defects.** Those abnormalities of structure and function which are present at birth are termed congenital. Such abnormalities may be inherited, which means they are passed on by the parents through their reproductive cells, or they may be acquired during the process of development within the mother's uterus (womb) (see Chap. 22).

6 **Degenerative process.** *Degeneration* (de-jen-er-a'shun) means breaking down. With aging, there is deterioration of tissue so that it becomes less active and less capable of performing its normal functions. Such degenerative processes may be caused by continuous infection, by repeated minor injuries to tissues by poisonous substances, or by the normal "wear and tear" of life. Thus degeneration is an anticipated result of aging.

7 **Neoplasms.** The word *neoplasm* (ne'o-plazm) means "new growth" and refers to cancer and other types of tumors (see Chap. 2).

Other factors that enter into the production of a disease are known as *predisposing causes*. While a predisposing cause may not in itself give rise to a disease, it increases the probability of a person's becoming ill. Examples of predisposing causes include the following:

Age. As we saw, the degenerative processes of aging can be a direct cause of disease. But a person's age also can be a predisposing factor. For instance, measles is more common in children than in adults.

Sex. Certain diseases are more characteristic of one sex than the other. Men are more susceptible to heart disease, while women are more prone to develop diabetes.

Heredity. Some individuals inherit a "tendency" to acquire certain diseases—particularly diabetes and many allergies.

Living conditions and habits. A person who habitually drives himself to exhaustion, does not have enough sleep, or pays little attention to his diet is highly vulnerable to the onslaught of disease. Overcrowding invites epidemics, and lack of sunshine can cause rickets in children. The use of narcotics and the abuse of alcohol and tobacco also can lower vitality and predispose to disease.

Occupation. A number of conditions are classified as "occupational diseases." For instance, coal miners are susceptible to lung damage caused by the constant inhalation of coal dust.

Physical exposure. Undue chilling of all or part of the body, or prolonged exposure to heat, can lower the body's resistance to disease.

Preexisting illness. Any preexisting illness, even the common cold, increases the chances of contracting another disease.

Psychogenic influences. "Psycho" refers to the mind, "genic" to origin. Some physical disturbances are due either directly or indirectly to emotional upsets caused by conditions of stress and anxiety in daily living. Peptic ulcers and so-called nervous indigestion are examples.

The Study of Disease

Our brief survey of the human body should give us a glimpse into three different studies which are considered the fundamentals of medical science. These are:

1 **Anatomy** (ah-nat′o-me)—the science of the structure of the body and the relationship of its parts to each other.
2 **Physiology** (fiz-e-ol′o-je)—the science that deals with the activities or dynamics (functions) of the body and its parts.
3 **Pathology** (pah-thol′o-je)—the science of the essential nature of disease, including the structural and functional changes produced by the disorders.

The modern approach to the study of disease emphasizes the close relationship of the pathologic and physiologic aspects and the need to understand the fundamentals of each in treating any body disorder. The term used for this combined study in medical science is *pathophysiology.*

Underlying the basic medical sciences are the still more fundamental disciplines of physics and chemistry. A knowledge of both of these is essential to any real understanding of the life processes.

It is interesting to note that many other sciences have grown up about the study of disease and that each has become a specialty in itself. Some examples of these more specialized sciences include the following:

1 **Bacteriology** (bac-te-re-ol′o-je), which includes a study of the many beneficial as well as disease-producing plantlike organisms called bacteria.
2 **Microbiology** (mi-kro-bi-ol′o-je), which is the science of microscopic plants and animals, usually emphasizing the bacteria. This term sometimes is synonymous with bacteriology.
3 **Protozoology** (pro-to-zo-ol′o-je), the study of one-celled animals.
4 **Parasitology** (par-ah-si-tol′o-je), the general study of parasites, a *parasite* being any organism that lives on or within another (called the *host*) at the host's expense.
5 **Helminthology** (hel-min-thol′o-je), the study of worms, particularly parasitic ones.

Disease Terminology

The study of the cause of any disease, or the theory of its origin, is *etiology* (e-te-ol′o-je). Any study of a disease usually includes some indication of its *incidence,* which means its range of occurrence and its tendency to affect certain groups of individuals more than others. Information about its geographic distribution and its tendency to appear in one sex, age group, or race more or less frequently than another is usually included in a presentation on disease incidence.

Diseases are often classified on the basis of severity and duration as

1 **Acute**—Those that are relatively severe but usually last a short time.
2 **Chronic**—Those that are often less severe but likely to be continuous or recurring for long periods of time.
3 **Subacute**—Those that are intermediate and fall between acute and chronic, not being quite so severe as acute infections nor as long lasting as chronic disorders.

Still another term used in describing certain diseases is *idiopathic* (id-e-o-path′ik), which means "self-originating" or "without a known cause."

A *communicable* disease is one that can be transmitted from one person to another. If many people in a given region acquire a certain disease at the same time, that disease is said to be *epidemic.* If a given disease is found to a lesser extent but continuously in a particular region, the disease is *endemic* to that area. A disease that is prevalent throughout an entire country or continent, or the whole world, is said to be *pandemic.*

Diagnosis, Treatment, and Prevention

In order to treat a patient, the doctor obviously must first determine the nature of the illness—that is, make a *diagnosis.* A diagnosis is the conclusion drawn from a number of facts put together. The doctor must know the *symptoms,* which are the changes in body function felt by the patient; and the *signs* (also called *objective symptoms*) which the doctor himself can observe. Sometimes a characteristic group of signs (or symptoms) accompanies a given disease. Such a group is called a *syndrome* (sin'drome). Frequently, certain laboratory tests are performed and the results evaluated by the physician in making his diagnosis.

Although nurses do not diagnose, they play an extremely valuable role in this process by observing closely for signs, encouraging the patient to talk about himself and his symptoms, and then reporting this information to the doctor. Once the patient's disorder is known, the doctor prescribes a course of treatment, also referred to as *therapy.* Many measures in this course of treatment are carried out by the nurse under the physician's orders.

In recent years physicians, nurses and other health workers have taken on increasing responsibilities in *prevention.* Throughout most of medical history, the physician's aim has been to cure a patient of an existing disease. However, the modern concept of prevention seeks to stop disease before it actually happens—to keep people well through the promotion of health. A vast number of organizations exist for this purpose, ranging from the World Health Organization (WHO) on an international level down to local private and community health programs. A rapidly growing responsibility of the nursing profession and of other health occupations is educating individual patients toward the maintenance of total health—physical and mental.

Infection

The predominant cause of disease in humans is the invasion of the body by disease-producing *microorganisms* (mi-kro-or'gan-izms). The word "organism" means "anything having life"; "micro" means "small." Hence, a microorganism is a tiny living thing, too small to be seen by the naked eye. Another term for microorganism is *microbe* or, more popularly, "germ."

Although the great majority of microorganisms are beneficial to man, or at the least are harmless, a certain few types cause illness; that is, they are pathogenic (path-o-jen'ic). Any disease-causing organism is a *pathogen* (path'o-jen). If the body is invaded by pathogens, with adverse effects, the condition is called an *infection.* If the infection is restricted to a relatively small area of the body, it is *local.* A generalized or *systemic* (sis-tem'ik) infection is one in which the whole body is affected. Systemic infections usually are spread by the blood stream.

Mode of Transmission

Microorganisms may be transmitted from an infected human, insect, or animal host to a susceptible human being; this transfer may be by direct or indirect contact. For example, infected human hosts may transfer their microorganisms to other individuals through direct personal contact such as shaking hands or kissing or during sexual intercourse. On the hand, indirect contact involves touching objects that have been contaminated by an infected person. For example, microorganisms may be transferred by bedding, toys, food, and dishes. Also, insects may deposit infectious material on food, skin, or clothing. Pets may be the source of a number of infections.

Portals of Entry and Exit

There are several avenues through which microorganisms may enter the body: the skin, respiratory tract, and digestive system, as well as the urinary and the reproductive systems. These portals of entry may also serve as exit routes. For example, discharges from the respiratory and intestinal tracts may spread infection through contamination of the air, through contamination of hands, and through contamination of food and water supplies. (Microbial control is discussed later in this chapter.)

The Microorganisms
Animal, Vegetable, or What?

Microorganisms are living things of a very primitive order. Because the early microscopes lacked high resolving power, many species of microorganisms such as rickettsias and viruses were unknown. These relatively simple organisms may be placed in a separate kingdom, called the Protista (pro-tis''tah) (Fig. 7-1).

Protista which means first, is a term used to designate a combination of one-celled organisms and certain very simple multicellular organisms. Among those microorganisms of medical interest are viruses, bacteria, protozoa, and some fungi. Viruses are mere particles comparable in size to molecules, but, unlike an ordinary molecule, they contain genetic material and are able to reproduce.

Higher forms of life, with which we are all familiar, are composed of vast numbers of cells

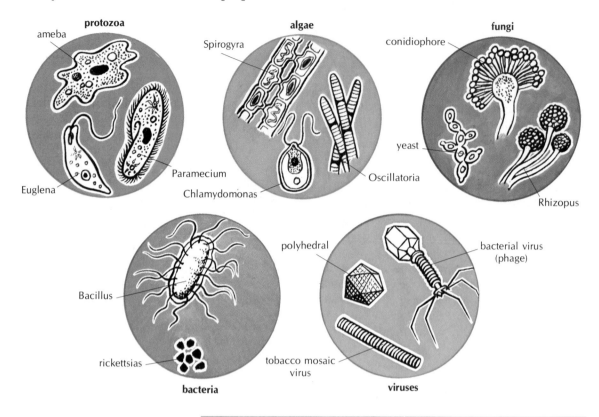

Fig. 7-1 *Some examples of protists.*

engaged to a greater or lesser degree in specialized tasks. Most microorganisms, however, are composed of but one cell in which all the processes of life are carried on—nutrition, growth, reproduction, response to environment, and so forth.

Bacteria

The bacteria are one-celled plants. Although they compose the largest group of pathogens, most bacteria are not only harmless to man but are absolutely essential to the continuation of all life on earth. It is through the action of bacteria that dead animals and plants are decomposed and transformed into substances that enrich the soil. Sewage is rendered harmless by bacteria. One type of bacterium transforms the nitrogen of the air into a form usable by plants, a process called *nitrogen fixation.* Farmers take advantage of this by allowing a field to lie fallow (untilled) so that the nitrogen of its soil can be replenished.

Bacteria can be seen only with the help of a microscope. Usually it is necessary to stain them with colored dyes in order to view their structures clearly. As a rough indication of their size, from 10 to 1000 bacteria (depending upon the species) could, if lined up, span a pinhead. Bacteria live in an environment of moisture and food materials. Bacterial spores are resistant forms that tolerate long periods of dryness or other adverse conditions. Some bacteria are capable of swimming rapidly about by themselves by means of threadlike appendages called *flagella* (flah-jel′ah). Their requirements as to water, food, oxygen, temperature, and other factors vary according to the species. Not surprisingly, the pathogenic bacteria are most at home within the "climate" of the human body. When living conditions are ideal, the organisms reproduce (by splitting in two) with unbelievable rapidity. If they succeed in overcoming the body's natural defenses, they can cause damage in two ways: by producing poisons, or *toxins,* and by entering the body tissues and growing within them. In Table 1 of the Appendix are listed some typical pathogenic bacteria and the diseases which they cause.

There are so many different types of bacteria that their classification is complicated. For our purposes, a convenient and simple grouping is based on the shape and arrangement of these organisms as seen with a microscope (Figs. 7-2 and 7-3):

1   **Rod-shaped cells**—*bacilli* (bah-sil'i). Cells are straight and slender, like match sticks. Some

are cigar-shaped, with tapering ends. Typical bacillary diseases include tetanus, diphtheria, tuberculosis, typhoid fever, and Legionnaire's (le'jun-nars) disease.

2   **Spherical cells**—*cocci* (kok'si). Cells resemble dots. Cocci are seen in characteristic arrangements. Some are in pairs and are called *diplococci* (diplo- meaning double). Another type is arranged in chains, like a string of beads. These are the *streptococci* (strepto- meaning chain). A third group is seen in large clusters and is known as *staphylococci* (staf-i-lo-kok'si) (staphlo-

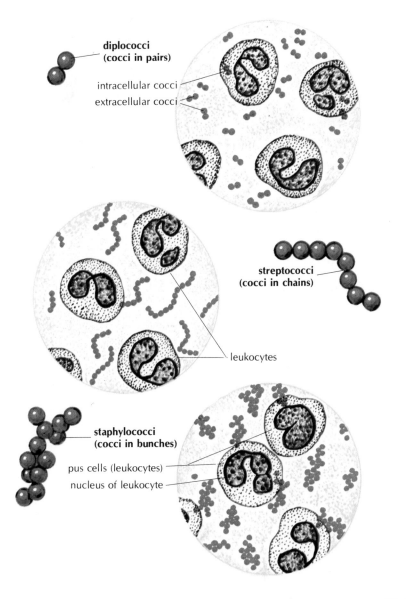

Fig. 7-2 *Bacteria of the spherical type.*

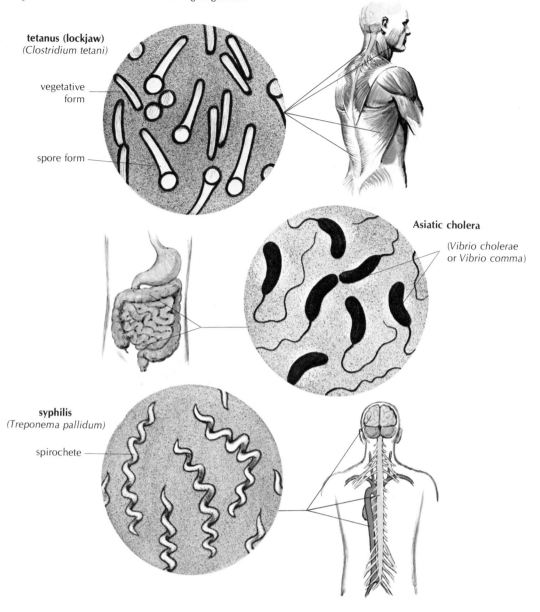

tetanus (lockjaw)
(Clostridium tetani)

vegetative form

spore form

Asiatic cholera

(Vibrio cholerae or Vibrio comma)

syphilis
(Treponema pallidum)

spirochete

Fig. 7-3   *Bacteria of the curved type. The illustration shows the areas of the body invaded by these pathogens.*

meaning bunch of grapes). Among the diseases caused by diplococci are gonorrhea and meningitis; streptococci and staphylococci are responsible for a wide variety of infections.

3 **Curved rods.** One type has only a slight curvature, like a comma, and is called *vibrio* (vib′re-o). Cholera is caused by a vibrio. Another form resembles a corkscrew and is known as

a *spirillum* (spi-ril′um) (plural *spirilla*). Bacteria very similar to the spirilla, but capable of waving and twisting motions, are called *spirochetes* (spi′ro-ketes). The most serious and widespread spirochetal infection is syphilis. In syphilis, the spirochetes enter the body at the point of contact through the genital skin or mucous membranes. They travel to the bloodstream and thus set up a systemic infection. (See Appendix, Table 1, for a summary of the three stages of syphilis.)

4 **Rickettsias** (ri-ket′se-ahs) and the **chlamydias** (klah-mid′e-ahs) (sometimes called rickettsiae and chlamydiae). Now classified as bacteria although considerably smaller. These microorganisms can exist only inside living cells. Because they exist at the expense of their host, they are *parasites;* and because they can grow only within living cells, they are referred to as *obligate parasites.*

The rickettsias are the cause of a number of serious diseases in man such as typhus and Rocky Mountain spotted fever. In almost every instance, these organisms are transmitted through the bites of such creatures as lice, ticks, and fleas. In Table 1 of the Appendix a few common rickettsial diseases are listed.

The chlamydias are smaller than the rickettsias. They are the causative organisms in trachoma (a serious eye infection that ultimately causes blindness), parrot fever or psittacosis, the venereal disease lymphogranuloma venereum, and some respiratory diseases (see Appendix, Table 1).

Fungi

The true *fungi* (fun′ji) are another large group of simple plants. Only a very few types are pathogenic. Although the fungi are much larger and more complicated than the bacteria, they are still a low order of plant life, lacking the green pigment chlorophyll which enables higher plants to utilize the energy of sunlight in carrying out their life processes. Like bacteria, the fungi prefer dark and damp places in which to grow. Reproductive cells of fungi include resistant "seeds" or spores.

Familiar examples of fungi are mushrooms, puffballs, bread molds, and yeasts (commercial yeast cakes used in baking and brewing). Diseases caused by fungi are called *mycotic* infections (myco- meaning fungus). Examples of these are athlete's foot and ringworm. Tinea capitis (tin′e-ah kap′′i-tis), which involves the scalp, and tinea corporis (kor-po′ris), which may be found almost anywhere on the nonhairy parts of the body, are common types of ringworm. Although few diseases are caused by fungi, some are very dangerous and all are difficult to cure. Pneumonia can be caused by

the inhalation of fungal spores contained in dust particles.

Table 2 of the Appendix is a list of typical fungous diseases.

Viruses

If the bacteria seem small, they are enormous in comparison to the *viruses.* These latter are so tiny as to be invisible in the ordinary light microscope and can be seen only in an electron microscope. Viruses are the smallest known infectious agents. They have some of the fundamental properties of living matter, but they are not cellular and they have no enzyme system. Like the rickettsias and the chlamydias, they can grow only within living cells—they are obligate parasites. Unlike these, the viruses are not usually susceptible to antibiotics.

At present there is no universally accepted classification of viruses. For our purpose, we can think of them in relation to the diseases that they cause. There is a considerable number of them—measles, poliomyelitis, hepatitis, chickenpox, and the common cold, to name a few. In Table 3 of the Appendix are listed representative viral diseases.

Protozoa

With the *protozoa* (pro-to-zo′ah) we come to the one and only group of microbes that can be definitely classed as animals because of their mode of nutrition. Although the protozoa are one celled, like the bacteria, they are much larger. Protozoa are found in almost any body of water from moist grass to mud puddles to the sea.

There are four main divisions of the protozoa:

1 **Amebae** (ah-me′bae). An ameba is an irregular blob of protoplasm which propels itself by extending a branch of itself (a "false foot") and then flowing over it. Amebic dysentery is caused by a pathogen of this group.

2 **Ciliates** (sil′e-ates). This type of protozoon is covered with tiny hairs called cilia which produce a wave motion to propel the organism.

3 **Flagellates** (flaj′e-lates). These organisms are propelled by the long whiplike filaments called flagella.

4 **Sporozoa** (spo-ro-zo′ah). Unlike other protozoa, the sporozoa cannot propel themselves. They are parasites, unable to grow outside the host. A member of this group causes malaria.

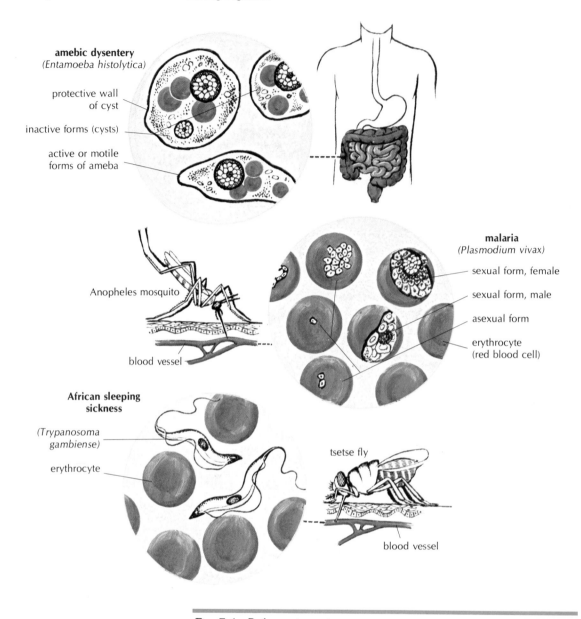

Fig. 7-4 *Pathogenic protozoa.*

Figure 7-4 illustrates some of the pathogenic protozoa and their portals of entry. Table 4 of the Appendix presents a list of typical pathogenic protozoa with the diseases for which they are responsible.

Parasitic Worms

Many species of worms (also referred to as *helminths*) are parasitic by nature and select the human organism as their host. Whereas invasion by any form of organism is usually called an infection, the presence of parasitic worms in the body also can be termed an *infestation* (Fig. 7-5). The microscope is required for the discovery of the eggs or larval forms of most worm infestations.

Roundworm

The most common of the intestinal worms is the large, rounded *ascaris* (as'kah-ris), which is very prevalent in many parts of Asia, where it is found mostly in the larval form. In the United States, it is found especially frequently in the children of the rural South. This worm resembles the earthworm (fishworm) in appearance and may be present in such large numbers that intestinal obstruction ensues. The eggs produced by the adult worms are very resistant so that they can live in soil during either freezing or hot, dry weather and cannot be destroyed even by strong antiseptics. The embryo worms develop within the eggs deposited with excreta in the soil, and later reach the digestive system of a victim by means of contaminated food. Discovery of this condition may be made by a routine stool examination.

Pinworms

Another fairly common infestation, particularly in children, is the seat or *pinworm* (*Enterobius vermicu-*laris), which is also very hard to control and eliminate. The worms average somewhat less than one half inch in length and live in the lower part of the alimentary tract. The adult female moves outside to the vicinity of the anus to lay its thousands of eggs. These eggs are often transferred by the child's fingers from the itching anal area to the mouth. In the digestive system of the victim the eggs develop to form new adult worms, and thus a new infestation is begun. The child also may infect others by this means. In addition, pinworm eggs that are expelled from the body also constitute a hazard, and they may live in the external environment for several months. Patience and every precaution, with careful attention to the doctor's instructions, are necessary if the patient is to be rid of the worms. Washing the hands, keeping fingernails clean, and avoiding finger sucking are all essential.

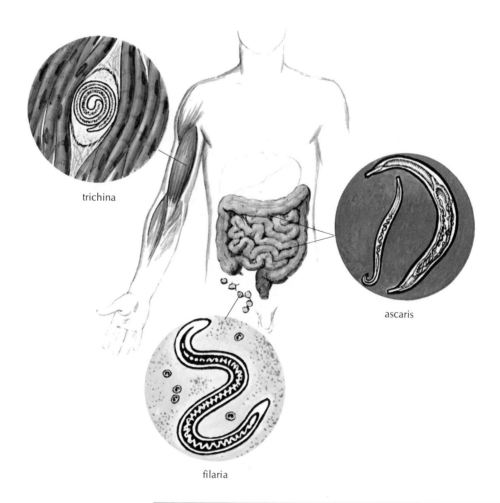

trichina

ascaris

filaria

Fig. 7-5 Common parasitic worms.

Hookworms

Hookworms are parasites that live in the small intestine. They are dangerous because they suck blood from the host, causing such a severe anemia (blood deficiency) that the victim becomes sluggish, both physically and mentally. Most victims become susceptible to various chronic infections because of extremely reduced resistance following such a great and continuous blood loss. Hookworms lay thousands of eggs, which are distributed in the soil by contaminated excreta. The eggs develop into small larvae which are able to penetrate the intact skin of bare feet. They enter the blood and, by way of the circulating fluids, the lungs and the upper respiratory tract, finally reach the digestive system. Prevention of this infestation is accomplished best by the proper disposal of excreta, attention to sanitation, and the wearing of shoes in areas where the soil is contaminated.

Other roundworms

While most roundworms are transmitted by excreta, the small *Trichinella* (trik-i-nel'ah), found in pork and other muscle foods, is an exception. These tiny round worms become enclosed in a cyst, that is, a sac, inside the muscles of the rat, the pig, and man. If pork is not well cooked, these sacs or cysts are dissolved by the host's digestive juices, and the tiny worms mature and travel to the muscles where they again become encased. This disease is known as *trichinosis* (trik-i-no'sis). Another threadlike worm causes *filariasis* (fil-ah-ri'ah-sis). This tiny worm is transmitted by such biting insects as flies and mosquitoes. The worms grow in large numbers, causing various body disturbances. If the lymph vessels become clogged by them, there results a condition called *elephantiasis* (el-e-fan-ti'ah-sis) in which the lower extremities and the scrotum may become tremendously enlarged. Filariasis is most common in tropical and subtropical lands, such as southern Asia and many of the South Pacific islands.

Flatworms

Some flatworms resemble long ribbons, while others have the shape of a leaf. Tapeworms may grow in the intestinal tract to a length of from 5 feet to 50 feet (1.5 meters to 15 meters) (Fig. 7-6). They are spread by infected, improperly cooked meats, including beef, pork, and fish. As is the case with most intestinal and worm parasites, the reproductive systems are very highly developed, so that each worm produces an almost unbelievable number of eggs which then may contaminate food, water, and soil. The leaf-shaped flatworms are known as flukes; they may invade various parts of the body including the blood, the lungs, the liver, and the intestine.

Microbial Control
The Spread of Microorganisms

There is scarcely a place on earth that is naturally free of microorganisms. One exception is the interior of normal body tissue. But on external body surfaces, on lining membranes and inside tubes and organs that are connected with the outside—such as the mouth, throat, nasal cavities, and large intestine—both harmless and pathogenic microbes live in abundance. As is explained in Chapter 23, the body has natural defenses against these organisms. If these natural defenses are sound, a person may harbor many microbes without ill effect. However, if his resistance becomes lowered, an infection can result.

Microbes are spread about through an almost infinite variety of means. The simplest way is by person-to-person contact. The more crowded the conditions, the greater the chances of epidemics breaking out. The atmosphere is a carrier of microorganisms. Although microbes cannot fly, the dust of the air is alive with them. In close quarters the atmosphere is further contaminated by bacteria-laden droplets discharged by sneezing, coughing, and even normal conversation. Pathogens also are spread by such pests as rats, mice, fleas, lice, flies, and mosquitoes. Microbial growth is further abetted by the prevalence of dirt and the lack of sunlight. In slum areas there is often a combination of crowded conditions and poor sanitation. In addition, many of the inhabitants have lowered resistance because of poor nutrition and other undesirable health practices. As a result, epidemics are apt to begin in these districts.

Microbes and Public Health

All civilized societies establish and enforce measures designed to protect the health of their populations. Most of these practices are concerned with

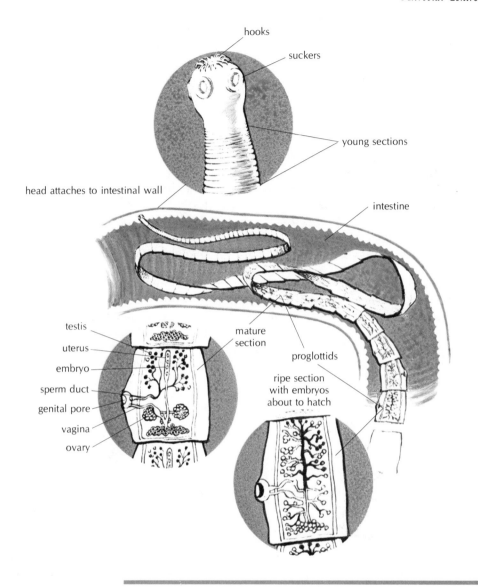

Fig. 7-6 *Tapeworm. Loss of segments (proglottids) will not cause injury to the parasite as long as the head remains attached to the host's intestine. Each proglottid contains testes and an ovary, so fertilization occurs between adjacent segments.*

preventing the spread of infectious organisms. A few examples of fundamental public health considerations are listed.

Sewage and garbage disposal. In times past, when people disposed of the household "slops" by the simple expedient of throwing them out the window, great epidemics were inevitable. Modern practice is to divert sewage into a processing plant in which harmless bacteria are put to work in destroying the pathogens. The resulting noninfectious "sludge" makes excellent fertilizer.

Purification of the water supply. Drinking water that has become polluted with untreated sewage may be contaminated with such dangerous pathogens as typhoid bacilli, the viruses of polio and hepatitis, and dysentery amebae. The municipal water supply usually is purified by a filtering process, and a close and constant watch is kept on its microbial population. Industrial and chemical wastes, such as asbestos fibers, acids and detergents from homes as well as from industry, and pesticides used in agriculture complicate the problems of obtaining pure drinking water.

Prevention of food contamination. Various national, state, and local laws all seek to prevent outbreaks of disease through contaminated food. Not only can certain animal diseases (tuberculosis, tularemia) be passed on, but food is a natural breeding place for many dangerous pathogens. Two organisms that cause food poisoning are the rod-shaped botulism bacillus (*Clostridium botulinum*) and the grapelike "staph" (*Staphylococcus aureus*). For further information, see Table 1 of the Appendix.

Most cities have sanitary regulations requiring, among other things, compulsory periodic inspection of food-handling establishments and medical examination of personnel.

Milk Pasteurization. Milk is rendered free of pathogens by pasteurization, a process in which it is heated to 145°F (63°C) for 30 minutes and then is allowed to cool rapidly before being bottled. Pasteurized milk still contains microbes, but no harmful ones. Sometimes slightly higher temperatures may be used for a shorter time with satisfactory results.

Aseptic Methods

In the practice of medicine, surgery, nursing, and other health fields, specialized procedures are performed for the purpose of reducing to a minimum the influence of pathogenic organisms. The word "sepsis" means "poisoning due to pathogens"; *asepsis* (ah-sep′sis) is its opposite: a condition in which no pathogens are present. Those procedures that are designed to kill, remove or prevent the growth of microbes are called aseptic methods.

There are a number of terms designating aseptic practices, many of which are often confused with one another. Some of the more commonly used terms and their definitions are as follows (Fig. 7-7):

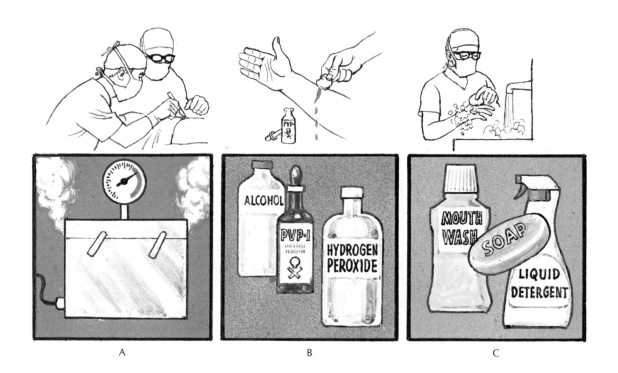

Fig. 7-7 *Aseptic methods—(A) sterilization, (B) disinfection, and (C) antisepsis.*

Sterilization. To sterilize an object means to kill *every* living microorganism on it. In operating rooms and delivery rooms especially, as much of the environment is kept sterile as is practicable—for instance, the gowns worn by operating room personnel and the instruments used. The usual sterilization agent is live steam under pressure, or else dry heat. Most pathogens can be killed by exposure to boiling water for 4 minutes. However,—and this is a vitally important fact to remember—a very few types of pathogenic bacteria are capable of developing a highly resistant, armorlike coat. The resulting stage is called a *spore.* Spores are very difficult to kill. To insure destruction of all spore-forming organisms, the time and temperature for sterilization are much greater than those required to kill most pathogens.

Disinfection. Disinfection refers to any measure that kills all pathogens (except spores), but not necessarily all harmless microbes as well. Most disinfecting agents (*disinfectants*) are chemical. Examples are iodine and phenol (carbolic acid). Two other terms for bacteria-killing agents, synonymous with disinfectant, are *bactericide* and *germicide.*

Antisepsis. This term refers to any process in which pathogens are not necessarily killed, but are prevented from multiplying, a state called *bacteriostasis* (bak-te-re-os′tah-sis). *Antiseptics* are less powerful than disinfectants.

Chemotherapy

Chemotherapy (ke-mo-ther′ah-pe) means the treatment of a disease by the administration of a chemical agent. This term has come to include the treatment of any disease by any natural or artificial (synthetic) substance.

Antibiotics

An antibiotic is a chemical substance, produced by *living* cells. It has the power to kill or arrest the growth of pathogenic microorganisms by upsetting vital chemical processes within them. Antibiotics that are nontoxic to the host are used for the treatment of infectious diseases. Most antibiotics are derived from molds and soil bacteria. Penicillin, the first widely used antibiotic, is made from a common blue mold, Penicillium. Another large group of antibiotics is produced by Streptomyces, a type of soil bacteria; a well-known example of this group is streptomycin.

Although the development of antibiotics has been of incalculable benefit to mankind, it has also given rise to serious complications. One danger is that of secondary infection. For example, an antibiotic may be given to combat the bacteria causing a specific disease. Now, it may well be that coexisting in the body with these pathogens is a second type of disease organism—say, a fungus. Up to the time of the administration of the drug the fungus had been no danger to the body because its growth was being suppressed by the bacteria. If the natural enemy of the fungus is now eliminated, and the fungus happens to be unaffected by the antibiotic, there is nothing to prevent it from growing unrestrainedly and setting up a new infection which is very difficult to cure.

Another danger in the use of antibiotics is the development of allergy (an abnormal reaction) to these substances within certain individuals. This complication can have very dangerous consequences.

Finally, the widespread use of antibiotics has resulted in the natural evolution of strains of pathogens that are resistant to such medications. One of the greatest problems in hospitals today is the prevalence of antibiotic-resistant ("drug-fast") staphylococci, which cause serious infections that may be unresponsive to chemotherapy.

Antineoplastic Agents

Antineoplastic agents are a group of chemotherapeutic drugs extensively employed to treat cancers. These agents are toxic to the host as well as to the tumor cells and must be administered by persons with an understanding of the complications caused by these drugs (see Chap. 2).

Laboratory Identification of Pathogens

The nurse, physician, or laboratory worker may obtain specimens from the patient in order to identify bacteria and other organisms. Specimens most frequently studied include blood, spinal fluid, feces, urine, and sputum, as well as swabbings from other areas. Swabs are used to collect specimens from the nose, throat, eyes, and cervix, and from ulcers or other infected areas.

There are so many different kinds of bacteria requiring identification that the laboratory must use a number of procedures for determining which organism is present in the material obtained from the patient. One of the most frequently used methods for beginning the process of identification involves the application of colored dyes, known as stains, to a thin smear of the specimen on a glass slide. After being stained with a reddish dye (carbolfuchsin), the smear may be treated with acid. Most bacteria quickly lose their stain upon application of the acid, but the organisms that cause tuberculosis and leprosy remain colored. Such organisms are said to be *acid-fast.*

Another commonly used procedure is known as the *Gram stain.* A bluish dye (such as methyl violet or gentian violet) is applied and then a weak solution of iodine is added. This causes a color-fast combination within certain organisms so that the use of alcohol or other solvents does not remove the dye. These bacteria are said to be *gram-positive.* Examples are the pathogenic staphylococci and streptococci, the cocci that cause certain types

of pneumonia, and the bacilli that produce diphtheria, tetanus, and anthrax. Other organisms are said to be *gram-negative* because the coloring can be removed from them by the use of a solvent, such as acetone or alcohol. Examples of gram-negative organisms are those diplococci that cause gonorrhea and epidemic meningitis, and the bacilli that produce typhoid fever, influenza, and one type of dysentery. The colon bacillus, normally found in the bowel, is also gram-negative, as is the cholera vibrio. A few organisms do not stain with any of the commonly used dyes, such as the spirochete of syphilis and the rickettsias. Special staining techniques must be used to identify those organisms.

In addition to the various staining procedures, other laboratory techniques include growing bacteria for study by culture, a process using substances called media (such as nutrient broth or agar) that bacteria can use as food; studying the ability of bacteria to act on (ferment) various carbohydrates (sugars); counting bacteria in a given specimen by specialized processes; inoculating animals and analyzing their reactions to the injections; and studying bacteria by serologic (blood) tests, mostly based on the antigen-antibody reaction (see Chap. 23). These are but a few of the many laboratory procedures that play a vital part in the process of diagnosing disease.

Summary

1 Disease—abnormal state of part or all of the body.
2 Direct causes of disease—disease-producing organisms, malnutrition, physical and chemical agents, congenital and inherited abnormalities, degeneration, neoplasms.
3 Predisposing factors—age, sex, heredity, living conditions and habits, occupation, physical exposure, preexisting illness, psychogenic influences.
4 Fundamental medical sciences—anatomy, physiology, pathology.
5 Terminology.
   A Etiology—study of causation.
   B Incidence—range of occurrence.
   C Disease description.
      (1) Acute—severe, short duration.
      (2) Chronic—less severe, long duration.
      (3) Subacute—intermediate between above in severity and duration.
      (4) Idiopathic—unknown cause.
      (5) Communicable—transmissible.
      (6) Epidemic—widespread in a given region.
      (7) Endemic—characteristic of a given region.
      (8) Pandemic—prevalent throughout an entire country.
   D Diagnosis—determination of the nature of an illness.
   E Symptom: change in body function felt by patient.
   F Sign—change in body function observable by others.
   G Syndrome—characteristic group of signs and symptoms.

H Therapy—course of treatment.

I Prevention—removing potential causes of disease.

6 Infection—invasion of the body by microorganisms.

A Mode of transmission—direct or indirect contact.

B Portals of entry and exit—skin, respiratory, digestive, and reproductive systems.

7 Microorganisms (also called microbes or germs)

A Microscopic living things.

B Disease-causing microorganisms are called pathogens.

8 Bacteria.

A One-celled plants.

B Classified according to shape.

(1) Bacilli (straight rods).

(2) Cocci (spherical).

(a) Diplococci—pairs.

(b) Streptococci—chains.

(c) Staphylococci—bunches.

(3) Curved rods.

(a) Vibrios—comma-shaped.

(b) Spirilla—corkscrew or wavy shaped.

(c) Spirochetes—like spirilla but flexible body.

(4) Modified bacteria, obligate parasites.

(a) Rickettsias.

(b) Chlamydias.

9 Fungi.

A Simple plants, larger than bacteria.

B Yeasts and molds include pathogenic species.

10 Viruses—smallest microorganisms, obligate parasites.

11 Protozoa.

A Only microbes in animal kingdom.

B Divisions—amebae, ciliates, flagellates, sporozoa.

12 Parasitic worms (helminths).

A Roundworms—ascaris, pinworms (both intestinal parasites); trichinella (encysted in muscle tissue); filariae (obstruct lymph vessels); hookworms (intestinal parasites).

B Flatworms—tapeworms (intestinal parasites); flukes (invade intestine, lungs, liver, etc.).

13 Microbial controls.

A Spread of microorganisms.

(1) Body normally harbors parasites.

(2) Microbes spread by direct contact, dust, droplets, vermin.

B Public health measures—sewage disposal, water purification, food inspection, milk pasteurization.

C Aseptic methods—sterilization (total removal of organisms); disinfection (destruction of pathogens except spores); antisepsis (bacteriostasis).

D Chemotherapy—includes drug treatment of any disease.

(1) Antibiotics—nontoxic treatment of infection.

(a) Derived from living cells.

(b) Disadvantages of antibiotics—allergy, secondary infection, drugfast strains.

(2) Antineoplastics for treatment of cancer.

14 Laboratory identification of pathogens.

A Examples of acid-fast organisms—those causing tuberculosis and leprosy.

B Examples of gram-positive organisms—those causing diphtheria, tetanus, anthrax, and certain types of pneumonia.

C Examples of gram-negtive organisms—those causing gonorrhea, epidemic meningitis, typhoid fever, influenza, and 1 type of dysentery.

Questions and Problems

1 What is disease? List 5 direct and 5 indirect causes.

2 Define etiology, incidence, acute, chronic, idiopathic, epidemic, endemic, diagnosis, symptom, sign, syndrome, therapy, infection, pathogen.

3 What are the 3 characteristic shapes of bacterial cells? Name a typical disease caused by each group. Name the portals of entry.

4 In what ways are bacteria beneficial to man?

5 How do the rickettsias and the chlamydias differ from other bacteria in size and living habits?

6 What is the typical mode of transmission of rickettsial infections?

7 What microbial group is classed as animals? Name 2 diseases caused by these.

8 Name 2 types of pathogenic fungi, and 1 common fungous infection.

9 Name 2 diseases caused by rickettsias and 2 due to chlamydias.

10 List 4 viral diseases. Describe the effects of antibiotics on these diseases.

11 Name 3 shapes of parasitic worms.

12 What are the most common ways by which disease organisms are spread? What measures do communities take to prevent outbreaks of disease?

13 Define: asepsis, sterilization, disinfection, antisepsis, chemotherapy.

14 What are some disadvantages in the use of antibiotics?

15 What are laboratory stains and why are they used? What are examples of acid-fast, gram-negative, and gram-positive organisms?

Chapter 8

The Skin
in Health
and Disease

8

Glossary

Ceruminous Pertaining to the waxlike secretion found in the external meatus of the ear.

Dermis The "true skin" that underlies the epidermis, having a framework of connective tissues, and many blood vessels, nerve endings, and glands.

Epidermis The outer epithelial layer of the skin, which contains no blood vessels and which rests on the dermis.

Erythema Skin redness usually due to congestion of the blood in the capillaries.

Excoriation Superficial loss of substance such as that produced on the skin by scratching.

Integument A covering, especially the skin.

Laceration A torn, ragged wound.

Macule A discolored spot on the skin that is not raised above the surrounding area, as seen in freckles or measles.

Melanin The dark pigment found in some parts of the body, such as the skin, the middle coat of the eye, and certain tissues in the brain.

Papule A small solid elevation on the skin; a pimple.

Pustule A small pus-containing elevation on the skin; a pimple that is filled with pus.

Sebaceous Secreting sebum, which is a greasy, lubricating substance.

Sudoriferous Secreting sweat.

Ulcer A lesion that causes or is associated with tissue death.

Vesicle A small sac or blister filled with fluid.

Is the skin merely a body covering, is it an organ, or is it a composite of parts that make it properly a system? Actually, it has some properties of each of these, and so may be classified in three different ways, namely:

1 It may be called an **enveloping membrane** because it is a rather thin layer of tissue covering the entire body.
2 It may be referred to as an **organ** (the largest one, in fact) because it contains several kinds of tissue, including epithelial, connective and nerve tissues.
3 The skin is also known as the **integumentary system,** "integument" (integ'u-ment) meaning "covering," because it includes sweat and oil

glands as well as other parts that work together as a body system.

Structure of the Skin
Layers Enveloping the Body

The skin covers the entire surface of the body. It consists of two main layers, different from each other in structure and function (Fig. 8-1). These are

1 The **epidermis** (ep-i-der′mis), or outermost layer, which is subdivided into *strata* (stra′tah), or layers, and is made entirely of epithelial cells with no blood vessels.

2 The **dermis,** or true skin, which has a framework of connective tissue, and contains many blood vessels, nerve endings, and glands.

The Epidermis

The epidermis is the surface layer of the skin, and the outermost cells are constantly being lost through the wear and tear of daily living. Since there are no blood vessels in the epidermis, the only living cells are in its deepest layer where nourishment is provided by capillaries in the underlying dermis. These cells are constantly dividing and producing daughter cells which are pushed upward toward the surface. As these cells die from the gradual loss of nourishment, they undergo changes. By the time they reach the surface they

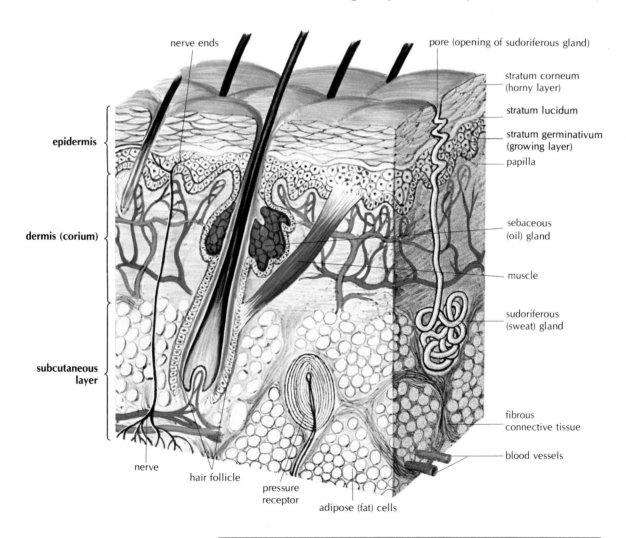

Fig. 8-1 Cross section of the skin.

have become flat and horny. Cells in the deepest layer of the epidermis also produce *melanin* (mel'ah-nin) the pigment that gives skin its color; irregular patches of melanin are called freckles. Ridges and grooves in the skin of the fingers, palms, toes, and soles form unchanging patterns peculiar to each individual; thus fingerprints and footprints are excellent means of identification. These ridges are due to elevations and depressions in the epidermis and the dermis. The deep surface of the epidermis is accurately molded upon the outer part of the dermis, which has raised and depressed areas.

The Dermis

The *dermis,* or *corium* (ko're-um), the so-called true skin, has a framework of elastic connective tissue and is well supplied with blood vessels and nerves. Involuntary muscle fibers also are found in the dermis, particularly where there are hairs. The thickness of the dermis as well as that of the epidermis varies so that some areas such as the soles of the feet and the palms of the hands are covered with very thick layers of skin, while the skin of the eyelids is very thin and delicate. Most of the appendages of the skin, including the sweat and oil glands, the nails, and the hairs, extend into the dermis and often deeper into the subcutaneous layer.

The Subcutaneous Layer

The dermis rests upon the *subcutaneous* (sub-ku-ta'ne-us) or under-the-skin layer. This layer contains parts of the sweat and oil glands as well as other skin appendages. Subcutaneous tissue is a combination of elastic and fibrous tissue as well as adipose tissue (fat). This layer sometimes is referred to as the superficial fascia (see Chap. 3) and is the means of connecting the skin proper to the surface muscles. The fat in this sheet of tissue serves as insulation as well as a reserve store for energy.

Glands of the Skin

The *sudoriferous* (su"do-rif'er-us) (sweat) glands are coiled, tube-like structures located largely in the subcutaneous tissue. These glands secrete a mixture of water and mineral salts. Their excretory ducts spiral upward and open as pores on the surface of the skin. Contrary to a popular notion, these pores do not open and close like a mouth, since

there is no muscle tissue associated with them. The *ceruminous* (se-roo'mi-nus) or wax glands, in the ear canal and the *ciliary* (sil'e-er''e) glands at the edges of the eyelids are modifications of sweat glands.

The *sebaceous* (se-ba'shus) *glands* are saclike in structure, and their oily secretion (called sebum) helps to keep the hair from becoming brittle. Their ducts often open into the hair follicles, but in some instances they open directly onto the skin surface. Before a baby is born these glands produce a covering that resembles cream cheese. This secretion is called the *vernix caseosa* (ver'niks ka-se-o'sah).

Blackheads consist of a mixture of dirt and sebum that may collect at the openings of the sebaceous glands. If these glands become infected, pimples result. If sebaceous glands of the scalp become blocked by accumulated sebum, a sac of this secretion may form and gradually become larger and larger. These sacs, or cysts, are referred to as sebaceous cysts. Usually it is not too difficult to remove such tumor-like cysts by surgery.

Functions of the Skin

Although the skin has several functions, the three that are by far the most important are:

1 Protection of deeper tissues against drying and against invasion by pathogenic organisms or their toxins by providing a mechanical barrier.
2 Regulation of body temperature by dissipating heat to the surrounding air.
3 Obtaining information about the environment by means of the nerve endings which are so profusely distributed in the skin. Some sensory information also has a protective function in that it enables one to withdraw from harmful stimuli, such as a hot stove.

The intact skin is incapable of defense against sharp objects, but it is an able defender against pathogens, toxins, and water loss. A break in the continuity of the skin by *trauma* (traw'mah), that is, a wound or injury of any kind, may be followed by serious infection. The care of wounds involves, to a large extent, the prevention of the entrance of pathogens and toxins into the deeper tissues and body fluids.

The regulation of body temperature is also a

very important function of the skin. The normal temperature may vary slightly, but we think of 98.6°F (37°C) as the standard when a thermometer is placed in the mouth for 3 to 5 minutes. The body temperature reading may be expected to be somewhat less if taken in the axilla and somewhat more if taken in the rectum. The skin forms a large surface for radiating body heat to the air. When the blood vessels dilate (enlarge), more blood is brought to the surface so that heat can be dissipated into the air. The evaporation of sweat from the surface of the body also helps to cool the body. As is the case with so many body functions, the matter of temperature regulation is complex and involves several parts of the body, including certain centers in the brain.

A child loses heat faster than does an adult since a higher proportion of the body is skin surface, and thus relatively more area is exposed. Therefore, it is important to prevent undue exposure to the elements in the case of infants and small children. The elderly do not produce heat in the body so easily nor to so great an extent; therefore, they also should be protected against cold.

Another important function of the skin is obtaining information from the environment. Because of the many receptors (nerve endings) for pain, touch, pressure, and temperature, which are located mostly in the dermis, the skin may be regarded as one of the chief sensory organs of the body. Many of the reflexes that make it possible for the human being to adjust himself to the environment begin as sensory impulses from the skin. Here, too, the skin works in cooperation with the brain and the spinal cord to make these important functions possible.

The functions of absorption and excretion are minimal as far as the skin is concerned. The absorbing power of the skin is very limited. Most medicated ointments used on the skin are for the treatment of local conditions. The injection of medication into the subcutaneous tissues is limited by the slow absorption that occurs here. Excretion by the skin includes water and mineral salts in perspiration. Even in disease the amount of waste products excreted from the body by the skin is negligible.

The human skin does not "breathe." The pores of the epidermis serve only as outlets for perspiration and oil from the sweat glands. The public is bombarded with misinformation about the skin,

sometimes merely for the purpose of selling lotions, potions, and all sorts of supposedly magical preparations. Breathing is a function of the respiratory system and not of the skin. Beware of cosmetics that purportedly aid the skin in breathing.

Observation of the Skin

What can the skin tell you? What do its color, texture, and other attributes indicate? Much can be learned by the astute observer.

In fact, the first indication of a serious systemic disease (such as syphilis) may be a skin disorder.

The color of the skin is dependent upon a number of factors, including the following:

1 The amount of pigment in the epidermis.
2 The quantity of blood circulating in the surface blood vessels.
3 The composition of the circulating blood
  a Presence or absence of oxygen.
  b Concentration of hemoglobin.
  c Presence of bile, silver compounds, or other chemicals.

Pigment of the Skin

The pigment of the skin, as we have noted, is called melanin. It is found also in the hair, the middle coat of the eyeball, the iris of the eye, and in certain tumors. Melanin is common to all races, but the darker peoples have a much larger quantity of it distributed in these tissues. A normal increase in this skin pigment occurs as a result of exposure to the sun. Abnormal increases in the quantity of melanin may occur either in localized areas or over the entire body surface. Diffuse spots of pigmentation may be characteristic of some endocrine disorders.

Discoloration of the Skin

A yellowish discoloration of the skin may be due to the presence of excessive quantities of bilirubin (bile pigment) in the blood. Such a condition is called *jaundice* (jawn'dis) and may be a symptom of a number of disorders such as

1 A tumor pressing on the common bile duct or a stone within the duct, either of which

would obstruct the flow of bile into the small intestine.

2 Inflammation of the liver (hepatitis).
3 Certain diseases of the blood in which red blood cells are rapidly destroyed.

Another cause of a yellowish discoloration of the skin is the excessive intake of carrots and other deeply colored vegetables. This condition is known as *carotinemia* (kar″o-tin-e′me-ah).

Chronic poisonings may cause grayish or brown discoloration of the skin. A peculiar bronze cast is present in Addison's disease (malfunction of the adrenal gland). So many other disorders cause discoloration of the skin that an entire chapter could be written on this topic alone.

Skin Injuries

A wound or local injury is called a *lesion* (le′zhun). Lesions of the skin that should be noted by those who care for the sick include

1 **Excoriations** (eks-ko-re-a′shuns) which may be evidence of scratching.
2 **Lacerations** (las″er-a′shuns) are rough, jagged wounds made by tearing the skin.
3 **Ulcers** (ul′sers) are sores associated with disintegration and death of tissue.
4 Areas of redness, called **erythema** (er-e-the′-mah), as well as other discoloration.
5 Spots of any kind.

Skin Eruptions

A skin rash (eruption) may be localized as in a diaper rash, or it may be generalized as in measles and other systemic infections. Some terms often used to describe skin eruptions are the following (Fig. 8-2):

1 **Macules** (mak′ules) or macular (mak′u-lar) rash, in which the spots are neither raised nor depressed, typical of measles and also descriptive of freckles.
2 **Papules** (pap′ules) or a papular (pap′u-lar) rash, in which there are firm raised areas, as in some stages of chickenpox and in the second stage of syphilis. Characteristic of pimples.
3 **Vesicles** (ves′e-kals) or vesicular (ve-sik′u-lar) eruptions, in which blisters or small sacs are

full of fluid, such as may be found in some of the eruptions of chickenpox.

4 **Pustules** (pus′tules) or pustular (pus′tu-lar) lesions, which may follow the vesicular stage of chickenpox.
5 **Crusts,** which are made of dried pus and blood and are commonly referred to by laymen as scabs.

Skin Diseases
Dermatosis and Dermatitis

Dermatosis (der″mah-to′sis) is a general term referring to any skin disease.

Inflammation of the skin is called *dermatitis* (der-mah-ti′tis). It may be due to many kinds of irritants, such as the oil of poison oak or poison ivy plants, detergents, and strong acids or alkalies or other chemicals. Prompt removal of the irritant is the most effective prevention and treatment. A thorough soap and water bath as soon as possible after contact with plant oils may prevent the development of the itching eruptions.

Sunburn and Its Complications

Sunlight may cause chemical and biological changes in the skin. The skin first becomes reddened (erythematous) and then may become swollen and blistered. Some people suffer from severe burns and become seriously ill. There is considerable evidence that continued excessive exposure to the sun is an important cause of skin cancer. The current fad for tanning requires the skin to protect itself by producing considerably more than usual amounts of melanin. This increase in pigmentation may have the effect of reducing the ability of the body to profit from the desirable smaller amounts of sun available during some parts of the year. A moderate amount of exposure to the sun enables the skin to convert certain substances into vitamin D, the so-called sunshine vitamin.

Eczema

Eczema (ek′ze-mah) is an unpleasant disease which may be found in all age groups and in both sexes. However, it is more common in the very young and in the elderly. Eczema may affect any and all parts of the skin surface. It is a noncontagious dis-

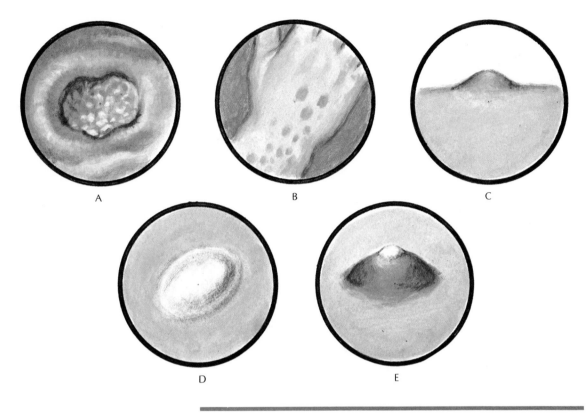

Fig. 8-2 *Some common skin eruptions—(A) ulcer, (B) macule, (C) papule, (D) vesicle, and (E) pustule.*

ease which may manifest itself by redness (erythema), blisters (vesicles), and pimple-like (papular) lesions. There also may be scaling and crusting of the skin surface. Eczema may be a manifestation of excessive sensitivity to detergents, soaps, and other chemicals. For example, if used frequently, even the mildest soap may cause irritation. The skin also may overreact to heat, dryness, rough fabrics (especially wool), and even to perspiration.

Common Acne

Acne (ak'ne) is usually a disease of the oil glands of the hair follicles of the skin called *acne vulgaris.* It is found most often in individuals between the ages of 14 and 25. The infection of the oil glands takes the form of pimples which generally surround blackheads. Acne is usually most severe at adolescence because certain endocrine glands in the body which control the secretions of the sebaceous

glands are then particularly active. Frequent, thorough cleansing of the skin with abrasive soaps and warm water, followed by the use of a clean pillow slip, changed daily, may be effective treatment in some cases. Occasionally antibiotics may prove useful, but should be taken only as prescribed by a physician.

Impetigo

Impetigo (im-pe-ti'go) is an acute contagious disease of staphylococcal or streptococcal origin that may be serious enough to cause the death of newborn infants. It takes the form of blister-like lesions which become filled with pus and contain millions of virulent bacteria. It is found most frequently among poor and undernourished children. A child may reinfect himself or infect others. Sometimes the infection is spread by contaminated linen or dishes. In a nursery, for example, utmost care in handling infants in order to prevent the spread from baby to baby is extremely important. Despite ordinary precautions, fatalities from impetigo have occurred at various times in the United States. Impetigo is so contagious that children who develop the disease should not be permitted to return to school until a health professional certifies that the condition is cured.

Baldness (Alopecia)

Alopecia (al-o-pe'she-ah) may be due to infection as well as to a number of other factors. It may be inherited, particularly in males. Baldness may be an expression of aging, in which case it usually begins at the crown of the head and is associated with atrophy of the structures of the scalp. It may be the result of such systemic diseases as syphilis and myxedema. A severe infection such as scarlet fever may cause the loss of hair, but in such cases recovery from the disease usually is accompanied by the regrowth of the hair. A chronic fungous infection which involves the oil glands and hair follicles may result in alopecia. In these cases frequent shampooing and constant attention to skin hygiene may prevent balding. Dandruff is often due to fungous disease of the scalp, and the assistance of a physician should be sought if one is to prevent alopecia. Baldness also is a common temporary side-effect of chemotherapeutic drugs used in treating neoplasms.

Athlete's Foot

Fungi are the usual cause of athlete's foot, also known as *epidermophytosis* (ep-e-der-mo-fi-to'sis). The disease involves the toes and the soles most commonly, but occasionally it may affect the fingers, the palms and the groin region. In acute cases the lesions may include vesicles, fissures, and ulcers. Predisposition to fungous infection varies. Some individuals may be exposed to pathogenic fungi with no ill effects, while in other people a mild exposure will cause a severe skin infection. Those who perspire a great deal are particularly susceptible to athlete's foot. Frequent changing of hose and of shoes together with thorough drying of the feet, with particular attention to the spaces between the toes, will discourage infection. Dusting powders in the shoes and on the feet will also deter fungous growth. Patent medicines may or may not be effective. It would be better to see a physician and then follow his instructions.

Other Disorders of the Skin

In addition to those disorders which have been discussed, other skin diseases include the following:

1 **Furuncles** (fu'rung-kls), or **boils,** which are localized collections of pus in cavities formed by the disintegration of tissue. They are caused by bacteria that enter hair follicles or sebaceous glands.
2 **Carbuncles** (kar'bung-kls) which are pus-producing lesions that result from extensions of infectious processes, such as boils. They involve both the skin and subcutaneous tissues and have numerous drainage channels that extend to the skin surface.
3 **Psoriasis** (so-ri'ah-sis) which is characterized by sharply outlined, red, flat areas (plaques) covered with silvery scales. The cause of this chronic, recurrent skin disease is unknown.
4 **Herpes** (her'pez) **simplex** which is characterized by the formation of watery vesicles (cold sores, fever blisters) on the skin and mucous membranes, including the genital area (see Appendix, Table 3, Viral Diseases).
5 **Cancer** of the skin which, in the United States is more common among those who have fair skin and who live in the southwestern part of the country, where exposure to the sun is consistent and may be intense. Early treatment in most cases means cure. Neglect can result in death.
6 **Urticaria** (ur"ti-ka're-ah) which is an allergic reaction characterized by the transient appearance of elevated red patches (hives) often accompanied by severe *pruritus* (proo-ri'tus) or itching.
7 **Scleroderma** (skle"ro-der'mah) and some of the metabolic diseases such as certain forms of lupus erythematosus cause thickening of the dermis.

Care of the Skin and Its Appendages
Cosmetics, Quackery, and Skin Care

It is rather ironic that more money is spent on skin, hair, and nail care than on a combination of all types of medical and health services. Yet authorities agree that the one most important factor in keeping the skin and the hair attractive is good general health. The person with even a slightly underactive thyroid gland (see Chap. 20) will have dry skin and hair, and no amount of creams could begin to take the place of taking thyroid extract tablets in proper amounts. The pallor of the anemia victim could be remedied much more effectively by appropriate health care than by any amount of cosmetics.

The normal skin secretions are slightly acid. Quacks have taken advantage of this fact by applying testing material (such as litmus paper) to the skin and then calling attention to the acid reaction with the warning that this "acid condition" should be corrected. Naturally they are selling the pills or potions for that purpose at a handsome profit. Actually the body protects itself against pathogens by producing this acid secretion. As the acid stomach juice kills bacteria in the food we eat, so the skin secretions tend to destroy or at least inhibit bacterial growth. Dirt and dead skin cells, however, dilute this acid; hence, cleanliness is important too. Careful handwashing with soap and water, with attention to the undernail areas, is a simple measure to reduce the spread of disease.

The cleansing soap and water bath or shower is an important part of good grooming and health. Here the individual should know himself and his peculiar personal needs. Those who have dry skins need to replace some of the oil that is removed by bathing if general health measures fail to remedy the dryness. For those who have very active sweat and oil glands, soap and water twice a day or more may be advisable, and creams and oily applications should be avoided. For most persons the so-called cleansing cream is not a proper substitute for soap and water.

Exposure to the elements, particularly to wind and sun, may call for applications of zinc ointment or some other fatty protective substance. Many sunburn lotions are of dubious value. A layer of an opaque ointment on the nose and other exposed surfaces will help to prevent overexposure to ultraviolet rays and may help to prevent undue drying of the skin.

Some of the newer sunscreening lotions have proved fairly effective. These contain a chemical known as PABA (para-aminobenzoic acid) or derivatives of this compound. They are clear liquids or creams, so they are not as visible as the zinc oxide ointments are. In any case, they all wash off during swimming and should be reapplied as may be indicated by conditions.

Even though a sun tan is regarded as a symbol of health, continued exposure to sunlight can cause premature aging and other undesirable changes in the skin.

Nails and Their Care

The nails are protective structures made of translucent (partly transparent) cells that originate from the outer part of the epidermis. Bacteria tend to collect under the nails and the cuticle, which should be kept pushed back. Hangnails should be removed after applying antiseptic. A clean manicure scissors should be used. Care should be taken to keep bacteria out of the deeper tissues and the blood vessels that are located in the root or nail bed. Toenails will have less tendency to become ingrown if they are cut straight across. Nails of both the toes and the fingers are affected by the general health. They may become discolored, dry, and cracked in chronic diseases of the nervous system and of the skin, and in conditions accompanied by prolonged fever.

Wanted and Unwanted Hair

Hair, like nails, is an appendage of the skin. It collects dirt easily and requires regular shampooing in order to be kept clean and healthy.

People seem to have formed a definite ideal as far as hair distribution is concerned, hence the universal concern over the vagaries of hair growth (or nongrowth). Much time and money are spent by men to check the relentless progress of baldness, and by women to correct an unfortunate excess of hair in the wrong places. Most of these expenditures are futile. Contrary to popular belief, shaving does not cause the hair to grow in more thickly, nor does it become coarser. Hair can be removed safely and effectively by electrolysis, one hair at a time, provided that it is done by an expert. It is an expensive and slow process. For the present it would seem advisable for women to shave if they wish to remove unwanted hair; and perhaps men can learn to accept baldness or wear an appropriate hairpiece.

Summary

1 Ways in which the skin can be classified.
A An enveloping membrane.
B The largest organ.
C A body system (integumentary).
2 Structure of the skin.
A Layers.
(1) Epidermis.
(a) Outermost layer of skin, stratified.
(b) Made of epithelial cells with no blood vessels.
(c) Undergoes constant cellular change.
(d) Contains pigment (melanin).
(2) Dermis.
(a) True skin, connective tissue framework.
(b) Contains blood vessels, nerves and glands.
(3) Subcutaneous layer.
(a) Contains parts of glands.
(b) Fat deposits are a reserve energy store.
B Glands of the skin.
(1) Sudoriferous—sweat glands.
(2) Ciliary and ceruminous—modified sweat glands.
(3) Sebaceous—oil glands.
3 Functions of the skin.
A Protection against pathogens, toxins, and drying of under tissues.
B Regulation of body temperature.
C Sensory organ for pain, touch, heat, cold, and pressure.
D Excretory function—limited to water and salt.
4 Observation of the skin.
A Pigmentation (melanin content).
(1) Melanin content varies with race.
(2) Sunlight causes increased pigmentation.
(3) Abnormal melanin content or distribution can be a sign of disease.
B Discoloration.
(1) Yellowish discoloration (jaundice)—bilirubin in the blood.
(2) Grayish or brown discoloration—chronic poisoning.

(3) Bronze discoloration—Addison's disease.
C Skin injuries—excoriations, lacerations, ulcers, erythema, spots.
D Skin eruptions; macules, papules, vesicles, pustules, crusts.
5 Skin disorders.
A Dermatitis (inflammation of the skin)—chemical irritants.
B Sunburn and complications.
(1) Severe burns.
(2) A possible cause of cancer.
(3) Pigmentation increase precludes benefit of small amounts of sunlight at other times.
C Eczema.
(1) Found mostly in the young and the aged.
(2) Erythema, blisters, papular lesions.
(3) Noncontagious.
D Acne.
(1) Most common at adolescence.
(2) Pimples and blackheads.
E Impetigo.
(1) Common in poor and malnourished children.
(2) Blisterlike lesions filled with pus and bacteria.
(3) Highly contagious
F Baldness.
(1) May be inherited.
(2) Can be caused by disease. Hair may grow back after a fever.
G Athlete's foot—a fungous infection.
H Other skin disorders—furuncles, carbuncles, psoriasis, herpes simplex, cancer, urticaria, scleroderma.
6 Care of the skin and its appendages.
A Cosmetics are of no value when the condition to be corrected is of pathologic origin.
B Nails must be kept free of bacteria.
C Most measures to check baldness or to remove unwanted hair are impractical or useless.

Questions and Problems

1 What characteristics of the skin classify it as a membrane, as an organ, as a system?

2 Of what type of cells is the epidermis composed?

3 Explain how the outermost cells of the epidermis are replaced.

4 What kind of tissue forms the framework of the dermis?

5 What glands extend down into the dermis and also into the subcutaneous layer, and what are their functions?

6 What is the subcutaneous layer made of and what is the importance of this layer?

7 Explain the 3 most important functions of the skin.

8 What are the facts about the skin as an organ of respiration and excretion?

9 What are the most important contributors to the color of the skin, normally?

10 What is the difference between a laceration and an ulcer?

11 Define acne. When is it usually most severe? Why?

12 What are some examples of irritants that frequently cause a dermatitis?

13 What are the dangers of overexposure to the sun, and what precautions need to be considered?

14 What is eczema? Name the most important causes.

15 At what ages are patients with impetigo in the most danger, and what are some of the precautions that need to be taken?

16 What are the most common causes of baldness?

17 What are the best measures to take to prevent and control athlete's foot?

18 Define furuncle, herpes simplex, and carbuncles.

19 Name some instances in which cosmetics are ineffective in remedying a basic defect. Why are they ineffective?

20 What is the value of the acid secretion of the skin?

Chapter 9

Bones and Joints

9

Glossary

Articulation Place of union; joint.

Endosteum A thin membrane that lines the marrow cavities of bone and is a source of cells that aid in growth and repair of bone tissue.

Foramen (foramina, pl.) A natural opening or passageway; a general term especially for a passage into or through a bone.

Ligament A band of fibrous tissue that connects bones or cartilages, whose function it is to support and strengthen joints.

Osteoblast A cell involved in production of bone.

Osteoclast A large cell involved in the absorption and removal of bone.

Process A prominence or part extending from an organ.

Resorption Loss or breakdown of substance; may be normal or pathologic (abnormal).

The Skeletal System

The bones are the framework of the body. They are a combination of several kinds of tissue and contain blood vessels and nerves. Bones are attached to each other at joints. The combination of bones and joints together with related connective tissues form the skeletal system.

The Bones
Bone Structure

In an earlier chapter we saw that the bones are composed chiefly of bone tissue, called osseous (os′e-us) tissue. It should be understood at the outset that a bone is anything but lifeless. Even though the spaces between the cells of bone tissue are permeated with stony deposits of calcium, these cells themselves are very much alive. Bones are organs, with their own system of blood and lymphatic vessels and nerves.

In the embryo (the early development stage of a baby) most of the bones-to-be are cartilage. Bone formation begins during the second and third months of embryonic life. At this time, bone-building cells, called *osteoblasts* (os′te-o-blasts″), become very active. First, they manufacture a substance, the intercellular (in″ter-sel′u-lar) material, which is located between the cells and contains large quantities of a protein called collagen. Then, with the help of enzymes, calcium compounds are deposited within the intercellular material. Other cells, called *osteoclasts* (os′te-o-klasts), are responsible for the process of *resorption,* or the breakdown of bone. Enzymes also implement this process. Thus, as a bone grows, alterations in its shape are the result of bone being added to some surfaces and resorbed from others. The processes of bone formation and bone resorption continue throughout life, more rapidly at some times than at others. The bones of small children are relatively pliable because they contain a larger proportion of cartilage and a smaller amount of the firm calcium salts than those of adults. In the elderly person there is much less of the softer tissues such as cartilage and a high proportion of calcium salts; therefore, the bones are brittle. Fractures of bones in older people heal with difficulty mainly because of this relatively high proportion of inert material and the small amount of the more vascular softer tissues.

There are two kinds of marrow: *red marrow,* found in certain parts of all bones, which manufactures most of the blood cells; and *yellow marrow* of the "soup bone" type, found chiefly in the central cavities of the long bones. Yellow marrow is largely fat.

Bones are covered on the outside (except at the joint region) by a membrane called the *periosteum* (per″e-os′te-um). The inner layer of this membrane contains osteoblasts which are essential in bone formation, not only during growth but in the repair of fractures as well. Blood and lymph vessels in the periosteum play an important role in nourishment of bone tissue. Nerve fibers make their presence known when one suffers a fracture, or when one receives a blow, such as striking the shinbone. A thinner membrane, the *endosteum* (en-dos′te-um), lines the marrow cavities of bone; it too contains cells that aid in growth and repair of bone tissue.

Main Functions of Bones

Bones have a number of functions, many of which are not at all obvious. Some of these are

1 To serve as a firm framework for the entire body.
2 To protect such delicate structures as the brain and the spinal cord.
3 To serve as levers, which are actuated by the muscles that are attached to them.
4 To serve as a storehouse for calcium, which may be removed to become a part of the blood if there is not enough calcium in the diet.
5 To produce blood cells.

Divisions of the Skeleton

The complete bony framework of the body is known as the *skeleton,* and it may be divided into two main groups of bones (Fig.9-1):

1 The *axial* (ak′se-al) *skeleton,* which includes the bony framework of the head and the trunk.
2 The *appendicular* (ap-en-dik′u-lar) *skeleton,* which forms the framework for those parts usually referred to as the arms and legs, but called the *extremities* by the biologists.

The Framework of the Head

The bony framework of the head is called the *skull,* and it is subdivided into two parts: the cranium and the facial portion (Figs. 9-2–9-5).

A The **cranium** is a rounded box that encloses the brain; it is composed of eight distinct cranial bones.
  1 The **frontal bone** forms the forehead, the front of the skull's roof, and helps in forming the roof over the eyes and the nasal cavities. The *frontal sinuses* (air spaces) communicate with the nasal cavities.
  2 The two **parietal** (pah-ri′e-tal) **bones** form most of the top and the side walls of the cranium.
  3 The two **temporal bones** form part of the sides and some of the base of the skull. Each one contains *mastoid sinuses* as well as the ear canal, eardrum, and the entire middle and internal ear.
  4 The **ethmoid** (eth′moid) **bone** is located between the eyes, in the orbital cavities. Its upper surface forms the roof of the nasal cavities and part of the base of the cranium. A thin plate of bone extends downward to form the upper part of the nasal septum.

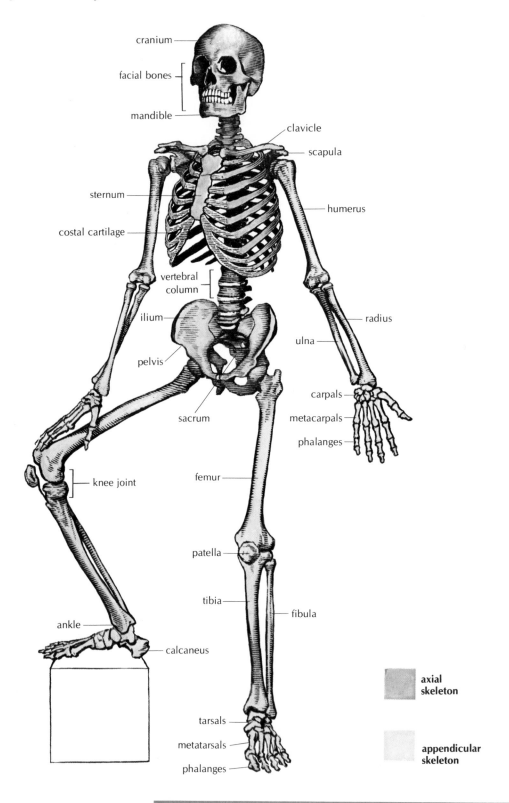

cranium

facial bones

mandible

clavicle

scapula

sternum

humerus

costal cartilage

vertebral column

radius

ilium

ulna

pelvis

sacrum

carpals

metacarpals

phalanges

knee joint

femur

patella

tibia

fibula

ankle

calcaneus

tarsals

metatarsals

phalanges

axial skeleton

appendicular skeleton

Fig. 9-1 The skeleton.

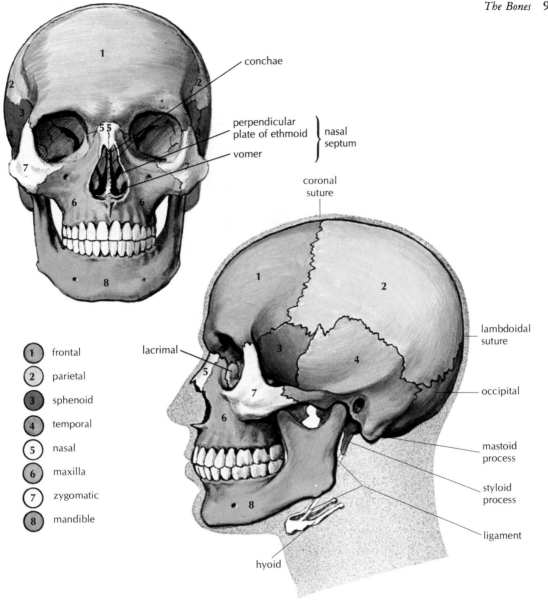

Fig. 9-2 *The skull, from the front and from the left.*

5 The **sphenoid** (sfe′noid) **bone,** when seen from above, resembles a bat with its wings extended. It lies at the base of the skull in front of the temporal bones.

6 The **occipital** (ok-sip′i′tal) **bone** forms the back and a part of the base of the skull.

B The **facial portion** of the skull is composed of 14 bones.

1 The **mandible** (man′di-b′l), or lower jaw bone, is the only movable bone of the skull.

2 The **maxillae** (mak-sil′e) fuse in the mid-line to form the upper jaw bone, including the front part of the hard palate (roof of the mouth). Each maxilla contains a large air space, called the *maxillary sinus,* that communicates with the nasal cavity.

3 The **zygomatic** (zi-go-mat′ik) **bones,** one on each side, form the prominence of the cheek.

4 Two slender **nasal bones** lie side by side, forming the bridge of the nose.

5 The **lacrimal** (lak′ri-mal) **bones,** about the

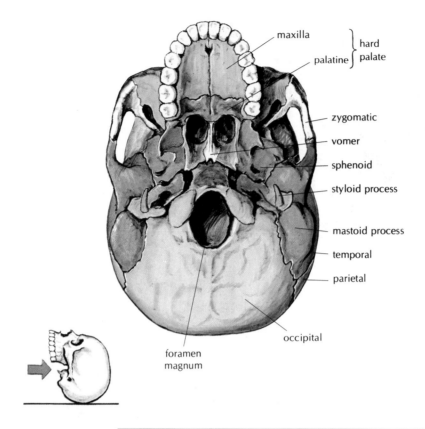

Fig. 9-3   *The skull from below, lower jaw removed.*

size of a fingernail, lie near the inside corner of the eye in the front part of the medial wall of the orbital cavity.

6   The **vomer** (vo′mer), shaped like the blade of a plow, forms the lower part of the nasal septum.

7   The paired **palatine bones** form the back part of the hard palate.

8   The two **inferior nasal conchae** (kon′ke) extend horizontally along the lateral wall (sides) of the nasal cavities. The paired superior and middle conchae are part of the ethmoid bone.

In addition to the bones of the cranium and the facial bones, there are three tiny bones or *ossicles* (os′sik′ls) in each middle ear (see Chap. 12) and a single horseshoe- or U-shaped bone that lies just below the skull proper, called the *byoid* (hi′oid) *bone,* to which the tongue is attached.

Openings in the base of the skull provide spaces for the entrance and exit of many blood vessels,

nerves, and other structures. Projections and slightly elevated portions of the bones provide for the attachment of muscles. Some portions contain delicate structures, as, for example, the part of the temporal bone that encloses the middle and internal sections of the ear. The air sinuses provide lightness and serve as resonating chambers for the voice.

The Framework of the Trunk

The bones of the trunk include the *vertebral* (ver′tebral) *column* and the bones of the chest or *thorax* (tho′raks). The vertebral column is made of a series of irregularly shaped bones, numbering 33 or 34 in the child; but because of unions that occur later in the lower part of the spine, there usually are just 26 separate bones in the adult column (Figs. 9-6 and 9-7). Each of these vertebrae (ver′te-bre), except the first two cervical, has a drum-shaped body located toward the front (anteriorly) which serves as the weight-bearing part; disks of cartilage between the vertebral bodies act as shock absorbers

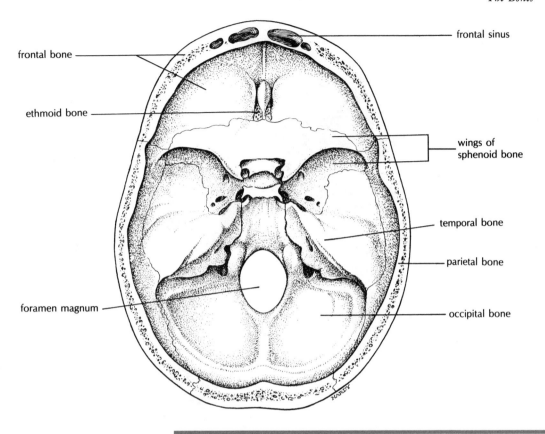

frontal sinus

frontal bone

ethmoid bone

wings of sphenoid bone

temporal bone

parietal bone

foramen magnum

occipital bone

Fig. 9-4 *Base of the skull as seen from above, showing the internal surfaces of some of the cranial bones. (Chaffee EE, Lytle IM: Basic Physiology and Anatomy, 4th ed. Philadelphia, JB Lippincott, 1980)*

and provide flexibility. In the center of each vertebra there is a large hole, or *foramen* (for-a'men), for the spinal cord. Projecting backward from the bony arch that encircles the spinal cord is the spinous process which usually can be felt just under the skin of the back. When all the vertebrae are linked in series by strong connective tissue bands (ligaments), the result is a bony cylinder that protects the spinal cord.

The bones of the vertebral column are named and numbered from above downward, on the basis of their location.

1 The **cervical** (ser'vi-kal) vertebrae, seven in number, are located in the neck. The first vertebra, called the *atlas,* supports the head; when one nods the head to indicate agreement, the skull (occipital bone) rocks back and forth on the atlas. The second cervical vertebra, called

the *axis,* serves as a pivot when the head is turned from side to side, as in indicating disagreement.

2 The **thoracic vertebrae,** 12 in number, are located in the thorax. The posterior ends of the ribs (12 pairs) are attached to these vertebrae.

3 The **lumbar vertebrae,** five in number, are located in the small of the back. They are larger and heavier than the other vertebrae.

4 The **sacral** (sa'kral) **vertebrae** are five separate bones in a child. However, these eventually fuse to form a single bone, called the **sacrum** (sa'krum), in an adult. Wedged between the two hip bones, the sacrum serves to complete the posterior part of the bony pelvis.

5 The **coccyx** (kok'siks), or tail bone, consists of four or five tiny bones in a child. These fuse to form a single bone in the adult.

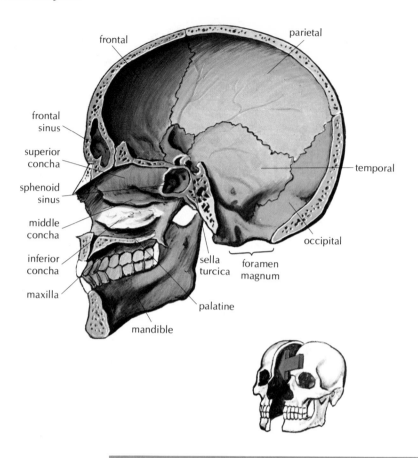

Fig. 9-5 *The skull, internal view.*

When viewed from the side, the vertebral column can be seen to have four curves, corresponding to the four groups of vertebrae. In a newborn infant the entire column is concave forward—the primary curve. When the infant begins to assume the erect posture, secondary curves, or those which are concave to the rear, may be noted. For example, the cervical curve appears when the infant begins to hold up his head at about three months; the lumbar curve appears when he begins to walk. The curves of the vertebral column provide some of the resilience and spring so essential in walking and running.

The bones of the thorax form a cone-shaped cage. Twelve pairs of *ribs* form the bars of this cage, assisted by the *sternum* (ster'num), or breastbone, anteriorly. The thorax serves to protect the heart, the lungs, and other organs.

All 24 of the ribs are attached to the vertebral column posteriorly. However, variations in the *an-terior* attachment of these slender, curved bones led to the following classification.

1 **True ribs,** the first seven pairs, are those that attach directly to the sternum by means of individual extensions called *costal* (kos'tal) *cartilages.*
2 **False ribs** include the remaining five pairs. Of these, the eighth, ninth, and tenth pairs attach to the cartilage of the rib above. The last two pairs have no anterior attachment at all and are known as *floating ribs.*

The spaces between the ribs, called *intercostal spaces,* contain muscles, blood vessels, and nerves.

The Bones of the Extremities

The framework of the extremities includes the longest bones in the body. A long bone has a shaft and two ends. The shaft contains a special hol-

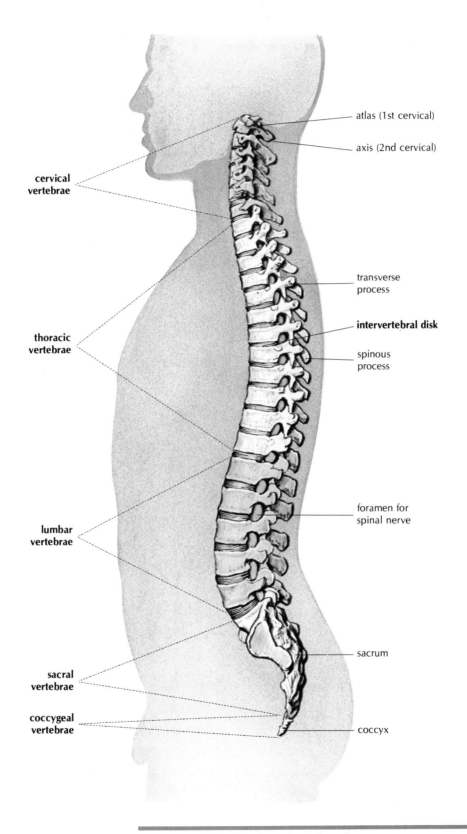

atlas (1st cervical)

axis (2nd cervical)

cervical vertebrae

transverse process

intervertebral disk

spinous process

thoracic vertebrae

foramen for spinal nerve

lumbar vertebrae

sacrum

sacral vertebrae

coccygeal vertebrae

coccyx

Fig. 9-6 *Vertebral column from the side.*

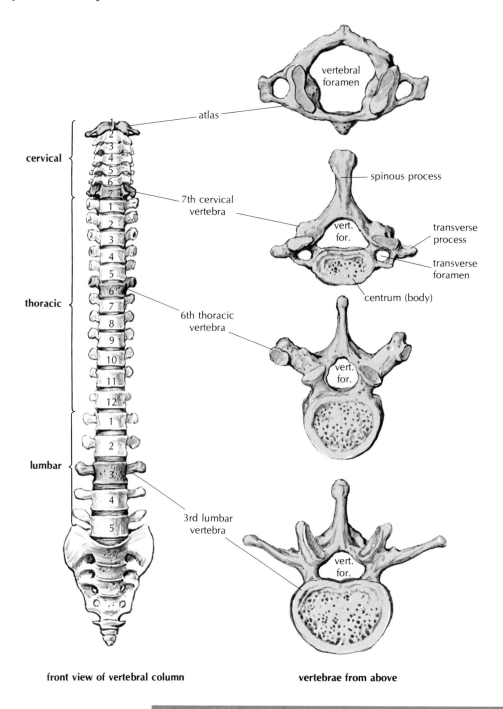

front view of vertebral column   **vertebrae from above**

Fig. 9-7   Front view of vertebral column; vertebrae from above.

lowed-out space called the *medullary* (med′u-lar-e) *cavity;* this space is filled with yellow marrow. The ends of long bones are honeycombed with tiny spaces that contain red marrow. This bone structure can be compared with a bamboo stick in its relative lightness and strength. Other bones of the extremities are flat, irregular, or short; and, like bones elsewhere in the body, contain red marrow.

The extremities are considered as having two divisions: upper and lower. The upper extremities include the shoulders, the arms (between the shoulders and the elbows), the forearms (between the elbows and the wrists), the wrists, the hands, and the fingers. The lower extremites include the hips (pelvic girdle), the thighs (between the hips and the knees), the legs (between the knees and the ankles), the ankles, the feet, and the toes.

The bones of the upper extremity may be divided into several groups for ease of study.

1 The **shoulder girdle** consists of two bones, the *clavicle* (klav′i-kle), or collar bone, and the *scapula* (skap′u-lah), or shoulder blade.
2 The arm bone is called the **humerus** (hu′mer-us). It forms a joint with the scapula above

and with the two forearm bones at the elbow.
3 The forearm bones are the **ulna** (ul′nah), which lies on the medial, or little finger side, and the **radius** (ra′de-us) on the lateral or thumb side. When the palm is up, or forward, the two bones are parallel; when the palm is turned down, or back, the lower end of the radius moves around the ulna so that the shafts of the two bones are crossed.
4 The wrist contains eight small **carpal** (kar′pal) bones arranged in two rows of four each. They are all different from each other and each has a name of its own (Fig. 9-8).
5 Five **metacarpal bones** are the framework for

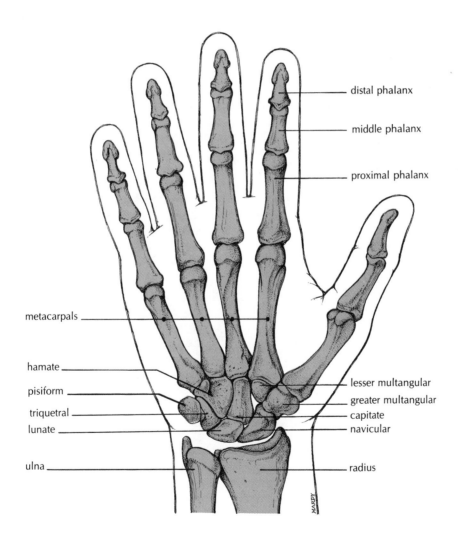

Fig. 9-8 *Bones of right hand, anterior view. (Chaffee EE, Lytle IM: Basic Physiology and Anatomy, 4th ed. Philadelphia, JB Lippincott, 1980)*

the body of each hand. Their rounded distal ends form the knuckles.

6   There are 14 **phalanges** (fa-lan′jez), or finger bones, in each hand, two for the thumb and three for each finger. Each of these bones is called a *phalanx* (fa′lanx). They are identified as the first, or proximal, which is attached to a metacarpal; the second, or middle; and the third, or distal phalanx. Obviously, the thumb has only a proximal and a distal phalanx.

The bones of the lower extremity are grouped together in a similar fashion.

1   The **pelvic girdle** is a strong bony ring that forms the walls of a basin called the pelvis. It is composed of two hip bones, which form the front and the sides of the ring, and the sacrum, which *articulates* (joins) with the hip bones to complete the ring at the back (posteriorly). Each hip bone (os coxae) begins its development as three separate parts; the *ilium* (il′e-um), which forms the upper, flared portion; the *ischium* (is′ke-um), which is the lowest and strongest part; and the *pubis* (pu′bis), which forms the anterior part. The joint formed by the union of the two hip bones anteriorly is called the *symphysis* (sim′fi-sis) *pubis.* The bony pelvis supports the trunk and the organs in the lower abdomen, or pelvic cavity, including the urinary bladder, the internal reproductive organs, and parts of the intestine. The female pelvis is adapted for pregnancy and childbirth; it is broader and lighter than that of the male (Fig. 9-9).

2   The thigh bone is called the **femur** (fe′mer). It is the longest and strongest bone in the body.

3   The **patella** (pah-tel′lah), or kneecap, is embedded in the tendon of the large anterior thigh muscle, the quadriceps femoris, where it crosses the knee joint. It is an example of a *sesamoid* (ses′ah-moid) bone, a type that develops within a tendon or a joint capsule.

4   There are two bones in the leg. Medially, (on the big toe side), the **tibia,** or shin bone, is the longer, weight-bearing bone. Laterally, the slender **fibula** (fib-u-lah) does not reach the knee joint; thus it is not a weight-bearing bone.

5   The structure of the foot is similar to that of the hand. However, the foot supports the weight of the body, so it is stronger and less mobile than the hand. There are seven **tarsal**

bones associated with the ankle and foot; the largest of these is the *calcaneus* (kal-ka′ne-us), or heel bone. Five **metatarsal bones** form the framework of the instep, and the heads of these bones form the ball of the foot.

6   The **phalanges** of the toes are counterparts of those in the fingers. There are three of these in each toe except for the great toe, which has but two.

Landmarks of Bones

The contour of bones resembles the topography of an interesting and varied landscape with its hills and valleys. The projections often serve as regions for muslce attachments. There are hundreds of these prominences or *processes* with different names. A few of the more important points of reference are identified below:

1   The **mastoid** process of the temporal bone projects downward immediately behind the external part of the ear. It contains the mastoid air cells and serves also as a place for muscle attachment.

2   The **acromion** (ah-kro′me-on) of the scapula forms the highest point of the shoulder. It overhangs the *glenoid cavity,* a smooth, shallow socket that articulates with the humerus to form the shoulder joint.

3   The **olecranon** (o-lek′rah-non) at the upper end of the ulna, forms the point of the elbow.

4   The **iliac** (il′e-ak) crest is the curved rim along the upper border of the ilium; it can be felt near the level of the waist. At either end of the crest there are bony projections, but the more prominent one is the *anterior superior iliac spine.* There are three other iliac spines on each hip bone, but the anterior superior spine is the most important. It is often used as a landmark, or reference point, in diagnosis and treatment.

5   The **ischial** (is′ke-al) **spine** at the back of the pelvic outlet is used as a point of reference during childbirth to indicate the progress of the presenting part (usually the baby's head) down the birth canal. Just below this spine is the large *ischial tuberosity* which helps to support the weight of the trunk when one sits down.

6   The **acetabulum** (as″e-tab′u-lum) is a deep socket in the hip bone; it receives the head of the femur to form the hip joint.

7   The **greater trochanter** (tro-kan′ter) of the

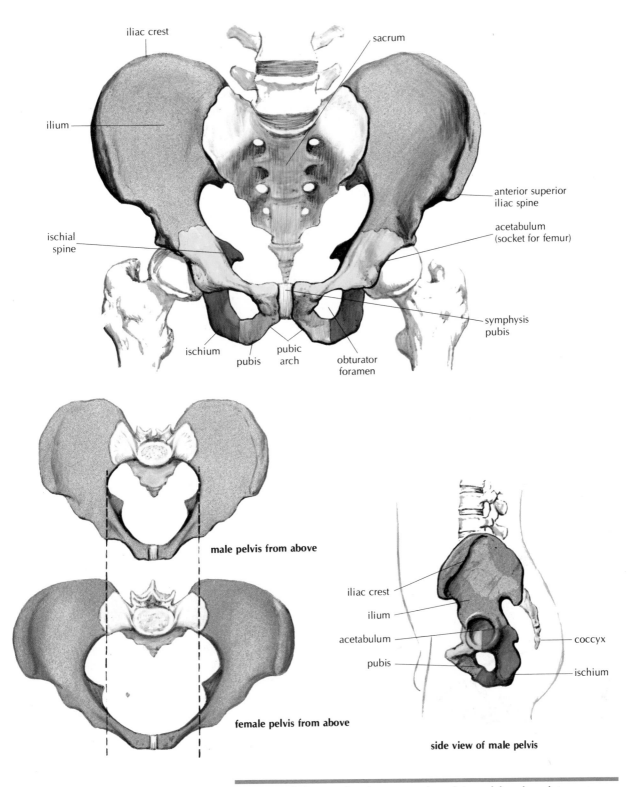

Fig. 9-9 *Pelvic girdle, showing male pelvis and female pelvis.*

femur is a very large protuberance located at the top of the shaft, on the lateral side. The **lesser trochanter,** a smaller elevation, is located on the medial side.

8   The **medial malleolus** (mal-le'o-lus) is a downward projection at the lower end of the tibia; it forms the prominence on the inner aspect of the ankle. The **lateral malleolus,** at the lower end of the fibula, forms the prominence on the outer aspect of the ankle.

The skull of the infant has areas in which the bone formation is incomplete, leaving so-called soft spots. Although there are a number of these, the largest and best known is near the front at the junction of the two parietal bones with the frontal bone. It is called the *anterior fontanel* (fon-tah-nel'), and it does not usually close until the child is about 18 months old (Fig. 9-10).

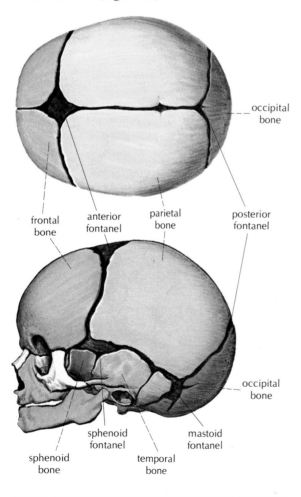

frontal bone   *anterior fontanel*   *parietal bone*   *posterior fontanel*   *occipital bone*

sphenoid fontanel   *mastoid fontanel*   *occipital bone*

sphenoid bone   *temporal bone*

Fig. 9-10   *Infant skull, showing fontanels.*

Holes that extend into or through bones are called *foramina* (fo-ram'i-nah). Numerous foramina permit the passage of blood vessels to and from the bone tissue and the marrow cavities. Larger foramina in the base of the skull and in other locations allow for the passage of cranial nerves, blood vessels, and other structures that connect with the brain. For example, the *foramen magnum,* located in the occipital bone, is a large opening through which the spinal cord communicates with the brain. When viewed from the side, the vertebral column can be seen to have a series of *intervertebral foramina,* the openings through which spinal nerves emerge as they leave the spinal cord. The largest foramina in the entire body are found in the pelvic girdle, near the front of each hip bone, one on each side of the symphysis pubis. These are called the *obturator* (ob'tu-ra-tor) *foramina,* and are partially covered by a membrane.

Valley-like depressions on a bone surface are called *fossae* (fos'se), the singular form being *fossa* (fos'sah). Some of these are filled with muscle tissue, as is the case with the large fossae of the two scapulae. Other depressions are narrow elongated areas called *grooves.* They may allow for the passage of blood vessels or nerves as in the case of the ribs, where grooves contain intercostal nerves and vessels.

Disorders of Bone

Cleft palate is a congenital deformity in which there is an opening in the roof of the mouth owing to faulty union of the maxillary bones. Infants born with this defect have difficulty in nursing, since their mouths communicate with the nasal cavities above, and air, rather than milk, is sucked in. Surgery is usually performed to correct the condition.

Osteomyelitis (os-te-o-mi-e-li'tis) is an inflammation of bone that is caused by *pyogenic* (py'o-jen'ik) (pus-producing) bacteria. It may remain localized or it may spread through the bone to involve the marrow and the periosteum as well. The bacteria may reach the bone through the bloodstream or by way of an injury in which the skin has been broken. Before the advent of antibiotic drugs, bone infection was very resistant to treatment and the outlook was poor. Now there are fewer cases in the first place because many of the bloodstream infections are prevented or treated early enough so that bone infection is less common. If those that do appear are treated promptly, the chance of a cure is usually excellent.

Tumors that develop in bone tissue may be benign, as is the case with certain cysts, or they may be malignant (osteosarcomas). In the latter case, the tumor originates most often in the bone tissue of a femur or a tibia usually in young persons. In older persons, metastases from epithelial tumors or carcinomas of various organs may spread to many bones.

Severe violence is capable of causing *fractures* in almost any bone (Fig. 9-11). The word "fracture" means "a break or rupture in a bone," and such injuries may be classified as follows:

1 **Compound** fractures, including those in which the skin and other soft tissues are torn and the bone protrudes through the skin.
2 **Simple** fractures, in which the break in the bone is not accompanied by a break in the skin.
3 **Greenstick** fractures, incomplete breaks in which the bone splits in much the same way

as a piece of green wood might. These are most common in children.
4 **Impacted** fractures, in which the broken ends of the bone are jammed into each other.
5 **Comminuted** (kom'i-noot-ed) fractures, those in which there is more than one fracture line with several fragments resulting.
6 **Spiral** fractures, in which the bone has been twisted apart. These are relatively common in skiing accidents.

The most important first aid care of fractures is to prevent movement of the affected parts. Protection by simple splinting after careful evaluation of the situation, leaving as much as possible "as is," and a call for expert help is usually safest. Those who have back injuries may be spared serious spinal cord damage if careful moving on a firm board or door can be done correctly. If a doctor or ambulance can reach the scene, a "hands off" rule for the untrained is strongly recommended. If there is no external bleeding, covering the victim with

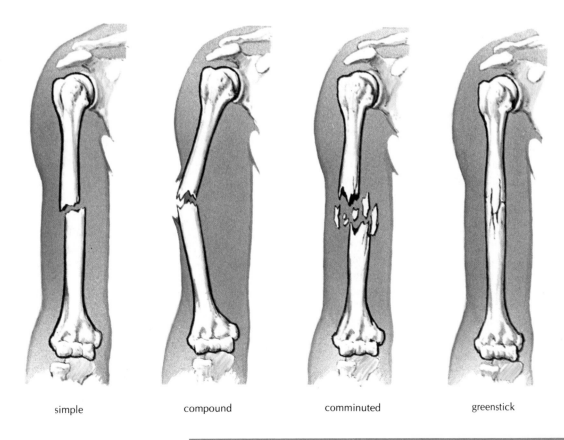

simple   compound   comminuted   greenstick

Fig. 9-11 *Types of fractures.*

blankets may help combat shock. First aid should always be immediately directed toward the control of hemorrhage.

Abnormal body chemistry involving calcium may cause various bone disorders. One of these is called Paget's disease, or *osteitis deformans* (os-te-i'tis de-for'mans). The bones undergo periods of calcium loss followed by times of excessive deposition of calcium salts. The bones become deformed. Cause and cure are not known at the present time. The bones also can become decalcified owing to the effect of a tumor of the parathyroid gland (see Chapter 20).

Rickets is primarily a disease of children, and is characterized by a hampering of growth and the failure of the bones to calcify sufficiently. The main cause of rickets is a deficiency of calcium and phosphorus. This can result directly from not having enough of these minerals in the diet. It can also result indirectly through a deficiency of vitamin D, a fat-soluble vitamin which is necessary in order that calcium and phosphorus may be absorbed by the body. Consequently, unless foods containing vitamin D are provided, the body will not be able to utilize these minerals, no matter how great the quantities of them taken in with food. Insufficient sunlight can be another predisposing factor in rickets, since the ultraviolet rays of the sun act on the skin to manufacture vitamin D. Rickets is most prevalent among children who grow up in the murk of city slums, and among those with heavy pigmentation.

The failure of the bones to calcify keeps them soft and easily bent. Certain deformities are a consequence, notably bowlegs.

There are also abnormalities of spinal curvature which include an exaggeration of the thoracic curve, resulting in *kyphosis* (ki-fo'sis) (hunchback) and the excessive concavity of the lumbar curve called *lordosis* (lor-do'sis). The most common disorder is *scoliosis* (sko-le-o'sis), a lateral curvature of the vertebral column. In extreme cases there may be compression of some of the internal organs. Scoliosis occurs in the rapid growth period of the teens, more often in girls. Early discovery and treatment produce good results.

The Joints

An *articulation,* or *joint,* is an area of junction or union between two or more bones.

Kinds of Joints

Joints are classified into three main groups on the basis of the degree of movement permitted:

1   **Synarthroses** (sin-ar-thro'sez), the immovable joints.
2   **Amphiarthroses** (am-fe-ar-thro'sez), the slightly movable joints.
3   **Diarthroses** (di-ar-thro'sez), the freely movable joints.

Joint Structure

Connective tissue bands, called *ligaments,* hold the bones together and are found in connection with all the freely movable joints and many of those that are less movable (Fig. 9-12). In some cases these completely enclose the joint and are called *capsular* (kap'su-lar) *ligaments.* Additional ligaments reinforce and help to stabilize the joints at various points. The contacting surfaces of each freely movable joint are covered by a smooth layer of gristle called the *articular* (ar-tik'u-lar) *cartilage.* Inside the joint space is the rather thick, colorless synovial fluid, which resembles uncooked egg white.

The slightly movable and immovable joints form continuous structures in which either cartilage or fibrous connective tissue fills the gap between the bones. These soft tissue areas are larger in the child, become smaller in the adult, and finally may be completely filled with bone in later life. The joints between the sacral vertebrae in the lower part of the spinal column are examples of immovable joints that completely disappear rather early in life. The sutures of the skull are held together by fibrous connective tissue aided by the dovetailing of the somewhat irregular sawtooth type of bone edges.

Joint Function

The chief function of the freely movable joints is to allow for changes of position and so provide for motion. These movements are given names to describe the nature of the change in the position of the body parts. For example, there are four kinds of angular movement, or movement that changes the angles between bones:

1 **Flexion** (flek′shun) is a bending motion that decreases the angle between bones, as in bending the fingers to close the hand.
2 **Extension** is a straightening motion that increases the angle between bones, as in straightening the fingers to open the hand.
3 **Abduction** (ab-duk′shun) is movement away from the midline of the body, as in moving the arms straight out to the sides.
4 **Adduction** is movement toward the midline of the body, as in bringing the arms back to their original position beside the body.

A combination of these angular movements enables one to execute a movement referred to as *circumduction* (ser″kum-duk′shun). To experience this movement, stand with your arm outstretched and draw a large imaginary circle in the air. Note the smooth combination of flexion, abduction, extension, and adduction that makes circumduction possible.

Rotation refers to a twisting or turning of a bone on its own axis, as in turning the head from side to side when saying "No."

There are special movements that are characteristic of the forearm and the ankle:

1 **Supination** (su″pĭ-na′shun) is the act of turning the palm up or forward; **pronation** (pro-na′shun) turns the palm down or backward.
2 **Inversion** (in-ver′zhun) is the act of turning the sole inward, so that it faces the opposite foot; **eversion** (e-ver′zhun) turns the sole outward, away from the body.

Disorders of Joints

Joints are subject to certain disorders of a mechanical nature, examples of which are *dislocations* and *sprains*. A dislocation is a derangement of the parts

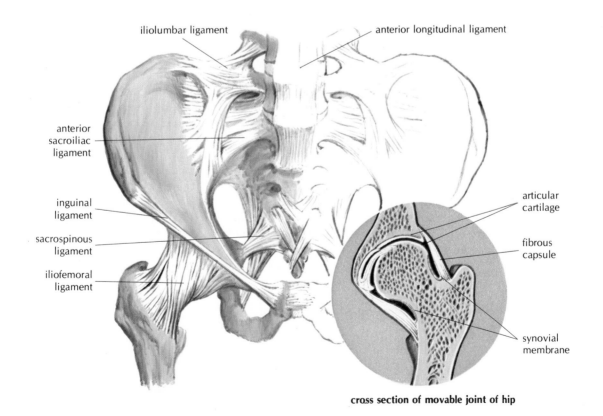

cross section of movable joint of hip

Fig. 9-12 Ligaments of hip and pelvis.

of the joint. A sprain is the name for the wrenching of a joint with rupture or tearing of the ligaments.

The most common type of joint disorder is *arthritis,* meaning "inflammation of the joints." There are many different kinds of arthritis, one familiar form being *rheumatoid arthritis.* This condition is a crippling one, characterized by swelling of the joints of the hands, the feet, and other parts of the body as a result of inflammation and overgrowth of the synovial membrane and other joint tissues. The articular cartilage is gradually destroyed, and the joint cavity develops adhesions— that is, the surfaces tend to stick together—so that the joints stiffen and are ultimately rendered useless. The cause of rheumatoid arthritis is uncertain, but it is now considered to be a disorder of metabolism. The administration of steroids and gold salts may provide some relief.

Arthritis also can be brought on by such infections as rheumatic fever and gonorrhea. Gonorrheal arthritis is becoming widespread as a result of the tremendous increase in cases of gonorrhea.

The joints as well as the bones proper are subject to attack by the tuberculosis organism, and the result may be a gradual destruction of parts of the bone near the joint. The organism is carried by the blood stream, usually from a focus in the lungs or lymph nodes, and may cause considerable damage before it is discovered. The bodies of several vertebrae sometimes are affected; or one hip or other single joint may be diseased. The patient may complain only of difficulty in walking, and diagnosis is difficult unless an accompanying lung tuberculosis has been found. This disorder is more common in children.

Degenerative joint diseases are a group which usually occur in older people. Sometimes such factors as obesity and repeated traumata can help to bring them about. Degenerative diseases occur mostly in joints involving weight bearing. Various degenerative changes in the joints include the formation of spurs at the edges of the articular surfaces, thickening of the synovial membrane, atrophy of the cartilages or calcification of the ligaments.

Gout is a kind of arthritis basically caused by a disturbance of metabolism. One of the products of metabolism is uric acid, which normally is excreted in the urine. If there happens to be an overproduction of uric acid, or for some reason not enough is excreted, the accumulated uric acid forms crystals which are deposited as masses about the joints and other parts of the body. The joints become inflamed and extremely painful. Any joint can be involved, but the one most commonly affected by gout is the great toe. Most victims of gout are men past middle life.

Backache is another common complaint. Some of its causes are

1   Diseases of the vertebrae, such as infections or tumors; and, in older people, degenerative arthritis or atrophy (wasting away) of the bone following long illnesses.
2   Disorders of the intervertebral disks, especially those in the lower lumbar region. Pain may be very severe, with muscle spasm and extension of symptoms along the course of the sciatic nerve (back of the thigh).
3   Abnormalities of the lower vertebrae or of the ligaments and other supporting structures.
4   Disorders involving organs of the pelvis or those in the retroperitoneal space (as the pancreas). Variations in the position of the uterus are seldom a cause.
5   Strains on the *lumbosacral* joint (where the lumbar region joins the sacrum) or strains on the *sacroiliac* joint (where the sacrum joins the ilium of the pelvis).

=================== *Summary*

1   Bones
   A   Structure—osseous tissue
      (1) Osteoblasts—build bone; osteoclasts— resorb bone.
      (2) Red marrow forms blood cells; yellow marrow is mostly fat.
      (3) Periosteum—covers bone; growth and repair.
   B   Functions—body framework; protect organs; serve as levers; calcium storage; form blood cells.
   C   Bones of axial skeleton.

(1) Cranial—frontal, 2 parietal, 2 temporal, ethmoid, sphenoid, occipital.

(2) Facial—mandible, 2 maxillae, 2 palatine, 2 nasal conchae, 2 nasal bones, ossicles (of ear), hyoid.

(3) Trunk.

(a) Vertebral column—7 cervical (C-1 atlas, C-2 axis), 12 thoracic, 5 lumbar, 1 sacrum and 1 coccyx in adult; curves—primary and secondary.

(b) Thorax—sternum; ribs—true (first 7 pairs), false (remaining 5 pairs—last 2 called floating ribs).

D Bones of appendicular skeleton.

(1) Upper extremity—shoulder girdle (clavicle, scapula), humerus, ulna, radius, 8 carpals, 5 metacarpals, 14 phalanges.

(2) Lower extremity—pelvic girdle (2 hip bones—divisions of each—ilium, ischium, pubis; anterior joint is symphysis pubis); femur, patella (sesamoid), tibia, fibula, 7 tarsals (calcaneus is heel bone), 5 metatarsals, 14 phalanges.

E Landmarks of bones.

(1) Processes—mastoid, acromion, glenoid cavity, olecranon, iliac crest, iliac spines, ischial spine and tuberosity, acetabulum, trochanters, malleoli.

(2) Anterior fontanel (and others) in infants.

(3) Foramina—foramen magnum, intervertebral foramina, obturator foramina.

(4) Fossae and grooves.

F Disorders—osteomyelitis, cleft palate, tumors, fractures, osteitis deformans, rickets, kyphosis, lordosis, scoliosis.

2 Joints.

A Types—immovable, slightly movable, freely movable.

B Structure—held together by ligaments; surfaces covered with articular cartilage, lubricated with synovial fluid.

C Movements—flexion, extension, abduction, adduction, rotation, circumduction, supination, pronation, inversion, eversion.

D Disorders—dislocations, sprains, arthritis, tuberculosis, degenerative diseases, gout, backache.

Questions and Problems

1 Distinguish between osteoblast and osteoclast; red marrow and yellow marrow; periosteum and endosteum.

2 Name 5 general functions of bones.

3 What are the main cranial and facial bones?

4 What are the main divisions of the vertebral column? The ribs?

5 Name the bones of the upper and lower extremities.

6 Name the bones on which you would find the following processes: mastoid, acromion, olecranon, iliac crest, trochanter, medial malleolus.

7 Define fontanel and name the largest one. What is a foramen? Give at least two examples of foramina.

8 Describe cleft palate, osteomyelitis, rickets, 5 types of fractures, and 2 abnormalities of spinal curvature.

9 Describe the structure of freely movable joints and describe the 4 angular movements; explain the difference between supination and pronation, between inversion and eversion.

10 Describe 3 joint diseases.

Chapter 10

The Muscular System

Glossary

Aponeurosis   A tendon-like expansion that connects a muscle with the parts that it moves.

Contractility   The capacity of a muscle fiber to become short in response to a stimulus.

Epimysium   A fibrous sheath surrounding a muscle.

Excitability, irritability   The capacity of a muscle to respond to a stimulus.

Insertion   The place of attachment of a muscle to the bone that it moves.

Origin   The less movable attachment of a muscle.

Tendon   A fibrous cord that attaches a muscle to a bone.

The muscular system is composed of more than 600 individual muscles, each of which is a distinct organ. However, muscles usually act in groups in order to execute a body movement.

Characteristics of Skeletal Muscle

As noted in Chapter 2, there are three basic kinds of muscle tissue: skeletal, smooth, and cardiac muscle. This chapter is concerned only with skeletal muscle, which is attached to the bones. Skeletal muscle also is known as voluntary muscle because it is normally under conscious control of the will (Figs. 10-1 and 10-2).

Skeletal muscles are regarded as organs because each muscle has, in addition to the specialized muscle cells which are capable of shortening or contracting, a connective tissue framework and is supplied with blood vessels and nerves. When seen through a microscope, the individual muscle cells are long and threadlike; thus they are usually referred to as muscle fibers. These fibers are arranged in bundles that are held together by connective tissue. Groups of these bundles are held together by additional connective tissue, and the entire muscle is encased in a tough connective tissue sheath called the *epimysium* (ep″i-mis′e-um) (Fig. 10-3).

Excitability, or *irritability,* is the capacity to respond to a stimulus, and it is an important property of muscle tissue. Muscle cells can be excited by chemical, electrical or mechanical means. Skeletal muscles usually are excited by nerve impulses that

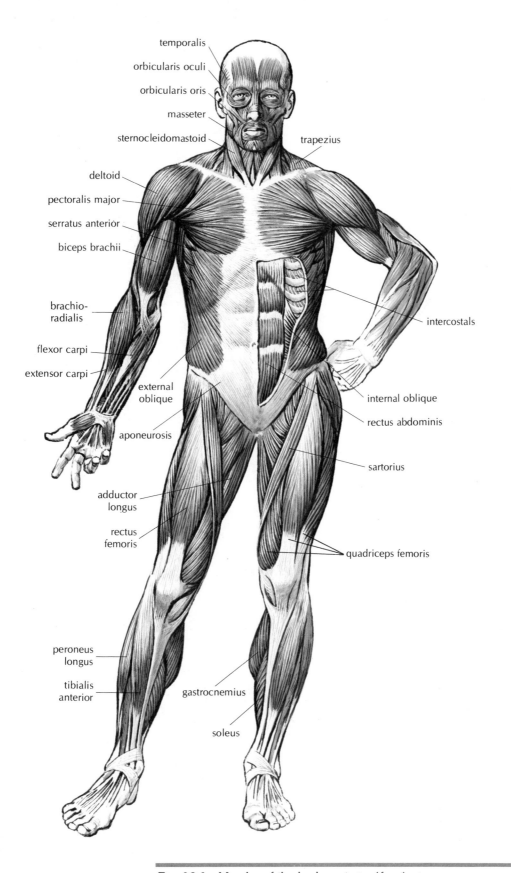

temporalis
orbicularis oculi
orbicularis oris
masseter
sternocleidomastoid
trapezius
deltoid
pectoralis major
serratus anterior
biceps brachii
brachio-
radialis
flexor carpi
extensor carpi
external
oblique
aponeurosis
adductor
longus
rectus
femoris
peroneus
longus
tibialis
anterior
intercostals
internal oblique
rectus abdominis
sartorius
quadriceps femoris
gastrocnemius
soleus

Fig. 10-1 *Muscles of the body, anterior (front) view.*

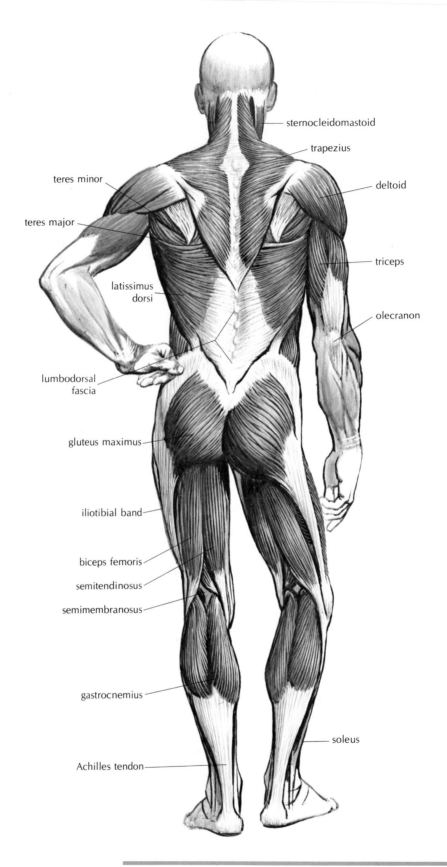

sternocleidomastoid

trapezius

teres minor

deltoid

teres major

triceps

latissimus dorsi

olecranon

lumbodorsal fascia

gluteus maximus

iliotibial band

biceps femoris

semitendinosus

semimembranosus

gastrocnemius

soleus

Achilles tendon

Fig. 10-2 Muscles of the body, posterior (back) view.

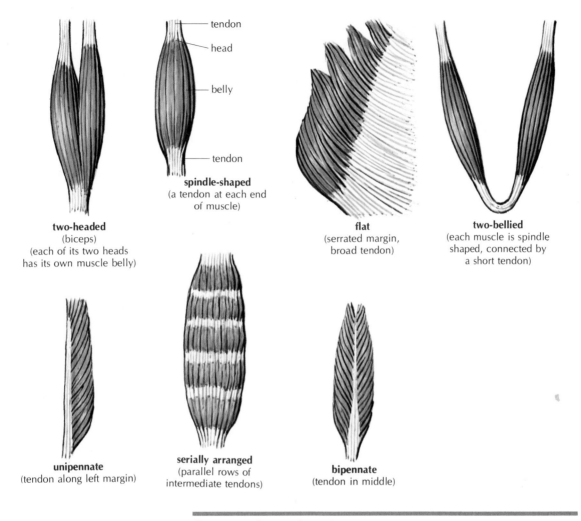

two-headed
(biceps)
(each of its two heads
has its own muscle belly)

spindle-shaped
(a tendon at each end
of muscle)

tendon
head
belly
tendon

flat
(serrated margin,
broad tendon)

two-bellied
(each muscle is spindle
shaped, connected by
a short tendon)

unipennate
(tendon along left margin)

serially arranged
(parallel rows of
intermediate tendons)

bipennate
(tendon in middle)

Fig. 10-3 *Types of muscles.*

are generated in the brain and the spinal cord (see Chap. 11). Nerve fibers carry impulses to the muscles, each fiber supplying from a few up to more than a hundred individual muscle cells. The endings of the motor nerve fibers are called *myoneural* (mi″o-nu′ral) junctions or motor end plates. The stimulus received by way of the end plate results in a change called an *action potential* that is transmitted along the cell membrane.

Contractility is the capacity of a muscle fiber to undergo shortening and to change its shape, becoming thicker. Studies with the electron microscope reveal that the cytoplasm of each skeletal muscle fiber contains special protein threads or filaments, called *actin* (ak′tin) and *myosin* (mi′o-sin). These filaments slide over each other in such a

way that the muscle fiber contracts, or becomes shorter and thicker. These contraction processes require energy; thus working muscles must have an adequate supply of oxygen and glucose. The immediate source of energy for muscle contraction is a substance called *adenosine* (ah-den′o-sin) *triphosphate* (tri-fos′fate) or simply *ATP*. It is a temporary energy store that acts as a go-between, since it transfers the energy released during chemical reactions, to the muscles or other tissues. Oxygen also plays an important role in preventing the accumulation of *lactic acid* waste products which can cause muscle fatigue. During strenuous activity, a person may not be able to breathe in oxygen rapidly enough to meet the needs of the hard-working muscles. If lactic acid accumulates, the person is said to develop an *oxygen debt*. After he has stopped his exercise he must continue to take in more oxygen until the debt is paid in full. Additional information on the effects of exercise are presented later in this chapter.

Muscle tone refers to a partially contracted state of the muscles which is normal even though the muscles may not be in use at the time. The maintenance of this tone or tonus (to′nus) is due to the action of the nervous system, and its effect is to keep the muscles in a constant state of readiness for action. Muscles that are little used soon become flabby, weak, and lacking in tone.

In addition to the partial contractions that are responsible for muscle tone, the body also depends on two other types of contractions:

1 **Isotonic** (i″so-ton′ic) **contractions** are those in which the tone or tension within the muscle remains the same, but the muscle as a whole shortens, producing movement. Lifting weights, walking, running, or any other activity in which the muscles become shorter and thicker (forming bulges) are examples of isotonic contractions.
2 **Isometric** (i″so-met′rik) **contractions** are those in which there is no change in muscle length, but there is a great increase in muscle tension. For example, if you push against a brick wall, there is no movement, but you can feel the increased tension within the arm muscles.

Most muscles may contract either isotonically or isometrically, but most of the movements of the body involve a combination of both types of contraction.

Attachments of Skeletal Muscles

Most muscles have two or more attachments to the skeleton. The method of attachment varies. In some instances, the connective tissue within the muscle ties directly to the periosteum of the bone. In other cases, the connective tissue sheath and partitions within the muscle all extend to form specialized structures that aid in attaching the muscle to bones. Such an extension may take the form of a cord, in which case it is called a *tendon*. (Fig. 10-4). In other cases a broad sheet called an *aponeu-*

rosis (ap″o-nu-ro′sis), may attach muscles to bones, or to other muscles.

Whatever the nature of the muscle attachment, the principle remains the same: to furnish a means of harnessing the power of the muscle contractions. A muscle has two (or more) attachments, one of which is more freely movable than the other. The less movable (more fixed) attachment is called the *origin;* the attachment to the part of the body which the muscle puts into action is called the *insertion.* When a muscle contracts, it pulls on both points of attachment, bringing the more movable insertion closer to the origin and thereby causing movement of the body part.

Muscle Movement

As we have noted, the human body contains more than 600 skeletal muscles, constituting between 35% and 40% of body weight. A large number of the skeletal muscles are arranged in pairs. A movement is initiated by one muscle or set of muscles called the *prime mover.* When an opposite movement is to be made, another muscle or set of muscles, known as the *antagonist,* takes over. In this way, body movements are coordinated, and a large number of complicated movements are carried out without the necessity of planning in advance the means of performing them. At first, however, any new, complicated movement must be learned. Think of a child learning to walk or to write, and consider the number of muscles which he uses unnecessarily or forgets to use when the situation calls for them.

Muscles of the Head and the Neck
Muscles of the Head

The principal muscles of the head are those of facial expression and of mastication (chewing) (Fig. 10-5).

The muscles of facial expression include the ring-shaped ones around the eyes and the lips. They are called the *orbicularis* (or-bik-u-la′ris) *muscles* because of their shape (think of "orbit"). The muscle surrounding each eye is called the *orbicularis oculi* (ok′u-li), while the muscle of the lips is the *orbicularis oris*. These muscles, of course, are all provided with antagonists. For example, the *levator*

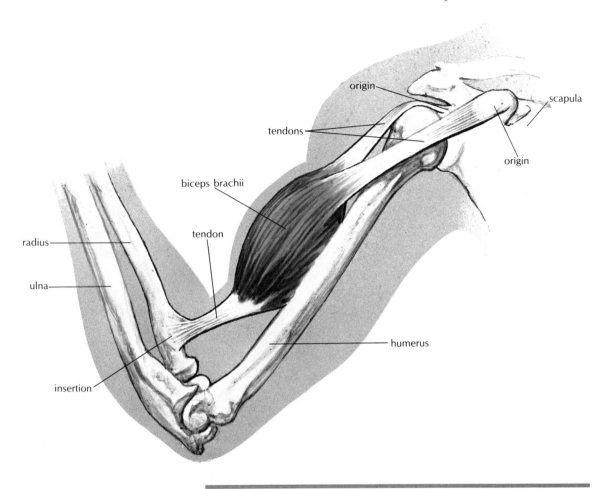

Fig. 10-4 *Diagram of a muscle, showing three attachments to bones—two by tendons of origin and one by a tendon of insertion.*

palpebrae (pal′pe-brae) *superioris,* or lifter of the upper eyelid, is the antagonist for the orbicularis oculi.

One of the largest muscles of expression forms the fleshy part of the cheek and is called the *buccinator* (buk′se-na-tor). It is used in whistling or blowing and is sometimes referred to as the trumpeter's muscle. You can readily think of other muscles of facial expression: for instance, the antagonists of the orbicularis oris which can produce a smile, a sneer, or a grimace. There are a number of scalp muscles by means of which the eyebrows are lifted or else drawn together into a frown.

There are four pairs of muscles of mastication, all of which insert on the mandible and move it. The largest are the *temporal* (tem′po-ral) *muscles,* located above and near the ear, and the *masseter* (mas-se′ter) *muscles* at the angle of the jaw.

The tongue has two groups of muscles. The first group, called the *intrinsic muscles,* are located entirely within the tongue. The second group, the *extrinsic muscles,* originate outside the tongue. It is because of these many muscles that the tongue has such remarkable flexibility and can perform so many different functions. Consider the intricate tongue motions involved in speaking, chewing, and swallowing.

Muscles of the Neck

The neck muscles tend to be ribbon-like and extend up and down or obliquely in several layers and in a complex manner. The ones that you will hear of most frequently are the *sternocleidomastoid* (sterno-kli-do-mas′toid) *muscles,* sometimes referred to simply as the *sternomastoids.* These strong muscles extend from the sternum upward, across either side of the neck, to the mastoid process. Working to-

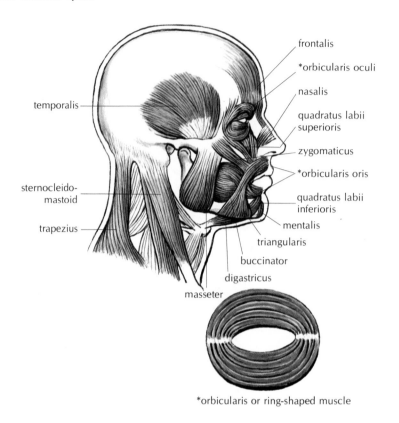

temporalis

frontalis

*orbicularis oculi

nasalis

quadratus labii
superioris

zygomaticus

*orbicularis oris

quadratus labii
inferioris

sternocleido-
mastoid

trapezius

mentalis

triangularis

buccinator

digastricus

masseter

*orbicularis or ring-shaped muscle

Fig. 10-5 *Muscles of the head.*

gether, they bring the head forward on the chest (flex-ion). Working alone, each muscle tilts and rotates the head so as to carry the face toward the opposite side. If the head is abnormally fixed in this position the person is said to have *torticollis* (wryneck); this condition may be due to injury or spasm of the muscle. A portion of the trapezius muscle (described later) is located in the back of the neck where it helps to hold the head up (extension). Other larger deep muscles are the chief extensors of the head and neck.

Muscles of the Upper Extremities
Movement of the Shoulder and Arm

The position of the shoulders depends to a large extent on the degree of contraction of the *trapezius* (trah-pe′ze-us) *muscles.* Each trapezius fans out like a pointed cape down the back of the neck and

over the back of the shoulders to insert on the scapula. These muscles enable one to raise the shoulders and to pull them back. The upper portion of each trapezius also can extend the head and turn it from side to side.

The *latissimus* (lah-tis′i-mus) *dorsi muscles* originate from the vertebral spines in the middle and lower back, and they cover the lower half of the thoracic region. The fibers of each muscle converge to a tendon that inserts on the humerus. The latissimus dorsi powerfully extends the arm, bringing it down forcibly as, for example, in swimming.

Moving around to the front of the body, we find a large *pectoralis* (pek-to-ra′lis) *major muscle* located on either side of the upper part of the chest. This muscle arises from the sternum, the upper ribs, and the clavicle, and forms the anterior ''wall'' of the arm pit or axilla; it inserts on the upper part of the humerus. The pectoralis major flexes and adducts the arm, pulling it across the chest.

Below the axilla, on the side of the chest, is the *serratus* (ser-ra′tus) *anterior.* It originates on the upper eight or nine ribs on the side and the front of the thorax and inserts in the scapula on the side toward the vertebrae. The serratus anterior muscle moves the scapula forward when, for example, one is pushing something. Also, it aids in raising the arm above the horizontal level.

The *deltoid muscle* covers the shoulder joint and is responsible for the roundness of the upper part of the arm just below the shoulder. This area is often used as an injection site. Arising from the shoulder girdle (clavicle and scapula), the deltoid fibers converge to insert on the lateral side of the humerus. Contraction of this muscle abducts the arm, raising it laterally to the horizontal position.

Movement of the Forearm and Hand

The *biceps brachii* (bra'ke-i) is often displayed by small boys as proof of their strength. It inserts on the radius and serves to flex the forearm. It is a supinator of the hand (see Fig. 10-4).

The *triceps brachii* is located on the back of the arm, and it inserts on the olecranon of the ulna. The triceps has been called the boxer's muscle, since it straightens the elbow when a blow is delivered. It is also important in pushing, since it converts the arm and forearm into a sturdy rod.

Most of the muscles that move the hand and fingers originate from the radius and the ulna; some of them insert on the carpal bones of the wrist, others have long tendons that cross the wrist and insert on bones of the hand and the fingers. The *flexor carpi* and the *extensor carpi muscles* are responsible for many movements of the hand. Muscles that produce finger movements are the several *flexor digitorum* (dij"e-to'rum) and the *extensor digitorum muscles.* Special groups of muscles in the fleshy parts of the hand are responsible for the intricate movements that can be performed with the thumb and the fingers. The position and freedom of movement of the thumb has been one of the most useful endowments of man.

Muscles of the Trunk
Muscles of Respiration

The most important muscle involved in the act of breathing is the diaphragm. This dome-shaped muscle forms the partition between the thoracic cavity above and the abdominal cavity below (Fig. 10-6). When the diaphragm contracts, the central dome-shaped portion is pulled downward, thus enlarging the thoracic cavity from top to bottom. The external *intercostal muscles* fill the spaces between, and are attached to, the ribs. Contraction of these muscles serves to elevate the ribs, thus enlarging the thoracic cavity from side to side and from front to back. The mechanics of breathing are described in Chapter 17.

Muscles of the Abdomen and Pelvis

The front and side (anterolateral) walls of the abdomen have three main muscles arranged in layers: the *external oblique* on the outside, the *internal oblique* in the middle, and the innermost layer called the *transversus abdominis.* The fibers of these three muscles all run in different directions. With these layers "glued" together, the total effect is like that of a piece of plywood; the result is a very strong abdominal wall. The front of the abdomen is closed in by the long, narrow *rectus abdominis,* which originates at the pubis and ends at the ribs. It is surrounded by connective tissue layers from the other three muscles.

The abdominal muscles have a number of functions in addition to protecting the underlying organs. One is to assist indirectly with the process of respiration, relaxing when the diaphragm contracts and vice versa. They also help in expelling substances from the body by compressing the abdominal cavity and increasing the pressure within that cavity (*e.g.,* coughing, vomiting, childbirth). Another function of the abdominal muscles is to help in bending the trunk forward and sideways.

The pelvic floor, or perineum (per-i-ne'um), has its own form of diaphragm, shaped somewhat like a shallow dish. One of the principal muscles of this pelvic diaphragm is the *levator ani* (le-va'tor-a'ni) which acts on the rectum and thus aids in defecation.

Deep Muscles of the Back

The deep muscles of the back, which act on the vertebral column itself, are thick vertical masses that lie under the trapezius and latissimus dorsi. The longest muscle is the *sacrospinalis* (sa"kro-spin-

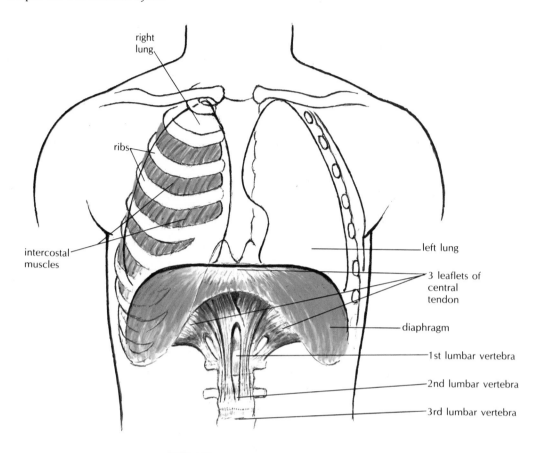

Fig. 10-6   *The diaphragm forms the partition between the thoracic cavity and the abdominal cavity.*

a'lis), and it helps to maintain the vertebral column in the erect posture.

Muscles of the Lower Extremities

The muscles in the lower extremities are among the longest and strongest in the body and are specialized for locomotion and balance.

Movement of the Thigh and Leg

The *gluteus maximus* (gloo'te-us mak'si-mus), which forms much of the fleshy part of the buttock, is relatively large in humans because of its function when a person is standing in the erect position. This muscle extends the thigh and is very important in walking and running. The *gluteus medius* is partially covered by the gluteus maximus and serves to abduct the thigh.

The *iliopsoas* (il-e-o-so'as) muscle arises from the ilium and the bodies of the lumbar vertebrae; it crosses the front of the hip joint to insert on the femur. It is a powerful flexor of the thigh and also helps to keep the trunk from falling backward when one is standing erect.

The *adductor muscles* are located on the medial part of the thigh. They arise from the pubis and ischium and insert on the femur. These strong muscles press the thighs together, as in grasping a saddle between the knees when one is riding a horse.

The *sartorius* is a long, narrow muscle that begins at the iliac spine, winds downward and inward across the entire thigh, and ends on the upper medial surface of the tibia. It is called the tailor's muscle because it is used in crossing the legs, in the manner of tailors, who in days gone by sat cross-legged on the floor.

The front and sides of the femur are covered by the *quadriceps femoris* (kwod're-seps fem'or-is), a large muscle that has four heads of origin (one from the ilium and three from the femur). However, all four heads have a common tendon of insertion on the tibia. You may remember that this is the tendon that encloses the knee cap or patella. This muscle extends the leg, as in kicking a ball.

The hamstring muscles are located in the posterior part of the thigh. Their tendons can be felt behind the knee as they descend to insert on the tibia and fibula. The hamstrings flex the leg on the thigh, as in kneeling.

Movement of the Foot

The *gastrocnemius* (gas-trok-ne'me-us) is the chief muscle of the calf of the leg. It has been called the toe dancer's muscle because it is necessary in order to stand on tiptoe. It ends near the heel in a prominent cord called the *Achilles tendon,* which then attaches to the calcaneus (heel bone). The Achilles tendon is the largest tendon in the body.

Another leg muscle that acts on the foot is the *tibialis* (tib-e-a'lis) *anterior,* located on the front of the leg. This muscle performs the opposite function of the gastrocnemius. Anyone who feels inclined to walk on his heels will use the tibialis anterior to raise the rest of the foot off the ground (dorsiflexion). This muscle also is responsible for inversion of the foot. The muscle for eversion of the foot is the *peroneus* (per-o-ne'us) longus, located on the lateral side of the leg.

The toes, like the fingers, are provided with sets of muscles called the *flexor digitorum muscles.* The former originate both at the tarsus and at the posterior surface of the tibia, and pass through the sole to the toes. The latter arise from both the tarsus and the anterior surface of the fibula, and pass over the top of the foot to the toes.

Applying Knowledge About the Muscles
Exercise

The rate of muscle metabolism increases during exercise, resulting in a relative deficiency of oxygen and muscle nutrients. In turn, this deficiency causes *vasodilation* (vas-o-di-la'shun)—an increase in caliber of blood vessels—thereby allowing blood to flow easily back to the heart. The temporarily increased load on the heart acts to strengthen heart muscle and to improve the circulation within the heart muscle. Regular exercise also improves respiratory efficiency; circulation in the capillaries surrounding the alveoli, or air sacs, is increased, and this brings about enhanced gas exchange and deeper breathing.

To begin with, the increased demands during muscular exercise are met by the energy-rich compounds that are stored in the tissues. Continual exercise depletes these stores. For a short period of time, glucose may be used without the benefit of oxygen, in which case lactic acid is formed. This anaerobic (without oxygen) process permits greater magnitude of activity than would otherwise be possible, as, for example, allowing sprinting instead of jogging. After a period of great exertion, extra oxygen is consumed to remove the lactic acid and replenish the energy-carrying compounds. As noted earlier in this chapter, the body has accumulated an oxygen debt which must be repaid by continued rapid breathing for some time after the activity has been completed. Training permits the more efficient distribution and utilization of oxygen so that less lactic acid is produced and the oxygen debt is smaller. The untrained person who has an excessive accumulation of lactic acid will suffer from such symptoms as muscle soreness and cramps.

Levers and Body Mechanics

Proper body mechanics helps to conserve energy and to ensure freedom from strain and fatigue; conversely, such ailments as lower back pain—a very common complaint—can be traced to poor body mechanics. Body mechanics has special significance to health workers, who are frequently called upon to move patients, handle cumbersome equipment, and so on. Maintaining the body segments in correct relation to one another has a direct effect on the working capacity of the vital organs that are supported by the skeletal structure.

If you have had a course in physics, recall your study of levers. A lever is simply a machine consisting of a rigid bar that moves about a fixed point, the fulcrum. There are three classes of levers, which differ only in the location of the fulcrum, the effort (force) and the resistance (weight). In a first-class lever, the fulcrum is located between the resistance and the effort; scissors, which you probably use every day, are an example of this class. The second-class lever has the resistance located between the fulcrum and the effort; turning a mattress, and lifting one end of a bed, are illustrations of this class. In the third-class lever, the effort is between the resistance and the fulcrum; your arm supporting an object held in your hand is an example of this class of lever. The musculoskeletal system can be considered a system of levers. By understanding and applying knowledge of levers to body mechanics, the health worker can improve his or her skill in carrying out numerous clinical maneuvers and procedures.

Disorders of Muscles

Atrophy (at′ro-fe) is a wasting or decrease in the size of a muscle when it cannot be used, such as when an extremity must be placed in a cast following a fracture. *Strains* and *sprains* are typical injuries that often affect muscles. Severe and excessive exertion can cause detachment of muscles from bones or tearing of some of the muscle cells. Sprains can involve damage to other structures besides the ligaments, namely blood vessels, nerves and muscles. Much of the pain and swelling accompanying a sprain can be prevented by the immediate application of ice packs, which will constrict some of the smaller blood vessels and reduce internal bleeding.

Two diseases that affect muscles are *muscular dystrophy* (dis′tro-fe) and *myasthenia gravis* (mi-as-the′ne-ah gra′vis). The cause and cure of these afflictions are not yet known but are the subject of intensive research. Muscular dystrophy appears most often in male children and is a progressive disorder ending in complete helplessness. Myasthenia gravis is characterized by chronic muscular fatigue brought on by the slightest exertion. It affects adults and begins with the muscles of the head. Drooping of the eyelids (*ptosis*) is a common early symptom.

Myalgia (mi-al′je-ah) means "muscular pain," whereas *myositis* (mi-o-si′tis) is a term that indicates actual inflammation of muscle tissue. *Fibrositis* (fi-bro-si′tis) means "inflammation of connective tis-

sues," particularly those connected with muscles and joints. Usually a combination disorder called *fibromyositis* is present. Such a condition is commonly referred to as rheumatism, lumbago, or charleyhorse. The disorder may be acute with severe pain on motion, or it may be chronic. Sometimes the application of heat together with massage and rest will relieve the symptoms.

Bursitis is inflammation of a *bursa,* a bursa being a cavity or sac filled with synovial fluid. The purpose of a bursa is to minimize friction. Some communicate with joints; others are closely related to muscles. Sometimes bursae develop spontaneously in response to prolonged friction.

Bursitis can be very painful, with swelling and limitation of motion. Some examples of bursitis are

1   **Students' elbow,** in which the bursa over the point of the elbow (olecranon) is inflamed owing to long hours of leaning on the elbow while studying.
2   **Ischial bursitis,** said to be common in those who must sit a great deal, such as taxicab drivers and truckers.
3   **Housemaid's knee,** in which the bursa in front of the patella is inflamed. This form of bursitis is found in those who must be on their knees a great deal.
4   **Subdeltoid bursitis** in the shoulder region, a fairly common and unpleasant form. In some cases a local anesthetic is injected to relieve the pain.

Bunions are enlargements commonly found at the base and medial side of the great toe. Usually, prolonged pressure has caused the development of a bursa, which has then become inflamed. Special shoes may be necessary if surgery is not performed.

Flatfoot is a common disorder in which the *arch* of the foot, the normally raised portion of the sole, breaks down so that the entire sole rests on the ground. This condition may be congenital, in which case it usually gives little trouble. However, flatfoot can result from a progressive weakening of the muscles that support the arch, and usually this condition is accompanied by a great deal of pain. Incorrect use of the muscles that support the arch (such as toeing out when walking), or lack of exercise, are thought to bring about flatfoot. Walking with the toes pointed straight forward, in properly fitted shoes, may help to prevent flat-foot and other painful foot disorders. Other exercises, under the supervision of a trained person can be helpful in strengthening the muscles that help maintain the foot arches.

Table 10-1   *Review of muscles*

Name	Location	Function
Muscles of the Head and Neck		
Orbicularis oculi	Encircles eyelids	Closes eye
Levator palpebrae superioris	Back of orbit to upper eyelid	Opens eye
Orbicularis oris	Encircles mouth	Closes lips
Buccinator	Fleshy part of cheek	Flattens cheek; helps in eating, whistling, and blowing wind instruments
Temporal	Above and near the ear	Closes jaw
Masseter	At angle of jaw	Closes jaw
Sternocleidomastoid	Along side of neck, to mastoid process	Flexes head; rotates head toward opposite side
Muscles of the Upper Extremities		
Trapezius	Back of neck and upper back, to scapula	Raises shoulders and pulls them back; extends head
Latissimus dorsi	Middle and lower back, to humerus	Extends and adducts arm behind back
Pectoralis major	Upper, anterior chest, to humerus	Flexes and adducts arm across chest; pulls shoulders forward and downward
Deltoid	Covers shoulder joint, to lateral humerus	Abducts arm
Biceps brachii	Anterior arm, to radius	Flexes forearm and supinates hand
Triceps brachii	Posterior arm, to ulna	Extends forearm
Flexor and extensor carpi groups	Anterior and posterior forearm, to hand	Flex and extend hand
Flexor and extensor digitorum groups	Anterior and posterior forearm, to fingers	Flex and extend fingers
Muscles of the Trunk		
Diaphragm	Dome-shaped partition between thoracic and abdominal cavities	Dome descends to enlarge thoracic cavity from top to bottom
External intercostals	Between ribs	Elevate ribs and enlarge thoracic cavity
Rectus abdominis, obliquus, transversus	Anterolateral abdominal wall	Compress abdominal cavity and expel substances from body; flex spinal column
Levator ani	Pelvic floor	Aid defecation
Sacrospinalis	Deep in back, vertical mass	Extends vertebral column; erect posture

(Continued)

Table 10-1 *Review of muscles (Continued)*

Name	Location	Function
Muscles of the Lower Extremities		
Gluteus maximus	Superficial buttock, to femur	Extends thigh
Gluteus medius	Deep buttock, to femur	Abducts thigh
Iliopsoas	Crosses front of hip joint, to femur	Flexes thigh
Adductor group	Medial thigh, to femur	Adduct thigh
Sartorius	Winds down thigh, ilium to tibia	Flexes thigh and leg (sit cross-legged)
Quadriceps femoris	Anterior thigh, to tibia	Extends leg
Hamstring group	Posterior thigh, to tibia and fibula	Flex leg
Gastrocnemius	Calf of leg, to calcaneus	Extends foot (as in tiptoeing)
Tibialis anterior	Anterior and laterial shin, to foot	Dorsiflexion of foot (as in walking on heels); inverts foot (sole inward)
Peroneus longus	Lateral leg, to foot	Everts foot (sole outward)
Flexor and extensor digitorum groups	Posterior anterior leg, to toes	Flex and extend toes

Summary

Muscles.

A Characteristics—bundles of fibers covered with epimysium; endings of nerve fibers at motor end plates; contractility—actin and myosin—oxygen debt; muscle tone; isotonic and isometric contractions.

B Attachments—tendons, aponeuroses; origin (fixed attachment); insertion (movable attachment).

C Individual muscles—see review chart.

D Practical application—value of exercise; importance of good body mechanics; bones and muscles as system of levers.

E Disorders—strains, sprains, muscular dystrophy, myasthenia gravis, myalgia, myositis, fibrositis, fibromyositis, bunions, flatfoot.

Questions and Problems

1 Give a general description of skeletal muscle in terms of its structure, contractility and tone. What is oxygen debt? Give examples of isometric and isotonic contractions.

2 Define tendon, aponeurosis, muscle origin, muscle insertion.

3 Name and define the principal muscles of the head and neck, upper extremities, trunk, lower extremities.

4 What are some valuable effects of exercise?

5 What are levers and how do they work? The forceps is an example of which class of levers?

6 Describe briefly and give at least one cause of atrophy, flatfoot.

Chapter 11

The Brain, the Spinal Cord, and the Nerves

- The nervous system and its parts
- Nerves and nerve cells
- The brain and its subdivisions
- Lobes and areas in the cerebral hemispheres
- Functions of various parts of the brain
- Speech centers and the process of learning
- Sleeping sickness and other brain infections
- Strokes, epilepsy, and brain tumors
- The structure and functions of the spinal cord
- Coverings of the brain and spinal cord
- Cranial nerves, spinal nerves, and their disorders
- The autonomic nervous system

Glossary

Afferent Carrying toward a center or main part; said of nerves that carry impulses toward the central nervous system, or toward ganglia.

Autonomic Pertaining to the division of the nervous system which controls more or less automatic activities.

Efferent Carrying away from a center.

Fissure, sulcus A cleft or groove.

Ganglion (ganglia, pl.) A group of nerve cell bodies located outside the central nervous system.

Lobe A fairly well-defined portion of an organ.

Nerve A collection of fibers that carry impulses between a part of the nervous system and another region of the body.

Plexus A network of vessels, nerves, or veins.

Receptor, sensory end organ A nerve ending that receives a stimulus.

Ventricle A small cavity, such as one of the several cavities of the brain.

None of the body systems is capable of functioning alone. All are interdependent and work together as one unit so that normal conditions (homeostasis) within the body may prevail. The nervous system serves as the chief coordinating agency. Conditions both within and outside the body are constantly changing; one purpose of the nervous system is to respond to these internal and external changes (known as stimuli) and so cause the body to adapt itself to new conditions. It is through the instructions and directions sent to the various organs by the nervous system that the person's internal harmony and the balance between him and the environment are maintained. The nervous system has been compared with a telephone exchange in that the brain and the spinal cord act as switching centers and the nerve trunks act as cables for carrying messages to and from these centers.

The Nervous System as a Whole

The parts of the nervous system may be grouped according to their structure or function. The anatomic or structural divisions of the nervous system are as follows:

1 The **central** nervous system includes the brain and spinal cord.
2 The **peripheral** nervous system is made up of *cranial* and *spinal* nerves.

Cranial nerves are those that carry impulses to and from the brain. Spinal nerves are those that carry messages to and from the spinal cord.

From the standpoint of structure, the central and peripheral nervous systems together include most of the nerve tissue in the body. However, certain peripheral nerves have a special function, and for this reason they are grouped together under the designation *autonomic* (aw''to-nom'ik) nervous system. The reason for this separate classification is that the autonomic nervous system has to do largely with activities that go on more or less automatically. This system carries impulses from the central nervous system to the glands, the involuntary muscles found in the walls of tubes and hollow organs, and the heart. Some of the nerves that carry autonomic nervous system impulses are cranial, and others are spinal. The autonomic nervous system is subdivided into the *sympathetic* and *parasympathetic* nervous systems, both of which will be explained later in this chapter.

On Nerves in General

As we said in Chapter 2, the nerve cell is a neuron. Each neuron is composed of a cell body, containing the nucleus, and of nerve fibers, which are thread-like projections of the cytoplasm. The covered or myelinated fibers are called white fibers and are found in the white matter of the brain and cord as well as in the nerve trunks in all parts of the body. The fibers (and cell bodies) of the gray matter are not covered with myelin. In addition to the myelin, nerve fibers in the nerves of the peripheral nervous system are covered by a thin, cellular sheath, the neurilemma. The neurilemma aids in the repair of damaged nerve fibers.

Nerve fibers are of two kinds: *dendrites* (den'-drites), which conduct impulses *to* the cell body; and *axons,* which conduct impulses *away from* the cell body (Fig. 11-1). The dendrites of sensory

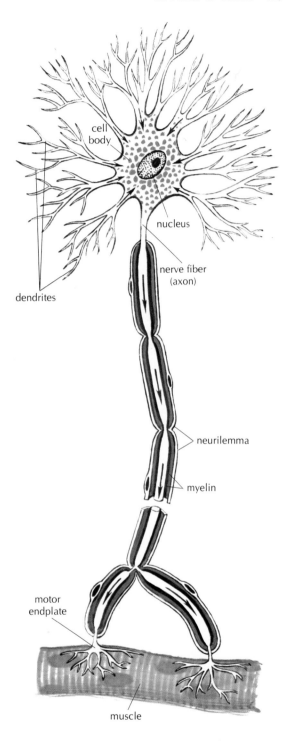

Fig. 11-1 Diagram of a motor neuron. The break in the axon denotes length.

neurons are very different from those of other neurons. They are usually single, and they may be very long (as much as 3 feet), or they may be short; but in any case, they do not have the treelike appearance so typical of other dendrites. Each sensory nerve fiber (dendrite) has a special structure called the *receptor,* or *end organ,* where the stimulus is received and the sensory impulse begins. Sensations such as pain, touch, hearing, and seeing which involve these sensory neurons are discussed in Chapter 12.

Each neuron is a separate unit, and there is no anatomic unity between neurons. It would be logical to ask how it is possible for neurons to be in contact; in other words, how the axon of one neuron can be in functional contact with the dendrite of another neuron. This is accomplished by the *synapse* (si′naps), from a Greek word meaning "to clasp." Synapses, then, are points of junction for transmission of nerve impulses. Certain chemicals, called neurotransmitters or transmitter substances, are released from the nerve fiber endings to enable the impulse to leap the synaptic junction. With the aid of chemical transmitters, impulses can be conducted between neurons and from a neuron or group of neurons to another type of cell. Like switches that open an electrical current to permit the passage of electricity, the synapses with the aid of the neurotransmitters allow the conduction of nerve impulses.

A *nerve* is a bundle of nerve fibers, located *outside* the central nervous system, which conducts impulses from one place to another. Bundles of nerve fibers *within* the central nervous system are *tracts* and are located within the spinal cord to conduct impulses to and from the brain. A nerve or tract can be compared with an electric cable made up of many wires. In the case of nerves the "wires," or nerve fibers, are bound together with connective tissue.

Nerve fibers that are connected with receptors (for receiving stimuli) conduct impulses *to* the brain and cord, and when grouped together form sensory or *afferent* nerves. Those fibers that carry impulses *from* the centers out to the muscles and glands form *efferent* nerves. The fibers of motor neurons, which carry impulses that lead to the contraction of skeletal muscles, are classified as efferent neurons (see Fig. 11-1). Some nerves contain a mixture of afferent and efferent nerve fibers and are often referred to as *mixed nerves.*

The Central Nervous System
The Brain

Main parts of the brain

The brain occupies the cranial cavity and is covered by bony tissue, the skull. The largest part of the brain is the *cerebrum* (ser′e-brum), which is divided into right and left *cerebral* (ser′e-bral) *hemispheres.* A second division of the brain is the *brainstem,* which connects the cerebrum with the spinal cord. The upper portion of the brainstem is the *midbrain.* Below it and plainly visible from the under view of the brain are the *pons* (ponz) and the *medulla oblongata* (me-dul′lah ob″long-ga′tah). The pons connects the midbrain with the medulla, while the medulla connects the brain with the spinal cord through a large opening in the base of the skull. The third main part of the brain is the *cerebellum* (ser″e-bel′um), a word meaning "little brain." It is located immediately below the back part of the cerebral hemispheres and is connected with the cerebrum, brainstem and spinal cord by means of the pons.

Structure of the Cerebral Hemispheres

The outer nerve tissue of the cerebral hemispheres is gray matter and is called the *cerebral cortex.* This gray cortex is arranged in folds forming elevated portions known as *convolutions* (kon-vo-lu′shuns), separated by depressions or grooves called *fissures,* or *sulci* (sul′si) (Fig. 11-2). Internally, the cerebral hemispheres are made largely of white matter and a few islands of gray matter. Inside the hemispheres are two spaces extending in a somewhat irregular fashion. These are the *lateral ventricles,* which are filled with a watery fluid common to both the brain and the spinal cord called *cerebrospinal* (ser-e-bro-spi′nal) *fluid,* to be discussed later.

Although there are many fissures (sulci), a few are especially important landmarks, as follows:

1   The **longitudinal fissure** is a deep groove that separates the cerebral hemispheres from each other.
2   A **central fissure** lies between the frontal and parietal lobes of each hemisphere at right angles to the longitudinal fissure.

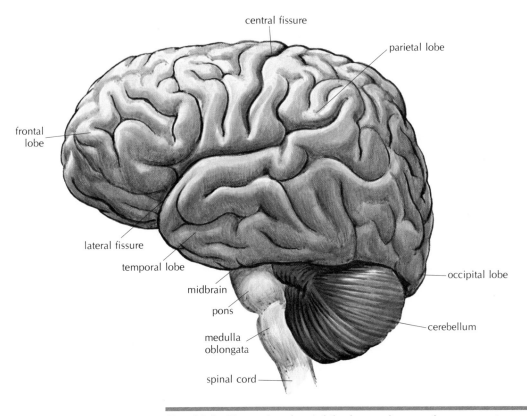

central fissure

parietal lobe

frontal lobe

lateral fissure

temporal lobe

midbrain

pons

medulla oblongata

spinal cord

occipital lobe

cerebellum

Fig. 11-2 *External surface of the brain, showing the main parts and some of the lobes and fissures of the cerebrum.*

3 A **lateral fissure** curves somewhat along the side of each hemisphere and separates the temporal lobe from the frontal and parietal lobes.

Let us examine the cerebral cortex, the layer of gray matter that forms the surface of each cerebral hemisphere. It is within the cerebral cortex that impulses are received and analyzed. These form the basis of knowledge; the brain "stores" information, much of which can be recalled on demand by means of the phenomenon that we call memory. It is in the cerebral cortex that thought processes, for example, association, judgment, and discrimination, take place. It is from the cerebral cortex, too, that the orders originating from conscious deliberation emanate; that is, voluntary actions are directed here.

Division and Functions of the Cerebral Cortex The cerebral cortex of each hemisphere is divided into four *lobes,* areas named from the overlying cranial bones. While coordination among the various areas of the brain occurs to produce human behavior, certain portions influence particular categories of function. The four lobes, with some of their characteristic functions, follow:

1 The **frontal lobe,** relatively larger in the human being than in any other organism, lies in front of the central fissure. This lobe contains the motor cortex which directs actions (Fig. 11-3). The left side of the brain governs the right side of the body and the right side of the brain governs the left side of the body (Fig. 11-4). The frontal lobe also contains two areas important in speech (the speech centers will be discussed later).

2 The **parietal lobe** occupies the upper part of each hemisphere and lies just behind the central fissure. This lobe contains the *sensory area,* in which impulses from the skin are interpreted, such as touch, pain, or temperature. Also such interpretations as the determination of distances, sizes, and shapes take place here.

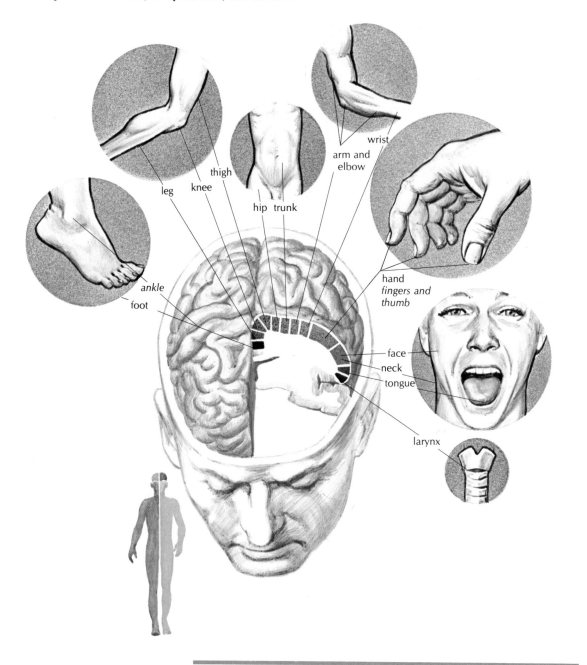

Fig. 11-3 *Controlling areas of the brain. The parts of the body are shown drawn in proportion to the area of control.*

3 The **temporal lobe** lies below the lateral fissure and folds under the hemisphere on each side. This lobe contains the *auditory area* for receiving and interpreting impulses from the ear. The *olfactory area,* concerned with the sense of smell, is located in the medial part of the temporal lobe. It is stimulated by impulses arising from receptors in the nose.

4 The **occipital lobe** lies behind the parietal lobe and extends over the cerebellum. This lobe contains the *visual area* for interpreting impulses arising from the retina of the eye.

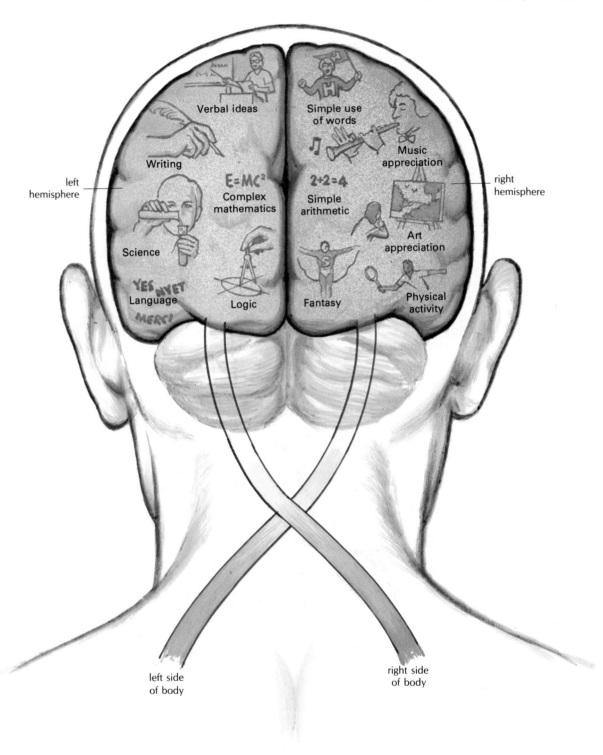

Fig. 11-4 Schematic representation of cerebral dominance, showing that the two sides of the cerebrum send impulses to, and receive impulses from, the opposite sides of the body. (*Chaffee EE, Lytle IM: Basic Physiology and Anatomy, 4th ed. Philadelphia, JB Lippincott, 1980*)

Beneath the gray matter of the cerebral cortex is the white matter, consisting of myelinated nerve fibers which connect the cortical areas with each other and with other parts of the nervous system. An important band of white matter is the *corpus callosum,* which acts as a bridge between the right and left hemispheres permitting impulses to cross from one side of the brain to the other. Another group of myelinated nerve fibers is the *internal capsule.* This is a crowded strip of white matter composed of many fibers (forming tracts). *Basal ganglia* are masses of gray matter located deep within each cerebral hemisphere. These groups of neurons help to regulate body movement and facial expressions communicated from the cerebral cortex. The transmitter substance, *dopamine* (do'pah-men) is secreted by the neurons of the basal ganglia.

Communication Areas   The ability to communicate by written and verbal means is an interesting example of the way in which areas of the cerebral cortex are interrelated (Fig. 11-5). The develop-

ment and use of these areas are closely connected with the process of learning.

1   The **auditory areas** are located in the temporal lobe. In one of these areas sound impulses, transmitted from the environment, are detected, while in the surrounding area (auditory speech center) the sounds are interpreted and understood. The beginnings of language are learned by auditory means, so the auditory area for understanding sounds is very near to the auditory receiving area of the cortex. Babies often seem to understand what is being said long before they do any talking themselves. It is usually several years before children learn to read or write words.

2   The **motor areas** for communication (for talking and writing) are located in front of the lowest part of the motor cortex in the frontal lobe. Since the lower part of the motor cortex controls the muscles of the head and neck, it seems logical to think of the motor speech cen-

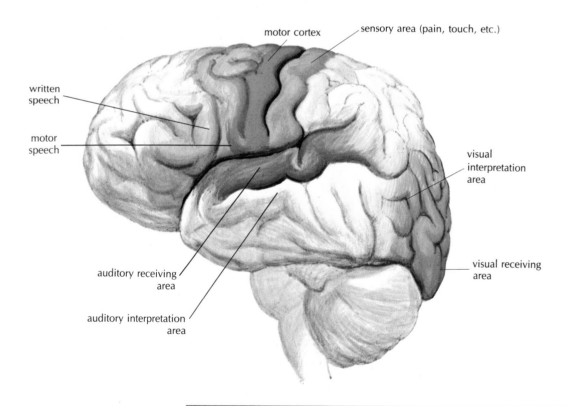

Fig. 11-5 Functional areas of cerebrum, including the communication areas.

ter as an extension forward in this area. Control of the muscles of speech (in the tongue, the soft palate, and the larynx) is carried out here. Likewise, the written speech center is located in front of the cortical area that controls the muscles of the arm and hand. The ability to write words is usually one of the last phases in the development of learning words and their meaning.

3 The **visual areas** of the cortex are involved in communication by receiving visual impulses in the occipital lobe. These images are interpreted as words in the visual area that lies in front of the receiving location. In this area the ability to read with understanding is developed. You may *see* writing in the Japanese language, for example, but this would involve only the visual receiving area in the occipital lobe unless you could *read* the words.

There is a functional relationship among areas of the brain. Numerous neurons must work together to enable the person to receive, interpret and respond to verbal and written messages as well as to touch (tactile) and other sensory stimuli.

The Diencephalon

The *diencephalon* (di-en-sef′ah-lon), or interbrain, can be seen by cutting into the central section of the brain. It includes the *thalamus* (thal′ah-mus) and the *hypothalamus.* Nearly all sensory impulses travel through the masses of gray matter that form the thalamus. The action of the thalamus is to sort out the impulses and direct them to particular areas of the cerebral cortex. The hypothalamus is located in the midline area below the thalamus and contains cells that help to control body temperature, water balance, sleep, appetite, and some emotions, such as fear and pleasure. Both the sympathetic and parasympathetic divisions of the autonomic nervous system are under the control of the hypothalamus. Thus, it influences the heart beat, the contraction and relaxation of the walls of blood vessels, and other vital body functions.

Division and Functions of the Brainstem and the Cerebellum

The brainstem is composed of the midbrain, the pons, and the medulla oblongata. These structures connect the cerebrum with the spinal cord.

The *midbrain* is located just below the center of the cerebrum. It forms the forward part of the brainstem. Four rounded masses of gray matter that are hidden by the cerebral hemispheres form the upper part of the midbrain. These four bodies act as relay centers for certain eye and ear reflexes. The white matter at the front of the midbrain conducts impulses between the higher centers of the cerebrum and the lower centers of the pons, medulla, cerebullum, and spinal cord. Cranial nerves III and IV originate from the midbrain.

The *pons* lies between the midbrain and the medulla, in front of the cerebellum. It is composed largely of myelinated nerve fibers which serve to connect the two halves of the cerebellum with the brainstem and also with the cerebrum above and the spinal cord below. The pons is an important connecting link between the cerebellum and the rest of the nervous system, and it also contains nerve fibers that carry impulses to and from the centers located above and below it. Certain reflex (involuntary) actions are integrated in the pons, for example, some of those occurring in respiration. Cranial nerves V through VIII originate from the pons.

The *medulla oblongata* of the brain is located between the pons and the spinal cord. It appears white externally because, like the pons, it contains many myelinated nerve fibers. Internally, it contains collections of cell bodies (gray matter) called *centers* or *nuclei.* Among these are vital centers such as the following:

1 The **respiratory center** controls the muscles of respiration in response to chemical and other stimuli.
2 The **cardiac center** helps to regulate the rate and force of the heart beat.
3 The **vasomotor** (vas-o-mo′tor) center regulates the contraction of smooth muscle in the blood vessel walls and thus helps to determine blood pressure.

The last four pairs of cranial nerves are connected with the medulla. The nerve fibers that carry messages through the spinal cord up to the brain continue through the medulla also, as do similar descending or *motor fibers.* These groups of nerve fibers form tracts (bundles) and are grouped together according to function. The motor fibers from the motor cortex of the cerebral hemispheres extend down through the medulla, and most of them cross from one side to the other (decussate) while going through this part of the brain. It is in the medulla that the shifting of nerve fibers occurs which causes the right cerebral hemisphere to control muscles in the left side of the body, and the upper portion of the cortex to control muscles in the lower portions of the person. The medulla is an important reflex center, and it is here that certain neurons end and impulses are relayed to other neurons. Cranial nerves IX through XII arise from the medulla.

The *cerebellum* is made up of three parts: the middle portion and two lateral hemispheres. As in the case of the cerebral hemispheres, the cerebellum has an outer area of gray matter and an inner portion that is largely white matter. The functions of the cerebellum are

1 To aid in the **coordination of voluntary muscles** so that they will function smoothly and in an orderly fashion. Disease of the cerebellum causes muscular jerkiness and tremors.
2 To help **maintain balance** in standing, walking and sitting, as well as during more strenuous activities. Messages from the internal ear and from the tendon and muscle sensory end organs aid the cerebellum.
3 To aid in **maintaining muscle tone** so that all muscle fibers are slightly tensed and ready to produce necessary changes in position as quickly as may be necessary.

Ventricles of the Brain

Within the brain are four fluid-filled spaces called the ventricles. These extend into the various parts of the brain in a somewhat irregular fashion. We have already mentioned the largest, the lateral ventricles in the two cerebral hemispheres. Their extensions into the lobes of the cerebrum are called *horns* (Fig. 11-6). These paired ventricles communicate with a midline space, the third ventricle, by means of the openings called *foramina* (fo-ram′i-nah). The third ventricle is bounded on each side by the two parts of the thalamus, while the floor is occupied by the hypothalamus. Continuing down from the third ventricle a small canal, called the *cerebral aqueduct,* extends through the midbrain into the fourth ventricle. The latter is continuous with the neural, or central, canal of the spinal cord. In the roof of the fourth ventricle are three openings that allow the escape of fluid to the area that

surrounds the brain and spinal cord. This fluid is called *cerebrospinal* (ser′e-bro′spi′nal) *fluid* and will be discussed later in this chapter.

Brain Studies

Diagnostic tests can be performed to examine the brain and related structures. One such test involves the removal of some of the cerebrospinal fluid. Air or other substances may be injected, and x-ray films called *encephalograms* (en-sef′ah-lo-grams) or *ventriculograms* (ven-trik′u-lo-grams) are taken.

Another kind of x-ray study available in larger medical centers is the CAT or CT scan (mentioned in Chap. 2). It provides multiple x-ray pictures taken from different angles simultaneously. By means of a computer, the information is organized and displayed as photographs of the bone, soft tissue, and cavities of the brain (Fig. 11-7). Anatomic lesions such as tumors or scar tissue accumulations are readily seen.

The interactions of the billions of nerve cells in the brain give rise to measurable electric currents. These may be recorded by an instrument called the *electroencephalograph* (e-lek′′tro-ensef′ah-lo-graf′′). The recorded tracings or brain waves produce an electroencephalogram, or EEG.

Disorders of the Brain

Since the scientific name for the brain is *encephalon* (en-sef′ah-lon), inflammation of the brain is known as encephalitis (en-sef′′ah-li′tis). There are many causes of such disease, but the two chief pathogens are as follows:

1 **Viruses** cause some of the epidemic types of sleeping sickness sometimes found in the United States and in other parts of the world.
2 Certain **protozoa** called *trypanosoma* (tri′′pan-o-so′mah), cause the so-called African sleeping sickness. These protozoa are carried by a kind of fly (tsetse) and are capable of invading the cerebrospinal fluid of man and infecting the surrounding tissue.

Stroke, or *cerebrovascular* (ser′′e-bro-vas′ku-lar) *accident* (CVA), is by far the most common kind of brain disorder. Rupture of a blood vessel (with a consequent *cerebral hemorrhage*), thrombosis, or embolism may cause destruction of brain tissue. Such disorders are more frequent in the presence of artery wall disease, and hence are more common

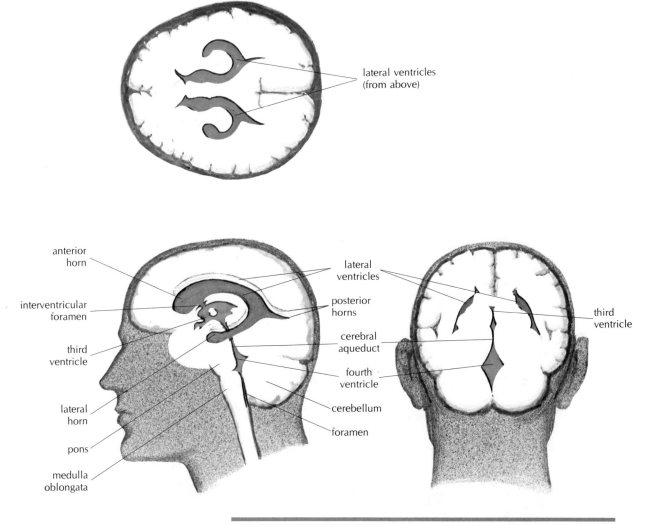

anterior horn

interventricular foramen

third ventricle

lateral horn

pons

medulla oblongata

lateral ventricles (from above)

lateral ventricles

posterior horns

cerebral aqueduct

fourth ventricle

cerebellum

foramen

third ventricle

Fig. 11-6 *Ventricles of the brain.*

after the age of 40. The effect of a stroke will depend on the location of the artery and the extent of the involvement. A hemorrhage into the white matter of the internal capsule in the lower part of the cerebrum may cause extensive paralysis of the side opposite to the affected area. Such a paralysis is called *hemiplegia* (hem''e-ple'je-ah), and the paralyzed person is called a hemiplegic (hem''e-ple'jik).

Cerebral palsy (pawl'ze) is a disorder caused by brain damage occurring before or during the birth process. It is characterized by diverse disorders of muscles varying in degree of disturbance from weakness to complete paralysis, and in extent from a slight disorder of the lower extremity muscles

to paralysis of all four extremities and the speech muscles as well. With muscle and speech training and other therapeutic approaches, these children can be helped.

Epilepsy is a chronic disorder in which there is abnormality of the electrical activity of the brain with or without apparent changes in the nerve tissues. One manifestation of epilepsy is seizure activity, which may be so mild as to be hardly noticeable, or so severe as to result in a loss of consciousness. In most cases the cause is not known. The study of brain waves obtained with the electroencephalograph (EEG) usually shows abnormalities and is helpful in both diagnosis and treatment. Many persons with epilepsy can lead

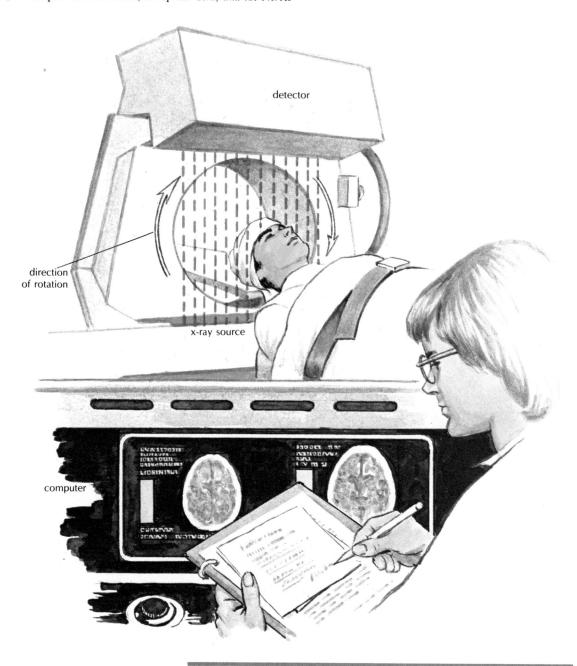

detector

direction
of rotation

x-ray source

computer

Fig. 11-7 CT scanner.

normal active lives if they use appropriate medication as outlined by a physician. Newer techniques of laser surgery may prove to be beneficial in controlling seizure activity.

Tumors of the brain may develop at any age, but are somewhat more common in young and middle-aged adults. The majority of brain tumors originate from the neuroglia and are called gliomas (see Chap. 2). The symptoms produced depend on the type of tumor, the location of the growth, its destructiveness, and the degree to which it compresses the brain tissue. Involvement of the frontal portion of the cerebrum often causes mental symptoms, such as changes in personality and in levels of consciousness. Early surgery, chemotherapy, and radiation therapy offer hope of cure in some cases.

Aphasia (ah-fa′ze-ah) is a term that refers to the loss of the ability to speak or write, or the loss of the understanding of written or spoken language. There are several different kinds of aphasia, depending on what part of the brain is affected. The lesion that causes aphasia is likely to be in the left cerebral hemisphere in the right-handed person. Often much can be done for these people by patient retraining and much understanding. The brain is an organ that has a marvelous capacity for adapting itself to different conditions, and its resources are tremendous. Often some means of communication can be found even though speech areas are damaged.

The Spinal Cord

Location of the Spinal Cord

In the embryo, the spinal cord occupies the entire spinal canal and so extends down into the tail portion of the vertebral column. However, the column of bone grows much more rapidly than the nerve tissue of the cord, so that the end of the cord no longer reaches the lower part of the spinal canal. This disparity in growth increases so that in the adult the cord ends in the region just below the area to which the last rib attaches (between the first and second lumbar vertebrae).

Structure of the Spinal Cord

Examination of the spinal cord reveals that it has a small, irregularly shaped internal section consisting of gray matter (nerve cell bodies), and a larger area surrounding this gray part that consists of white matter (nerve fibers). A cross section of the cord shows that the gray matter is so arranged that a column of cells extends up and down dorsally, one on each side; another column is found in the ventral region; while a third, less conspicuous part is situated on each side. These three pairs of columns of gray matter give this cross section an H-shaped appearance (Fig. 11-8). The white matter consists of thousands of nerve fibers arranged in three areas external to the gray matter on each side.

Functions of the Spinal Cord

The functions of the cord may be divided into three aspects:

1   **Reflex activities,** which involve the transfer and integration of messages that enter the cord, so that a sensory (afferent) impulse entering the center will become a motor (efferent) message leaving the cord.
2   A pathway for **conducting sensory impulses** from afferent nerves upward through ascending tracts to the brain.
3   A pathway for **conducting motor** (efferent) **impulses** from the brain down through descending tracts to the nerves that will supply muscles or glands.

The reflex pathway through the spinal cord usually involves three or more neurons, as illustrated in Figure 11-8 and listed here:

1   The **sensory neuron,** which has its beginning in a receptor and its nerve fiber in a nerve that leads to the cord.
2   One or more **central neurons,** which are entirely within the cord.
3   The **motor neuron,** which receives the impulse from a central neuron and then carries it by way of its long axon through a nerve to a muscle or a gland.

The knee jerk is an example of a spinal reflex. The pathway for the impulses that make this reflex possible includes a sensory neuron that has its receptor in the tendon just below the knee, its sensory nerve fiber in the nerves that extend to the spinal cord, central neurons inside the lower part of the cord, and motor neurons that send processes through nerves from the cord to the effectors in the quadriceps femoris (the thigh's kicking muscle).

Lumbar Puncture

Since the cord is only about 18 inches long and ends some distance above the level of the hip line, a lumbar puncture or spinal tap is usually done between the third and fourth lumbar vertebrae, at about the level of the top of the hipbone. During this procedure, a small amount of cerebrospinal

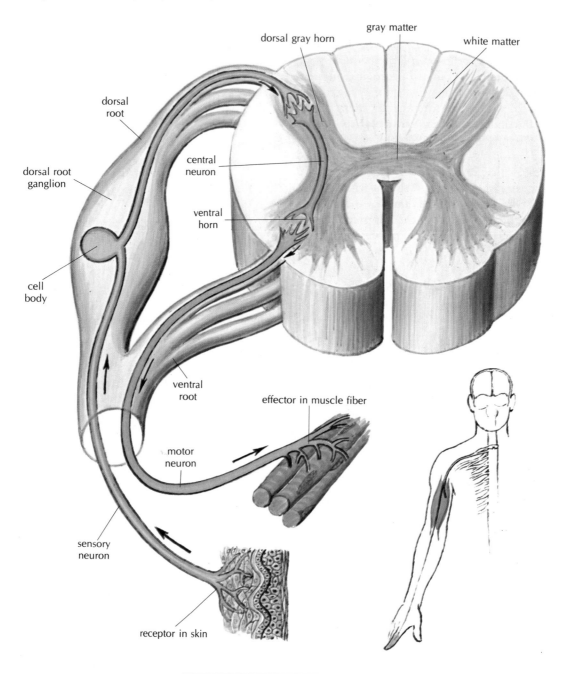

Fig. 11-8 Reflex arc showing pathway of impulses and cross section of spinal cord.

fluid may be removed from the space below the spinal cord. The fluid can then be studied in the laboratory for evidence of disease or injury.

Anesthetics or medications are sometimes injected into the space below the cord. The anesthetic agent will temporarily block all sensation from the lower part of the body. This method of giving anesthesia has an advantage for certain types of procedures or surgery; the patient is awake, but feels nothing in his lower body.

Disorders Involving the Spinal Cord

An acute viral disease affecting both the spinal cord and the brain is *poliomyelitis* ("polio"), which occurs most commonly in children. The polio virus enters the body through the nose and the throat; it multiplies in the gastrointestinal tract and then travels to the central nervous system, possibly by way of the blood. The virus may destroy the motor nerve cells in the spinal cord, in which case paralysis of one or more limbs results. The virus also can attack some of the cells of the brain and cause death. Prevention of poliomyelitis by means of the oral Sabin vaccine is one of the many significant advances in preventive medicine.

Injuries to the spinal cord occur in instances in which bones of the spinal column are broken or dislocated, such as in swimming and diving accidents. Gunshot or shrapnel wounds may damage the cord in varying degrees. Since the nerve tissue of the brain and cord cannot repair itself, severing the cord causes paralysis of the muscles supplied by nerves, below the level of the injury. Loss of sensation and motion in the lower part of the body is called *paraplegia* (par''ah-ple'je-ah).

Other disorders of the spinal cord include tumors that grow from within the cord or that compress the cord from outside.

Multiple sclerosis (sclerosis means hardening) involves the entire spinal cord as well as the brain. In this disease the myelin, a fatlike substance that forms a sheath around certain nerve fibers, disappears and the nerve axons themselves degenerate. It is an extremely disabling disease; however, it usually progresses very slowly so that the patient may have many years of relatively comfortable life remaining to him.

Amyotrophic (ah-mi''o-trof'ik) *lateral sclerosis* is a disorder of the nervous system in which motor neurons are destroyed. The progressive destruction causes muscle atrophy and loss of motor control until finally the person is unable to swallow, or to talk.

Coverings of the brain and the spinal cord

The *meninges* (me-nin'jez) are three layers of connective tissue that surround the brain and the spinal cord to form a complete enclosure. The outermost of these membranes is called the *dura mater* (du'rah ma'ter). It is the thickest and toughest of the meninges. Inside the skull, the dura mater splits in certain places to provide venous channels for the blood coming from the brain tissue. The second layer around the brain and the spinal cord is the *arachnoid* (ah-rak'-noid) membrane. This membrane is loosely attached to the deepest of the meninges by web-like fibers allowing a space for the movement of cerebrospinal fluid between the arachnoid and the innermost membrane. The third layer around the brain, the *pia mater* (pi'ah-ma'-ter), is attached to the nerve tissue of the brain and spinal cord and dips into all the depressions (Fig. 11-9). It is made of a delicate connective tissue in which there are many blood vessels. The blood supply to the brain is carried, to a large extent, by the pia mater.

Inflammation of the Meninges

Meningitis (men-in-ji'tis) is an inflammation of the brain and spinal cord coverings caused by pathogenic bacteria, notably a diplococcus called the meningococcus (me-ning''o-kok'us). If this organism attacks only the membranes around the spinal cord, the condition is called spinal meningitis; whereas, if it attacks the entire membranous enclosure, it is called cerebrospinal meningitis. Occasionally, other bacteria or viruses cause inflammation of the meninges. Sometimes the inflammatory processes may be so severe as to cause permanent brain damage or even death. Squeezing a pimple or a boil in the area of the nose or forehead may result in the spread of staphylococci or streptococci through associated veins to the meninges, causing a serious meningitis.

Trauma to the Meninges

Trauma to the head may cause bleeding between the skull and the brain. Arterial bleeding outside the dura causes *epidural hematomas* with rapidly progressing symptoms (such as coma and dilated pupils). Tears in the dural walls of the venous sinuses cause *subdural hematomas,* with a slow leak and less dramatic symptoms. Frequent observation of the level of consciousness, pupil response, and extremity reflexes are important for patients with head injuries.

Cerebrospinal Fluid

Cerebrospinal fluid (CSF) is a clear liquid formed inside the ventricles of the brain, mostly by structures called the *choroid plexuses;* some may be

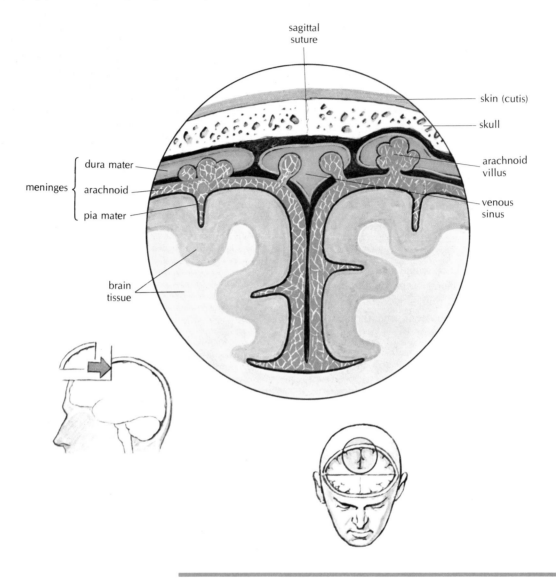

Fig. 11-9 *Frontal (coronal) section of top of head, showing meninges and related parts.*

formed by filtration from the capillaries. The function of CSF is to cushion shocks that would otherwise injure the delicate structures of the central nervous system. This fluid also carries nutrients to the cells and transports waste products from the cells. The CSF normally flows freely from ventricle to ventricle and finally out into the subarachnoid space, which surrounds the brain and spinal cord. Much of the fluid is returned to the blood in the venous sinuses through projections called the arachnoid villi (Fig. 11-10).

Any obstruction to the flow of CSF, as for example in injury to the membranes around the three exit openings, may cause the condition called *hydrocephalus* (hi-dro-sef'ah-lus). As the fluid accumulates, the mounting pressure can squeeze the brain against the skull and destroy the brain tissue.

Hydrocephalus is more common in infants than in adults, and if the fontanels of the infant skull have not closed, the cranium itself can become greatly enlarged. Since cranial enlargement cannot occur in the adult, a slight increase in fluid will result in symptoms of increased pressure within the skull as brain tissue is damaged.

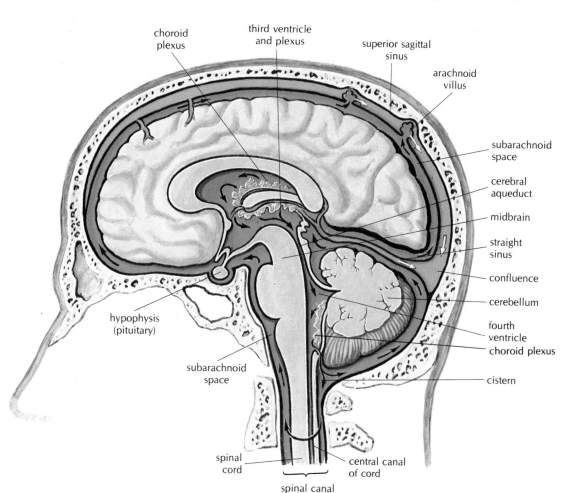

Fig. 11-10 *Flow of cerebrospinal fluid from choroid plexuses back to blood in venous sinuses is shown by black arrows; blood flow is shown by white arrows.*

A treatment for hydrocephalus involves the creation of a shunt to drain excess CSF from the brain.

The Peripheral Nervous System
Cranial Nerves
Location of the Cranial Nerves

There are 12 pairs of cranial nerves (henceforth, when a cranial nerve is identified, a pair is meant). The cranial nerves are numbered according to their connection with the brain, beginning at the front and proceeding back (Fig. 11-11). The first nine pairs of cranial nerves and the 12th pair supply structures in the head.

General Functions of the Cranial Nerves

From a functional point of view, we may think of the kinds of messages that the cranial nerves handle as belonging to one of four categories.

1 Special sensory impulses, such as for smell, vision, and hearing.

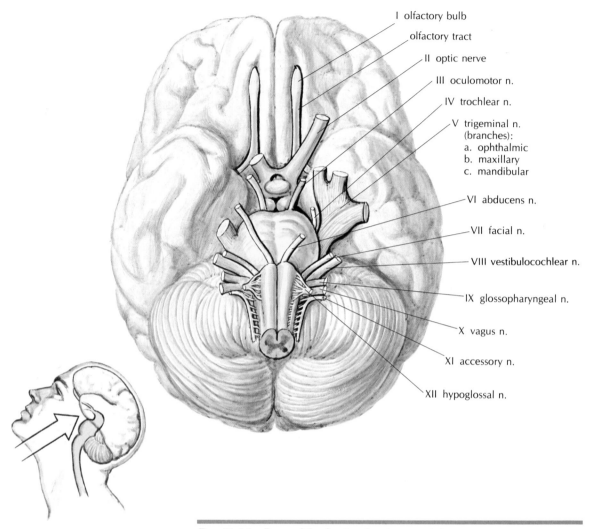

I olfactory bulb
olfactory tract
II optic nerve
III oculomotor n.
IV trochlear n.
V trigeminal n.
(branches):
a. ophthalmic
b. maxillary
c. mandibular
VI abducens n.
VII facial n.
VIII vestibulocochlear n.
IX glossopharyngeal n.
X vagus n.
XI accessory n.
XII hypoglossal n.

Fig. 11-11 *Base of the brain, showing cranial nerves.*

2 General sensory impulses, such as for pain, touch, temperature, deep muscle sense, pressure, and vibrations.
3 Voluntary muscle control or somatic motor impulses.
4 Involuntary control or visceral effector messages to glands and involuntary muscles.

Names and Functions of the Cranial Nerves

A list of the 12 cranial nerves follows (numbered according to the traditional Roman style, which is always used):

I The **olfactory nerve** carries smell impulses from receptors in the nasal mucosa to the brain.
II The **optic nerve** carries visual impulses from the eye to the brain.
III The **oculomotor nerve** is concerned with the contraction of most of the eye muscles.
IV The **trochlear** (trok′le-ar) **nerve** supplies one eyeball muscle on each side.
V The **trigeminal** (tri-jem′i-nal) **nerve** is the great sensory nerve of the face and head. It has three branches that carry general sense impulses, (*e.g.,* pain, touch, temperature)

from the face to the brain. The third branch is joined by motor fibers to the muscles of mastication (chewing).

VI The **abducens** (ab-du′senz) nerve is another nerve sending controlling impulses to an eyeball muscle.

VII The **facial nerve** is largely motor. The muscles of facial expression are all supplied by branches from the facial nerve. This nerve also includes special sensory fibers for taste (anterior two thirds of the tongue) and contains secretory fibers to the smaller salivary glands (the submaxillary and sublingual), and to the lacrimal gland.

VIII The **vestibulocochlear (acoustic) nerve** contains special sensory fibers for hearing as well as those for balance from the semicircular canals of the internal ear.

IX The **glossopharyngeal** (glos-o-fah-rin′ge-al) **nerve** contains general sensory fibers from the back of the tongue and the pharynx (throat). This nerve also contains sensory fibers for taste from the posterior third of the tongue, secretory fibers that supply the largest salivary gland (parotid), and motor nerve fibers to control the swallowing muscles in the pharynx.

X The **vagus** (va′gus) **nerve** is the longest cranial nerve. It supplies most of the organs in the thoracic and abdominal cavities. This nerve also contains secretory fibers to glands that produce digestive juices and other secretions.

XI The **accessory nerve** (formerly called the spinal accessory nerve) is made up of motor nerve fibers controlling two muscles of the neck (trapezius and sternocleidomastoid).

XII The **hypoglossal nerve,** the last of the 12 cranial nerves, carries impulses controlling the muscles of the tongue.

Disorders Involving the Cranial Nerves

Destruction of optic nerve (II) fibers may result from increased pressure of the eye fluid on the nerves, as occurs in glaucoma, the influence of poisons, and certain infections. Certain medications, when used in high doses for a long period of time, can damage the branch of the vestibulocochlear nerve responsible for hearing.

Injury to a nerve that contains motor fibers causes paralysis of the muscles supplied by these fibers. The oculomotor nerve (III) may be damaged by certain infections or various poisonous substances. Since this nerve supplies so many muscles connected with the eye, including the levator, which raises the eyelid, injury to it will cause a paralysis that usually interferes with eye function. Bell's palsy is a facial paralysis due to damage to the facial (VII) nerve usually on one side of the face. This injury results in distortion of the face because of one-sided paralysis of the muscles of facial expression.

Neuralgia (nu-ral′je-ah) means ''nerve pain.'' It is used particularly to refer to a severe spasmodic pain affecting the fifth cranial nerve, and goes by various names, including *trigeminal neuralgia, trifacial neuralgia,* and *tic douloureux* (tik doo-loo-roo′). At first the pain comes at relatively long intervals; but as time goes on, it is likely to appear at shorter intervals with the attacks of pain of longer duration. Newer treatments include microsurgery and high frequency current.

Spinal Nerves
Location and Structure of the Spinal Nerves

There are 31 pairs of spinal nerves, each pair numbered according to the level of the spinal cord from which it arises. Each nerve is attached to the spinal cord by two roots, the dorsal root and the ventral root. On each dorsal root there is a marked swelling of gray matter called the dorsal root ganglion, which contains the cell bodies of the sensory neurons. A ganglion (pl. ganglia) is a collection of nerve cell bodies located outside the central nervous system.

Nerve fibers from the sensory receptors of various areas of the body lead to these ganglia. A sensory receptor is a nerve ending that responds to stimuli. There are two categories of receptors. Those for general sensation are located in the skin and the body wall. They respond to stimuli that give rise to sensations of pain, touch, and temperature and of the location and position of body parts. The second category includes receptors for the special senses—taste, vision, and hearing. Impulses from these receptors are carried by cranial nerves from the organ involved to the brain. These organs of special sense will be taken up in the next chapter.

While sensory fibers form the dorsal roots, the

ventral roots of the spinal nerves are a combination of motor (efferent) nerve fibers supplying voluntary muscles, involuntary muscles, and glands. The cell bodies for the voluntary fibers are located in the ventral part of the cord gray matter (anterior or ventral gray horn), while the cell bodies for the involuntary fibers are to be found in the lateral gray horns.

Branches of the Spinal Nerves

Each spinal nerve continues only a very short distance away from the spinal cord and then branches into small posterior divisions and rather large anterior divisions. The larger anterior branches interlace to form networks called *plexuses* (plex′sus-es) which then distribute branches to the body parts. The three main plexuses are described as follows:

1 The **cervical plexus** supplies motor impulses to the muscles of the neck and receives sensory impulses from the neck and the back of the head. The phrenic nerve, which activates the diaphragm, arises from this plexus.
2 The **brachial** (bra′ke-al) **plexus** sends numerous branches to the shoulder, the arm, the forearm, the wrist, and the hand. The radial nerve emerges from the brachial plexus.
3 The **lumbosacral** (lum-bo-sa′kral) **plexus** supplies nerves to the lower extremities. The largest of these branches is the *sciatic* (si-at′ik) nerve, which leaves the dorsal part of the pelvis, passes beneath the gluteus maximus muscle, and extends down the back of the thigh. At its beginning it is nearly an inch thick, but it soon sends branches to the thigh muscles; and near the knee it divides into two subdivisions that supply the leg and the foot.

Disorders of the Spinal Nerves

Neuritis (nu-ri′tis) means "inflammation of a nerve." The term is also used to refer to degenerative and other disorders that may involve nerves. It may affect a single nerve, or many nerves throughout the body, as a result of blows, bone fractures, or other mechanical injuries. Nutritional deficiency, as well as various poisons such as alcohol, carbon monoxide, and barbitals, are causative agents.

Neuritis is fairly common in chronic alcoholic persons and is thought to be related to the severe malnourished state these persons display. B vitamin deficiencies, especially of thiamin (thi′ah-min), are related to both the malnourished state and chronic alcoholism. Neuritis is really a symptom rather than a disease, so that thorough physical and laboratory studies may need to be made to discover the cause.

Sciatica (si-at′e-kah) is a form of neuritis characterized by severe pain along the sciatic nerve and its branches. There are many causes of this disorder, but probably the most common are rupture of a disk between the lower lumbar vertebrae and arthritis of the lower part of the spinal column.

Herpes zoster, commonly known as shingles, is characterized by numerous blisters along the course of certain nerves, most commonly the intercostal nerves, which are branches of the thoracic spinal nerves in the waist area. The cause is the chicken pox virus that attacks the sensory cell bodies inside the spinal ganglia. Recovery in a few days is usual, but neuralgic pains may persist for years and be very distressing. This infection also may involve the first branch of the fifth cranial nerve and cause pain in the eyeball and surrounding tissues.

The Autonomic Nervous System
Parts of the Autonomic Nervous System

Although the internal organs such as the heart, the lungs, and the stomach contain nerve endings and nerve fibers for conducting sensory messages to the brain and cord, most of these impulses do not reach consciousness. These *afferent* impulses from the viscera are translated into reflex responses without reaching the higher centers of the brain. The sensory neurons from the organs are grouped with those that come from the skin and voluntary muscles. On the other hand, the *efferent* neurons that supply the glands and the involuntary muscles are arranged very differently from those that supply the voluntary muscles. This variation in the location and arrangement of the *visceral efferent* neurons has led to their classification as part of a separate division called the autonomic nervous system (Fig. 11-12).

The autonomic nervous system has many ganglia that serve as relay stations. In these ganglia each message is transferred at a synapse from the

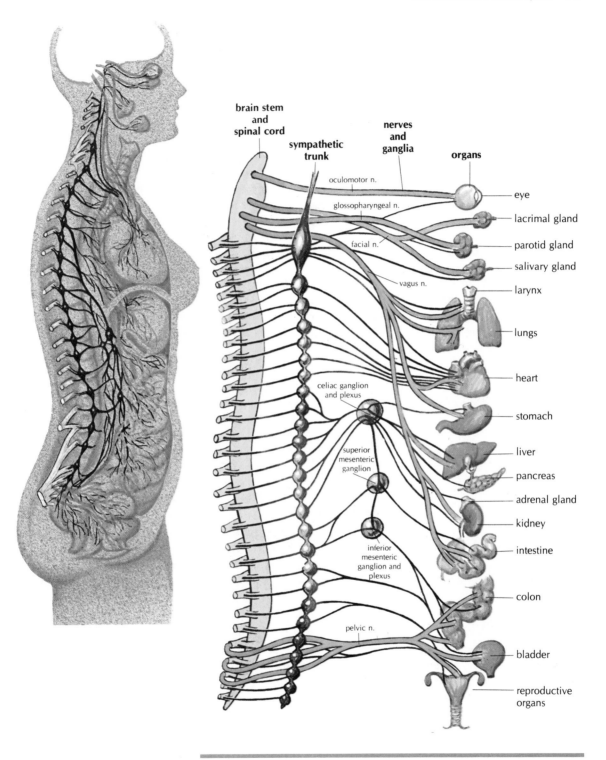

Fig. 11-12   Topography of the autonomic nervous system.

first neuron to a second one which then carries the impulse to the muscle or gland cell. In the case of voluntary muscle cells each nerve fiber extends all the way from the spinal cord to the muscle with no intervening relay station. The location of parts of the autonomic nervous system is roughly as follows:

1 The sympathetic pathway begins in the spinal cord with cell bodies of the **thoracolumbar** (tho-rah-ko-lum′bar) area, which serves numerous organs located in the head region through those in the lower extremities. The sympathetic fibers arise from the spinal cord level of the first thoracic nerve down to the level of the second lumbar spinal nerve. From this part of the cord, nerve fibers extend to the ganglia of one of the sympathetic trunks. These trunks are two cordlike strands that extend up and down on either side of the spinal column from the lower neck to the upper abdominal region. The beadlike enlargements of this trunk are called the **lateral ganglia**. These ganglia contain the cell bodies of the second set of neurons whose fibers then extend to the glands and involuntary muscle tissues.

2 The parasympathetic pathway begins in the **craniosacral** areas; this means that fibers arise from cell bodies of the midbrain, medulla and lower (sacral) part of the spinal cord. From these centers the first set of fibers extends to autonomic ganglia that are usually located near or within the walls of the organs. The pathway then continues along a second set of neurons that stimulate the visceral tissues.

Functions of the Autonomic Nervous System

The autonomic nervous system regulates the action of the glands, the smooth muscles of hollow organs, and the heart. These actions are all carried on automatically; and whenever any changes occur which call for a regulatory adjustment, this is done without our being conscious of it. The sympathetic part of the autonomic nervous system tends to act largely as an accelerator, particularly under conditions of stress. If you will think of what happens to a person who is frightened or angry, you can easily remember the effects of impulses from the sympathetic nervous system.

1 Stimulation of the adrenal gland produces hormones, including *epinephrine* (ep-e-nef′rin), that prepare the body to meet emergency situations in many ways (see Chap. 20). The sympathetic nerves and hormones from the adrenal reinforce each other.

2 Dilation of the pupil and decrease in focusing ability (for near objects).

3 Increase in the rate and forcefulness of heart contractions.

4 Increase in blood pressure due partly to the more effective heartbeat and partly to constriction of small arteries in the skin and the internal organs.

5 Dilation of the bronchial tubes in order to allow for more oxygen to enter.

6 Inhibition of peristalsis and of secretory activity so that digestion is slowed.

If you have tried to eat while you were angry, you may have noted that the saliva was thicker and so small in amount that the food was swallowed with difficulty. Then when the food does reach the stomach, it seems to remain there longer than usual.

Once the crisis has passed, the parasympathetic part of the autonomic nervous system normally acts as a balance for the sympathetic system. The parasympathetic system brings about constriction of the pupil, slowing of the heart rate, and constriction of the bronchial tubes; and stimulation of peristaltic and secretory activities. The saliva, for example, flows more easily and profusely as its quantity and fluidity increases.

Disorders of the Autonomic Nervous System

Injuries due to wounds by penetrating objects, or due to tumors, hemorrhage, or spinal column dislocations or fractures, may cause damage to the sympathetic trunk. In addition to these rather obvious kinds of disorders, there are a great number of conditions in which symptoms such as heart palpitations, increased blood pressure, and stomach aches suggest autonomic malfunction but in which the method of operation is not so well understood. These disorders are related to the part that psychological problems play in the functioning of the viscera, owing to the close interrelationships between the brain, brain stem, and spinal cord and the autonomic nervous system.

Summary

1 Nervous system as a whole.
  A Function—coordinating system of the body.
  B Divisons.
    (1) Central nervous system—brain, spinal cord.
    (2) Peripheral nervous system—cranial and spinal nerves.
    (3) Autonomic nervous system (functional classification of a certain group of peripheral nerves).
2 Nerves—bundles of nerve fibers, carrying impulses. Nerve tissue is made of nerve cells (neurons) whose components are cell body, nerve fibers (axons, dendrites). Afferent nerves to central nervous system; efferent nerves from central nervous system.
3 Brain.
  A Main parts—cerebrum (2 hemispheres), midbrain, pons, medulla, cerebellum.
  B Fissures (sulci)—longitudinal fissure, central fissure, lateral fissure.
  C Cerebral cortex—highest functions of brain performed here.
    (1) Frontal lobe (motor cortex).
    (2) Parietal lobe (sensory area).
    (3) Temporal lobe (auditory center).
    (4) Occipital lobe (visual area).
  D Communication areas—auditory, visual, motor, written.
  E Interbrain (thalamus and hypothalamus) and midbrain.
  F Midbrain.
  G Pons—links parts of brain; some reflex action.
  H Medulla—contains respiratory, cardiac, vasomotor centers.
  I Cerebellum—aids in muscle coordination, balance, muscle tone.
  J Ventricles of the brain.
  K Brain studies.
  L Brain disorders—encephalitis, abscess, stroke, cerebral palsy, epilepsy, tumors, aphasia.
4 Spinal cord.
  A Structure—H-shaped gray matter, surrounded by white matter; all inside spinal canal.
  B Function—reflexes, conducts sensory impulses to brain, conducts motor impulses from brain to organs. Reflex pathway—nerve cells are sensory (outside cord in ganglia), central, motor.
  C Disorders—poliomyelitis, injuries (paraplegia).
5 Coverings of brain and spinal cord.
  A Meninges—dura mater, arachnoid, pia mater.
  B Disorders—cerebrospinal meningitis.
6 Cerebrospinal fluid.
  A Cushions shocks.
  B Accumulation in brain—hydrocephalus.
7 Cranial nerves.
  A General functions—special sense impulses, general sense impulses, voluntary muscle control, involuntary control.
  B Names—olfactory, optic, oculomotor, trochlear, trigeminal, abducens, facial, vestibulocochlear, glossopharyngeal, vagus, accessory, hypoglossal.
  C Disorders—infections, Bell's palsy, injury, neuraglia.
8 Spinal nerves.
  A Attached to spinal cord by dorsal and ventral roots. Dorsal roots conduct sensory impulses, ventral roots supply muscles and glands.
  B Branches (plexuses)—cervical, brachial, lumbosacral.
  C Disorders—neuritis, sciatica, shingles.
9 Autonomic nervous system.
  A Regulates action of glands, smooth muscles, heart.
  B Divisions.
    (1) Sympathetic nervous system—origin in thoracolumbar area. Accelerates some body processes.
    (2) Parasympathetic nervous system—some originate in cranial, others in spinal (sacral) region. Balances action of sympathetic system.
  C Disorders—some irregularities complicated by psychological influences.

Questions and Problems

1 What is the main function of the nervous system?
2 Name the 3 divisions of the nervous system.
3 Describe a neuron and name its parts.
4 What is a transmitter substance?
5 Name and locate the main parts of the brain and briefly describe the main functions of each.
6 Name 4 divisions of the cerebral cortex and state what each does.
7 Name and describe the speech centers.
8 Describe the thalamus; where is it located? What are its functions?
9 What activities does the hypothalamus regulate?
10 Name and describe 6 typical brain disorders.
11 Locate and describe the spinal cord. Name 3 of its functions.
12 Describe a typical reflex action.

13 Name and describe 2 spinal cord disorders.
14 Name the covering of the brain and the spinal cord and its divisions. What is an infection of this covering called?
15 What is the purpose of the cerebrospinal fluid? Describe hydrocephalus.
16 Name 4 general functions of the cranial nerves.
17 Name and describe the functions of the 12 cranial nerves.
18 Locate the spinal nerves and name 3 main branches of each of them.
19 Name 2 disorders of the spinal nerves.
20 Describe the function of the autonomic nervous system.
21 Name the 2 parts of the autonomic nervous system, and show how they work during and following a moment of extreme fear.

Chapter 12

The Sensory System

Glossary

Accommodation A change in the shape of the eye lens so that vision is more acute; an adjustment of the eye lens for various distances; the focusing process.

Adaptation Adjustment of an organism to its environment.

Anorexia Extreme loss of appetite.

Choroid Pertaining to the thin, dark brown, vascular middle coat of the eyeball; also relating to the capillary fringelike parts of the pia mater that extend into the brain ventricles and produce cerebrospinal fluid.

Conjunctiva The thin delicate membrane that lines the eyelids and is reflected over the front of the eyeball.

Cornea The transparent front part of the eyeball; the forward continuation of the outer coat (sclera).

Lens Transparent part of the eye located between the posterior chamber and the vitreous humor, part of the refracting mechanism of the eye.

Presbyopia A visual change due to advancing age; loss of elasticity of the lens in the eye.

Proprioceptor A receptor that gives information about movements and position of the body.

Sclera The tough opaque white coat that forms the outer protective layer of the eyeball. It is continuous with the transparent, colorless cornea at the front.

Senses and Sensory Mechanisms

The word "sense" might be defined as "the interpretation, by the specialized areas of the cerebral cortex, of an impulse arising from the receptors which are designed to report changes taking place either within the body or outside of it." Sensory receptors are specialized tissues on the endings of the dendrites of afferent neurons. Some receptors are designed to respond only to special stimuli (sound waves, light rays) while others respond to such general sensations as pain or pressure.

There is no completely satisfactory classification of the senses. A partial list includes the following:

1 **Visual** sense from receptors in the eye.
2 **Hearing** sense from receptors in the ear.

3 **Taste** sense from the tongue receptors.
4 **Smell** sense from receptors in the upper nasal cavities.
5 **Pressure, heat, cold, pain,** and **touch** senses from the skin.
6 **Position** and **balance** sense from the muscles, the joints, and the semicircular canals in the ear.
7 **Hunger** and **thirst** senses from various internal parts of the body.

The Eye
Protection of the Eyeball and Its Parts

In the embryo, the eye develops as an outpocketing of the brain. The eye is a delicate organ, and nature has carefully protected it by means of the following structures:

1 The skull bones form the eye orbit (cavity) and serve to protect more than half of the dorsal part of the eyeball.
2 The lids and the eyelashes aid in protecting the eye anteriorly.
3 The tears wash away small foreign objects that may enter the eye.
4 A sac lined with an epithelial membrane separates the front of the eye from the eyeball proper and aids in the destruction of some of the pathogenic bacteria that may enter from the outside.

Coats of the Eyeball

The eyeball has three separate coats or tunics (Fig. 12-1). The outermost layer is called the *sclera* (skle'rah) and is made of firm tough connective tissue. It is commonly referred to as the white of the eye. The second tunic of the eyeball is the *choroid* (ko'roid) coat. Composed of a delicate network of connective tissue interlaced with many blood vessels, this layer contains much dark brown pigment. The choroid may be compared to the dull black lining of a camera. It prevents incoming light rays from scattering and reflecting off the inner surface of the eye. The innermost coat, called the retina (ret'i-nah), includes ten layers of nerve cells, including the end organs commonly called the rods and cones (Fig. 12-2). These are the re-ceptors for the sense of vision. The rods are sensitive to white and black. The cones are sensitive to color. As far as is known, there are three types of cones, each of which is sensitive to red, green, or blue. Persons who completely lack cones are totally color blind; those who lack one type of cone are partially color blind. Color blindness is an inherited condition and occurs almost exclusively in males.

Pathway of Light Rays

Light rays pass through a series of transparent, colorless eye parts. On the way they undergo a process of bending known as *refraction.* This refracting of the light rays makes it possible for light from a very large area to be focused upon a very small surface, the retina, where the receptors are located. The following are, in order from outside in, the transparent refracting parts, or *media,* of the eye:

1 The **cornea** (kor'ne-ah) is a forward continuation of the outer coat, but it is transparent and colorless, whereas the sclera is opaque and white.
2 The **aqueous humor,** a watery fluid which fills much of the eyeball in front of the lens, helps to maintain the slight forward curve in the cornea.
3 The **crystalline lens** is a circular structure made of a jelly-like material.
4 The **vitreous body** is a jelly-like substance that fills the entire space behind the lens and keeps the eyeball in its spherical shape.

The cornea is referred to frequently as the "window" of the eye. It bulges forward slightly and is the most important refracting structure. Injuries caused by foreign objects or by infection may result in scar formation in the cornea, leaving an area of opacity through which light rays cannot pass. If such an injury involves the central area in front of the pupil (the hole in the center of the colored part of the eye), blindness may be the result. Eye banks store corneas obtained from donors, and corneal transplantation is a fairly common procedure.

The next light-bending medium is the aqueous humor, followed by the crystalline lens. The lens has two bulging surfaces, so it may be best described as biconvex. During youth, the lens is elas-

(*Text continues on p. 156.*)

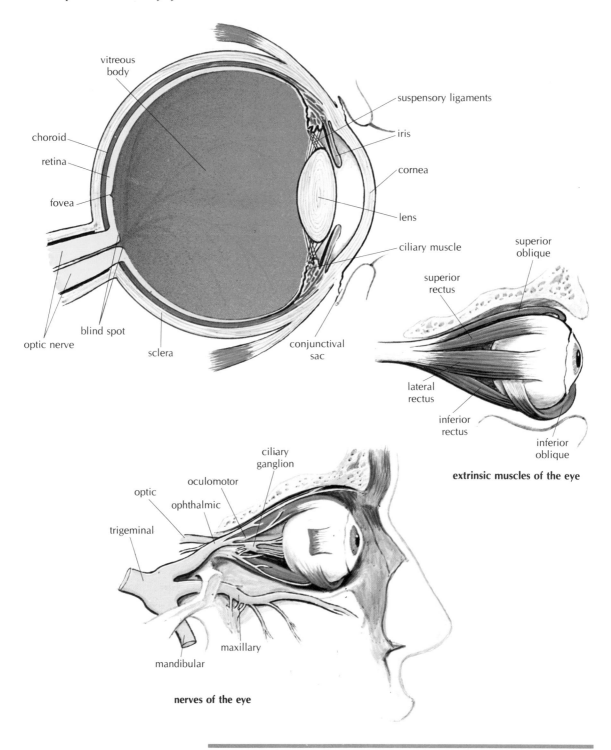

Fig. 12-1   The eye.

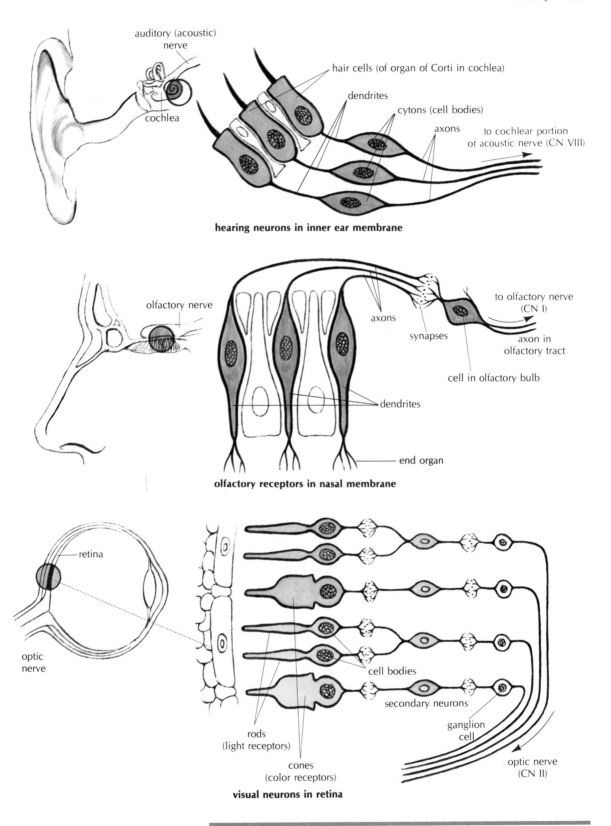

Fig. 12-2 Diagram of neurons for receiving impulses from the special sense organs.

tic, and therefore its thickness can be readily adjusted according to the need for near or distance vision. With aging, the lens loses its elasticity and therefore its ability to adjust by thickening, resulting in what is known as *presbyopia* (pres''be-o'pe-ah).

The last of these transparent refracting parts of the eye is the vitreous body. Like the aqueous humor, it is important in maintaining the ball-like shape of the eyeball as well as aiding in refraction. The vitreous body is not replaceable; an injury that causes loss of an appreciable amount of the jelly-like vitreous material will cause collapse of the eyeball. This will require the removal of the eyeball, an operation called *enucleation* (e-nu-kle-a'shun).

Muscles of the Eye

The muscles inside the eyeball itself are *intrinsic* (in-trin'sik) muscles, while others, attached to bones of the eye orbit as well as to the sclera, are *extrinsic* (eks-trin'sik) muscles.

The intrinsic muscles are found in two circular structures as follows:

1 The **iris** is the colored or pigmented part of the eye and is composed of two types of muscles. The iris has a central opening called the pupil. The size of the pupil is governed by the action of these two sets of muscles, one of which is arranged in a circular fashion, while the other extends in a radial manner resembling the spokes of a wheel.
2 The **ciliary body** is shaped somewhat like a flattened ring with a hole that is the size of the outer edge of the iris. This muscle alters the shape of the lens during the process of accommodation.

The purpose of the iris is to regulate the amount of light entering the eye. If a strong light is flashed in the eye, the circular muscle fibers of the iris, which form a sphincter, contract and thus reduce the size of the pupil. On the other hand, if the light is very dim, the radial involuntary iris muscles, which are attached at the outer edge, contract; the opening is pulled outward and thus enlarged. This pupillary enlargement is known as *dilation* (di-la'shun).

The pupil changes size, too, according to

whether one is looking at a near object or a distant one. Viewing a near object causes the pupil to become smaller; a far view will cause it to enlarge.

The muscle of the ciliary body is similar in direction and method of action to the radial muscle of the iris. When the ciliary muscle contracts, it removes the tension on the suspensory ligament of the lens. The elastic lens then recoils and becomes thicker in much the same way that a rubber band would thicken if a pull on it were released. When the ciliary body relaxes, the lens becomes flattened. These actions change the refractive ability of the lens.

The process of *accommodation* involves coordinated eye changes to enable one to focus on near objects. The ciliary body contracts, thereby thickening the lens, and the circular muscle fibers of the iris contract to decrease the size of the pupillary opening.

The six extrinsic muscles connected with each eye are ribbon-like and extend forward from the apex of the orbit behind the eyeball (see Fig. 12-1). One end of each muscle is attached to a bone of the skull, while the other end is attached to the sclera. These muscles pull on the eyeball in a coordinated fashion that causes the two eyes to move together in order to center on one visual field. There is another muscle located within the orbit which is attached to the upper eyelid. When this muscle contracts, it keeps the eye open.

Nerve Supply to the Eye

Two sensory nerves supply the eye (see Fig. 12-1):

1 The **optic nerve** (cranial nerve II) carries visual impulses initiated by the rods and cones in the retina to the brain.
2 The **ophthalmic** (of-thal'mic) **branch** of the trigeminal (tri-jem'i-nal) **nerve** (cranial nerve V) carries impulses of pain, touch, and temperature from the eye and surrounding parts.

The optic nerve arises from the retina a little toward the medial or nasal side of the eye. Visual impulses are transmitted from the retina, ultimately to the occipital lobe of the cortex. There are no rods and cones in the retina near the area of the optic nerve fibers; and so this part, which is a circular white area, is the blind spot, known as the *optic disk.* There is a tiny depressed area in the retina called the *fovea centralis* (fo've-ah sen-tra'lis), which is the point of most acute vision.

There are three nerves that carry *motor fibers* to the muscles of the eyeball. The largest is the oculomotor nerve (cranial nerve III) which supplies motor fibers, voluntary and involuntary, to all the muscles but two. The other two nerves, the *trochlear* (cranial nerve IV) and the abducens (cranial nerve VI) supply one voluntary muscle each.

The Conjunctival Sac and the Lacrimal Apparatus

The *conjunctiva* (kon-junk-ti'vah) is a sac that lines the eyelid and covers the anterior part of the sclera in order to protect the eyeball from drying. Tears, produced by the *lacrimal* (lak'ri-mal) *gland* serve to keep the conjunctival sac moist. Also, as tears flow from the lacrimal gland, located in the upper part of the orbit, across the eye, the fluid carries away small particles that have entered the conjunctival sac. The tears are then carried into ducts near the nasal corner of the eye, and drain into the nose by way of the *nasolacrimal* (na''zo-lak'ri-mal) *duct* (Fig. 12-3). Any excess of tears causes a "runny nose"; and a greater overproduction of them results in tears spilling over onto the cheeks.

Eye Infections

Inflammation of the membrane that lines the eyelids and covers the front of the eyeball is called *conjunctivitis* (kon-junk''te-vi'tis). It may be acute or chronic, and may be caused by a variety of irritants and pathogens. "Pinkeye" is an acute conjunctivitis that is highly contagious and is caused by cocci or bacilli in most cases. Sometimes irritants such as wind and excessive glare may cause an inflammation that then may cause a susceptibility to bacterial infection. In the case of the contagious epidemic form, children should be kept home until the infection has subsided.

Trachoma (trah-ko'mah), sometimes referred to as *granular conjunctivitis,* is caused by the *Chlamydia trachomatis* (klah-mid'e-ah trah-ko'mah-tes) bacterium. This disease was formerly quite common in the mountains of the southern United States, and among native Americans. It is still prevalent in the Far East, in Egypt, and in southern Europe. Trachoma is characterized by the formation of granules on the lids, which may cause such serious irritation of the cornea that blindness can result. Better hygiene and the use of antibiotic drugs have reduced the prevalence and seriousness of this infection.

If a woman has a gonococcal infection, an eye infection of her newborn infant may result; this infection is called *ophthalmia neonatorum* (of-

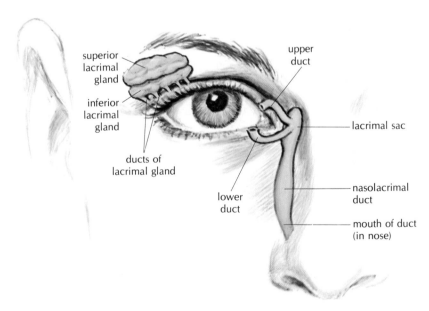

Fig. 12-3 Lacrimal apparatus.

thal'me-ah ne-o-na-to'rum). The bacterium enters the conjunctival sac of the fetus as it proceeds through the birth canal during the process of delivery. Prevention in those babies at risk for the development of ophthalmia neonatorum is achieved by the instillation of an appropriate antiseptic solution, such as silver nitrate, to the conjunctiva just after birth.

The iris, the choroid coat, the ciliary body, and other parts of the eyeball may become infected by various organisms. Such disorders are likely to be very serious; fortunately, they are not very common. Syphilis spirochetes, tubercle bacilli, and a variety of cocci may cause these painful infections. They may follow sinus infections, tonsillitis, conjunctivitis and other disorders in which the infecting agent can spread from nearby structures. The care of these conditions usually should be in the hands of an *ophthalmologist* (of''thal-mol'o-jist), a physician who specializes in the diagnosis and treatment of disorders of the eye.

Eyestrain and Eye Defects

Eyestrain, or fatigue of the eye, may result from overuse; improper conditions for reading, such as poor lighting or very small print; or from disturbances in the focusing ability of the eye.

Some of the symptoms of eyestrain include the following:

1 Inflammation and infection of structures in the eyelids, as, for example, sty formation, in which oil glands on the lid edges become infected.
2 Excessive tear formation and pain in the eyes.
3 Pain in the orbit and forehead.
4 Digestive disturbances and loss of appetite.

Eyestrain is so common that people need to give more attention to proper eye care. Some points to remember are

1 Smaller children should begin reading books in which the type is larger than is customary and the letters are spaced relatively far apart to make them easier to differentiate.
2 Be certain that there is enough light without glare.
3 The table or desk on which the work is being done should be of proper height.
4 Proper examination of the eyes and the use

of adequate lenses are very important. The notion that glasses will weaken the eyes has absolutely no basis in fact.

Several disorders of the eye can lead to eyestrain. *Hyperopia* (hi''per-o'pe-ah), or farsightedness, is due to the eyeball being too short (Fig. 12-4). In this situation, the focal point is behind the retina because light rays cannot bend sharply enough to focus on the retina. This is normal in the infant but usually corrects itself by the time the child uses his eyes more for near vision. To a certain extent, the ciliary muscle will thicken the lens and enable the person to focus objects on the too-near retina. However, this effort causes eyestrain and its symptoms of pain in the eye and forehead. Visual tests may not show that the condition exists unless drops that temporarily paralyze the ciliary muscle are instilled before the examination. Glasses that aid in refracting light rays—convex lenses—will alleviate the symptoms of eyestrain by decreasing the amount of work that the ciliary muscle must do.

Myopia (mi-o'pe-ah), or nearsightedness, is another defect of the eye and is also related to development. In this case the eyeball may be too long, or the bending of the light rays may be too sharp, so that the focal point is in front of the retina (see Fig. 12-4). Objects that are a distance away appear blurred, and may appear clear only if brought very near the eye. Only by wearing concave lenses that alter the angle of refraction so that the focal point is moved backward will myopia be corrected. In a young person, nearsightedness becomes worse each year until the person reaches his twenties. By wearing appropriate eyeglasses the person can avoid development of eyestrain.

Another rather common visual defect is *astigmatism* (ah-stig'mah-tism). This condition is due to irregularity in the curvature of the cornea or the lens (see Fig. 12-4). As a result the light rays are incorrectly bent, causing blurred vision and severe eyestrain. Astigmatism is often found in combination with hyperopia or myopia, so a careful eye examination and properly fitted glasses will reduce or prevent eyestrain.

Strabismus (strah-biz'mus) means that the muscles of the eyeballs do not coordinate, so that the two eyes do not work together (see Fig. 12-4). There are several types of strabismus. One common type is *convergent* strabismus, in which the eye

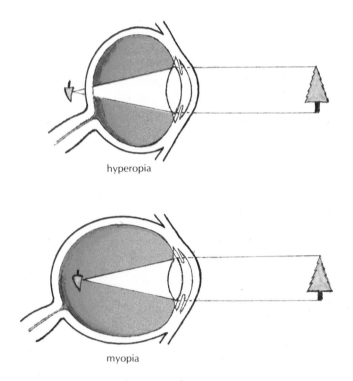

hyperopia

myopia

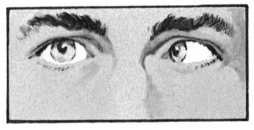

convergent strabismus

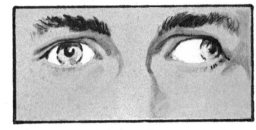

divergent strabismus

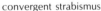

Fig. 12-4 *Disorders of the eye.*

deviates toward the nasal side, or medially. This disorder gives an appearance of cross-eyedness. A second type of strabismus is *divergent* strabismus in which the affected eye deviates laterally. If correction of these disorders is not accomplished early, the transmission and interpretation of visual impulses from the affected eye to the brain will be decreased. The brain will not develop ways to "see" images from the eye. Care by an ophthalmologist as soon as the condition is detected may result in restoration of muscle balance. In some cases, glasses and exercises will correct the defect, while, in others, surgery may be required.

Blindness and Its Causes

The most frequent cause of blindness is *cataract* formation. A cataract is an opacity of the lens or its capsule. Sometimes the areas of opacity can be seen through a pupil that becomes greatly enlarged because of the reduction in the amount of light that can reach the retina. In other cases, there is very gradual loss of vision, and frequent changes in glasses may aid in maintaining useful vision for some time. Removal of the lens may restore some vision, but the addition of eyeglasses or a contact lens usually is required to achieve satisfactory visual acuity, as well as binocular vision which is needed for driving a car, for example. Most affected persons will need reading glasses for close work. Surgical techniques are now available to implant an artificial lens, and this procedure has been successful in restoring normal vision.

A second very important cause of blindness is *glaucoma,* a condition characterized by excess pressure of the aqueous humor. This fluid is being produced constantly from the blood; and after circulation it is reabsorbed into the bloodstream. Interference with the normal reentry of this fluid to the bloodstream leads to an increase in pressure inside the eyeball. As in the case of cataract, glaucoma usually progresses rather slowly, with vague visual disturbances and gradual impairment of vision. Halos around lights, headaches, and the need for frequent changes of glasses (particularly by people over 40) are symptoms that should be investigated by an ophthalmologist. There are different forms of glaucoma, some occurring in the very young; and each type requires a different management. Since continued high pressure of the aqueous humor may cause destruction of the optic nerve fibers, it is important to obtain continuous treatment, beginning early in the disease, to avoid blindness.

Diabetes as a cause of blindness is increasing in the United States. Disorders of the eye directly related to diabetes include optic atrophy in which the optic nerve fibers die, cataracts, which occur earlier and with greater frequency among diabetics, and diabetic *retinopathy* (ret''i-nop'ah-the), in which the retina can be damaged by blood vessel hemorrhages and other causes. Diabetics also are extremely susceptible to *atherosclerosis* (ath-er-o-skle-ro'sis), fatty deposits in the arteries (see Chap. 15).

Another cause of blindness is retinal detachment. This may be a slowly developing disorder or may occur suddenly. In this condition, the retina becomes detached from the underlying layer as a result of trauma or an accumulation of fluid or tissue between the layers. If left untreated, complete detachment can occur, resulting in blindness. Surgical treatment includes a sort of "spot welding" with an electric current or a weak laser beam. A series of pinpoint scars (connective tissue) develop to reattach the retina.

There are many other causes of blindness, and frequently these could have been prevented. Injuries by pieces of glass and other sharp objects are an important cause of eye damage. Industrial accidents involving the eye have been greatly reduced by the use of protective goggles. If an injury should occur, it is then very important to prevent infection. Even a tiny scratch can become so seriously infected that blindness will result.

The Ear

The ear is a sense organ, related to both hearing and equilibrium (Fig. 12-5). It may be divided into three main sections:

1 The **external ear** includes the outer projection and a canal.
2 The **middle ear** is an air space containing three small bones.
3 The **internal ear** is the most important part, since it contains the sensory end organs or receptors for hearing and equilibrium.

The External Ear

The projecting part of the ear is known as the *pinna* (pin'nah), or the *auricle* (aw're-kl). From a functional point of view it is probably of little importance in the human. Then follows the opening itself, the *external auditory canal,* which extends medially for about 1 inch or more, depending upon which wall of the canal is measured. The skin lining this tube is very thin, and in the first part of the canal contains many *ceruminous* (ce-roo'me-nus) glands. The *cerumen* (se-roo'men), or wax, may become dried and impacted in the canal and must be removed. The same kinds of disorders that involve the skin elsewhere also may affect the skin of the external auditory canal: eczema, boils, and other infections.

At the end of the auditory canal is the *tympanic* (tim-pan'ik) *membrane,* or eardrum. It serves as a boundary between the external auditory canal, or *meatus* (me-a'tus), and the middle ear cavity. It may be injured by bobby pins or toothpicks inserted into the ear. Normally the air pressure on the two sides of the tympanic membrane is equalized by means of the *eustachian* (u-sta'ke-an) *tube* connecting the middle ear cavity and the throat, or pharynx (far-inks), allowing the eardrum to vibrate freely with the incoming sound waves.

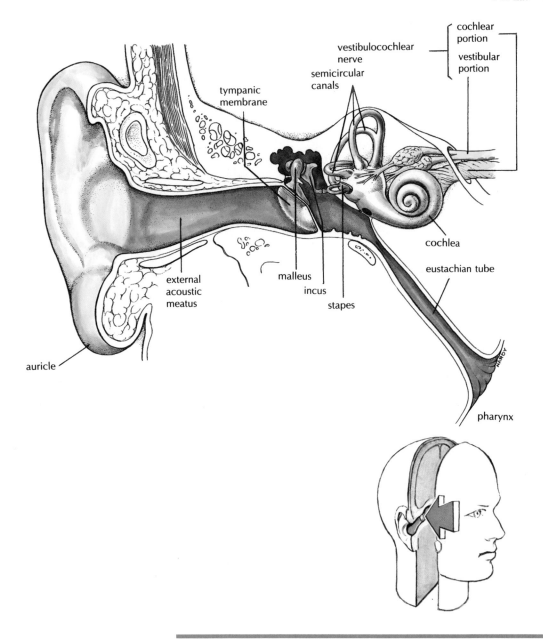

Fig. 12-5 *The ear, showing the external, middle, and internal subdivisions. (Chaffee EE, Lytle IM: Basic Physiology and Anatomy, 4th ed. Philadelphia, JB Lippincott, 1980)*

The Middle Ear

The middle ear cavity is a small, flattened space that contains air and three small bones, or *ossicles* (os′e-kles). Air enters the cavity from the pharynx through the eustachian, or auditory, tube. The mucous membrane of the pharynx is continuous through the eustachian tube into the middle ear cavity, and infection may travel along the membrane, causing middle ear disease. At the back of the middle ear cavity is an opening into the mastoid air cells, which are spaces inside the mastoid process of the temporal bone.

The three ossicles are joined in such a way that they amplify the sound waves received by the tympanic membrane (eardrum) and then transmit the sounds to the fluid in the internal ear. The handle-like part of the first bone, or *malleus* (mal'e-us), is attached to the tympanic membrane, while the headlike portion connects with the second bone, which is called the *incus* (ing'kus). The innermost of the ossicles is shaped somewhat like a stirrup and is called the *stapes* (sta'pez). It is connected with the membrane of the *oval window* which, in turn, vibrates and transmits these waves to the fluid of the internal ear.

The Internal Ear

The most complicated and important part of the ear is the internal portion, consisting of three separate spaces hollowed out inside the temporal bone. This part of the ear is called the *bony labyrinth* (lab'i-rinth), and it consists of three divisions. One is the vestibule, next to the oval window. The second and third divisions of the bony labyrinth are the *cochlea* (kok'le-ah) and the *semicircular canals.* All three divisions contain a fluid called perilymph (per'i-limf). The cochlea is a bony tube shaped like a snail shell toward the front, and the semicircular canals are bony processes toward the back. In the fluid of the bony semicircular canals are the *membranous* (mem'brah-nus) *canals,* which contain another fluid called *endolymph* (en'do-limf) (Fig. 12-6). In a similar fashion, a *membranous cochlea* is situated in the perilymph of the bony cochlea, and it also is filled with endolymph. The organ of hearing consists of receptors connected with nerve fibers in the *cochlear nerve* (a part of the acoustic nerve); it is located inside the membranous cochlea, or *cochlear duct.* The sound waves enter the external auditory canal and cause the tympanic membrane to vibrate. These vibrations are amplified by the ossicles and transmitted by them to the perilymph. They then are conducted by the perilymph through the membrane to the endolymph.

The waves of the endolymph stimulate the tiny hairlike receptors which then initiate nerve impulses that are conducted to the brain.

Other sensory receptors in the internal ear include those related to equilibrium, which are in the semicircular canals. The membranous canals are connected with two small sacs in the vestibule, and one of these sacs contains sensory end organs for obtaining information with relation to the position of the head. Nerve fibers from these sacs and from the canals form the vestibular (ves-tib'u-lar) nerve which joins the cochlear nerve to form the *vestibulocochlear* (acoustic) *nerve,* the latter being the eighth cranial nerve (see Chap. 11).

Disorders of the Ear

Sudden great changes in the pressure on either side of the typanic membrane may cause excessive stretching and inflammation of the membrane. There may even be perforation of the tympanic membrane to relieve the pressure.

Infection of the middle ear cavity is rather common and is called *otitis media* (o-ti'tis me'de-ah). A variety of bacteria as well as viruses may cause otitis media. It is also a frequent complication of measles, influenza, and other infections, especially those of the pharynx. Transmission of pathogens from the pharynx to the middle ear happens more often in children, partly because the eustachian tube is shorter and more horizontal in the child, while in the adult the tube is longer and tends to slant down toward the pharynx. Antibiotic drugs have reduced complications and have caused a marked reduction in the amount of surgery done to drain middle ear infections. However, in some cases, pressure from pus or exudate in the middle ear can be relieved only by cutting the tympanic membrane, a procedure called a *myringotomy* (mir''in-got'o-me).

Another disorder of the ear is hearing loss, which may be partial or complete. When the loss is complete, the condition is called deafness. The two main types of hearing loss are *conduction* deafness and *nerve* deafness. Conduction deafness is due to interference with the passage of the sound waves from the outside to the inner ear. There may be obstruction of the external canal by wax or a foreign body. Blockage of the eustachian tube prevents the equalization of air pressure on both sides of the tympanic membrane, thereby decreasing the ability of the membrane to vibrate. Another cause of conduction deafness is damage to the tympanic membrane and ossicles resulting from chronic otitis media or from *otosclerosis* (o''to-skle-ro'sis), an hereditary disease that causes bone changes in the stapes that prevent its normal vibration. Surgical removal of the diseased stapes and its replacement with an artificial device will allow

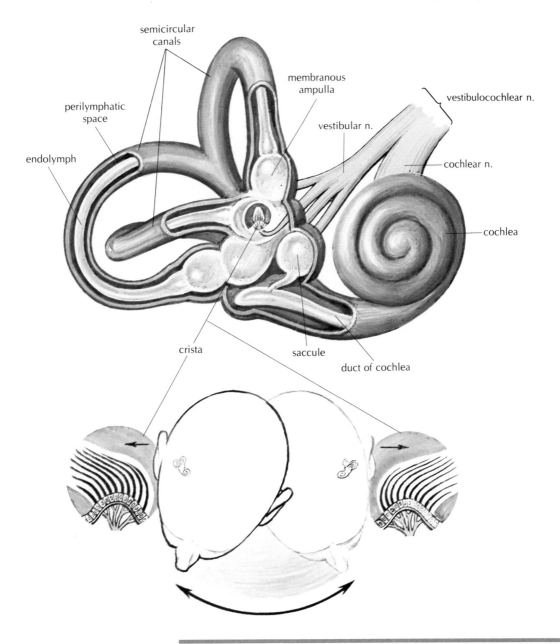

semicircular
canals

membranous
ampulla

vestibulocochlear n.

perilymphatic
space

vestibular n.

endolymph

cochlear n.

cochlea

crista

saccule

duct of cochlea

Fig. 12-6 *The internal ear, including a section showing the crista where the sensory receptors for balance are located.*

conduction of sound from the ossicles to the oval window and the cochlea. *Nerve deafness* is due to disorders of the sensory mechanism affecting the cochlea, the vestibulocochlear nerve or the brain areas concerned with hearing. It may result from prolonged exposure to loud noises, to the use of certain drugs for long periods of time, or to various infections and toxins.

Other Organs of Special Sense

Taste Sense

The sense of taste involves receptors in the tongue and two different nerves that carry taste impulses to the brain. The taste receptors are known as *taste buds* and are located along the edges of small depressed areas called *fissures.* Taste buds are stimulated only if the substance to be tasted is in solution. Tastes have been described as essentially of four kinds:

1 **Sweet** tastes are most acutely experienced at the tip of the tongue.
2 **Sour** tastes are most effectively detected by the taste buds located at the sides of the tongue.
3 **Salty** tastes, as in the case of sweet tastes, are most acute at the tip of the tongue.
4 **Bitter** tastes are detected at the back part of the tongue.

The nerves of taste include the facial and the glossopharyngeal (cranial nerves VII and IX). The interpretation of taste impulses probably is accomplished by the lower front portion of the brain, although there may not be a sharply separate taste or *gustatory* (gus'tah-to-re) center (Fig. 12-7).

Sense of Smell

The sensory end organs, or receptors, for smell are located in the olfactory *epithelium* of the upper part of the nasal cavity. Because they are high in the nasal cavity, an animal or a person "sniffs" in order to bring the gases responsible for an odor upward in the nose. The pathway of the impulses from the receptors for smell is the *olfactory nerve* (cranial nerve I). This leads to the olfactory center in the brain. The interpretation of smell is closely related to the sense of taste. The smell of foods is just as important in stimulating appetite and the flow of digestive juices as is the sense of taste.

Hunger and Appetite

Hunger is the desire for food and can be satisfied with the ingestion of a filling meal. Hunger is regulated by centers in the hypothalamus which can be modified by input from higher brain centers. Therefore, cultural factors and memories of past food intake can influence hunger. Strong, mildly painful contractions of the empty stomach may stimulate a feeling of hunger. Messages received by the hypothalamus reduce hunger as the food is chewed and swallowed, and begins to fill the stomach. The short-term regulation of food intake works to keep the amount of food taken in within

the limits of that which can be processed by the intestine. The long-term regulation of food intake maintains appropriate blood levels of certain nutrients. Appetite differs from hunger in that although it is basically a desire for food, it often has no relationship to the need for food. Hunger may have been relieved by an adequate meal, but the person may still have an appetite for additional food. A loss of appetite is called *anorexia* (an''o-rek'se-ah), and may be due to a great variety of physical and mental disorders. Since the hypothalamus and the higher brain centers are involved in the regulation of hunger, it is likely that emotional and social factors contribute to the development of anorexia.

Sense of Thirst

Depletion of body water and changes in the concentration of body fluids lead to stimulation of the thirst center in the hypothalamus. The individual becomes aware of a desire for water. Dryness of the mouth also causes a sensation of thirst. When excessive thirst is due to excessive urine loss, as in diabetes, the condition is called *polydipsia* (pol-e-dip'se-ah).

General Senses

As opposed to the *special* senses, in which the receptors are limited to a relatively small area in the body, the *general* sensory receptors are scattered throughout the body. These include pressure, heat, cold, pain, touch, position, and balance senses, all of which are rather widely distributed (Fig. 12-8).

Pressure Sense

It has been found that even though the skin is anesthetized, there still is consciousness of pressure. These end organs for deep sensibility are located in the subcutaneous and deeper tissues. They are sometimes referred to as receptors for deep touch.

Temperature Sense

Heat and cold receptors have separate nerve fiber connections. Each has its type of end organ structure peculiar to it, and the distribution of each

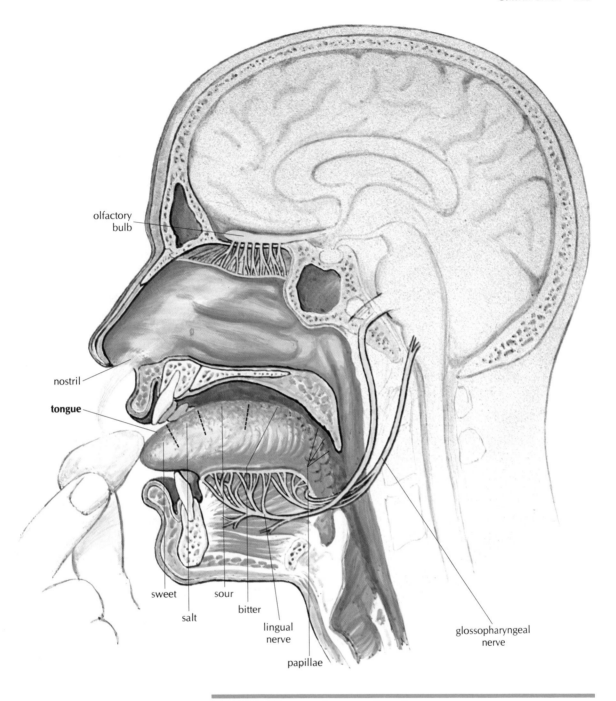

Fig. 12-7 Organs of taste and smell.

varies considerably. A warm object will stimulate only the heat receptors, while a cool object affects only the cold terminals. As in the case of other sensory receptors, continued stimulation results in *adaptation;* that is, the receptors adjust themselves in such a way that one does not feel a sensation so acutely if the original stimulus is continued. For example, the initial immersion of a hand in hot water may give rise to an uncomfortable sensation; however, if the immersion is prolonged, the water

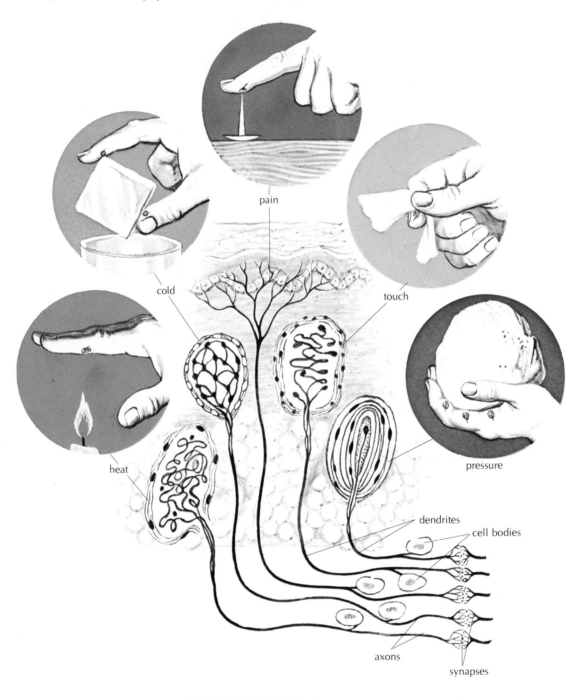

Fig. 12-8 Diagram showing the superficial receptors and the deeper cell bodies and synapses to suggest the continuity of sensory pathways into the central nervous system.

very soon will not feel as hot as it did at first (even if it has not cooled appreciably).

Sense of Touch

The touch receptors are small rounded bodies called *tactile* (tak'til) *corpuscles.* They are found mostly in the dermis and are especially numerous and close together in the tips of the fingers and the toes. The tip of the tongue also contains many of these receptors and so is very sensitive to touch, whereas the back of the neck is relatively insensitive.

Pain Sense

Pain is the most important protective sense. The receptors for pain are the most widely distributed sensory end organs. They are found in the skin, the muscles, and the joints, and to a lesser extent in most internal organs (including the blood vessels and viscera). Pain receptors are not oval bodies as are many of the other sensory end organs, but apparently are merely branchings of the nerve fiber, called *free nerve endings. Referred pain* is a term used in cases in which pain that seems to be in an outer part of the body, particularly the skin, actually originates in an internal organ located near that particular area of skin. These areas of referred pain have been mapped out on the basis of much experience and many experiments. It has been found, for example, that liver and gallbladder disease often cause referred pain in the skin over the right shoulder. Spasm of the coronary arteries that supply the heart may cause pain in the left shoulder and the left arm. One reason for this is that some neurons have the twofold duty of conducting impulses both from visceral pain receptors and from pain receptors in neighboring areas of the skin. The brain cannot differentiate between these two possible sources; but since most pain sensations originate in the skin, the brain automatically assigns the pain to this more likely place of origin.

Pain sense differs from other senses in that continued stimulation does not result in adaptation. This is nature's way of being certain that the warnings of the pain sense are heeded. Sometimes the cause cannot be remedied quickly, and occasionally not at all. Then it is necessary to relieve pain. Some pain relief methods that have been found to be effective include the following:

1. **Application of cold,** especially crushed ice in ice caps, for headaches; or in bags for localized areas of injury or inflammation; or cold compresses made by wringing out a towel (or gauze for small compresses) in cold water.
2. **Pressure,** applied to the site of pain or to certain other locations in the body can provide pain relief.
3. **Analgesic** (an-al-je'zik) **drugs,** which are mild pain relievers. Examples are *acetaminophen* (as'et-am'i-no-fen) and aspirin.
4. **Narcotic** drugs, which produce stupor and sleep. These are often very effective pain relievers. An example of a narcotic drug is morphine.
5. **Anesthetics,** which may be either local (*i.e.,* that render only a certain area insensitive) or general, producing total unconsciousness. These are used largely to prevent pain during surgery.
6. **Endorphins** (en-dor'fins) and **enkephalins** (enkef'ah-lins) are substances that are associated with the control of pain. The endorphins and enkephalins are under intensive study, and several theories have been proposed about the circumstances that can cause them to be released from the hypothalamus and the pituitary.

Sense of Position

Receptors located in muscles, tendons and joints relay impulses that aid in judging the position and changes in the locations of parts with respect to each other. They also inform the brain of the amount of muscle contraction and tendon tension. These rather widely spread end organs, which are known as *proprioceptors* (pro-pre-o-sep'tors), are aided in this function by the semicircular canals and related internal ear structures. Information received by these receptors is needed for coordination of muscles and is important in such activities as walking, running, and many more complicated skills such as playing a musical instrument. These muscle sense end organs also play an important part in maintaining muscle tone and good posture, as well as allowing for the adjustment of the muscles for the particular kind of work to be done. The nerve fibers that carry impulses from these receptors enter the spinal cord and ascend to the brain in the posterior part of the cord.

Summary

1 Senses—sight, hearing, taste, smell, pressure, heat, cold, pain, touch, position, balance, hunger, thirst.
2 Eye.
  A Parts and purposes.
    (1) Protection—orbits, lids, eyelashes, tears, conjunctiva.
    (2) Coats—sclera, choroid, retina.
    (3) Light path—cornea, aqueous humor, lens, vitreous body.
    (4) Muscles—intrinsic (iris, ciliary body); 6 extrinsic.
    (5) Nerves—optic (visual impulses from rods and cones of retina); ophthalmic (pain, touch, temperature impulses from eye and surrounding parts); 3 motor nerves.
    (6) Lacrimal apparatus—lacrimal gland produces tears which moisten conjunctiva.
  B Disorders—infections (conjunctivitis, trachoma, ophthalmia neonatorum); defects (hyperopia, myopia, astigmatism, strabismus). Causes of blindness—cataracts (lens loses transparency); glaucoma (excess pressure of eye fluid); diabetic retinal disease; retinal detachment.
3 Ear.
  A Parts and purposes.
    (1) Divisions—external, middle, internal.
    (2) External—pinna, auditory canal, tympanic membrane.
    (3) Middle—ossicles (malleus, incus, stapes) amplify sounds from tympanic membrane, transmit them to oval window. Eustachian tube connects to pharynx, equalizes pressure, pathway for infection.
    (4) Internal—bony labyrinth. Oval window, vestibule, cochlea, semicircular canals, which contain perilymph. Membranous canals (in semicircular canals), membranous cochlea (in cochlea) both filled with endolymph. Receptors in cochlear duct make up the organ of hearing.
    (5) Path for sound—eardrum vibrates, vibrations amplified by ossicles, transmitted to perilymph, to endolymph, to nerve receptors, to nerves, to brain.
    (6) Equilibrium—membranous canals connected with 2 sacs, 1 sac containing sensory nerves indicating position of head.
  B Disorders—otitis media; hearing loss of 2 types—conduction, obstruction in external canal or eustachian tube, otitis media or otosclerosis; nerve deafness, damage to sensory mechanisms such as cochlea, nerves, brain.
4 Other special sense organs.
  A Taste—receptors (taste buds on tongue). Four tastes (sweet, sour, salty, bitter).
  B Smell—receptors (olfactory epithelium of nasal cavity).
  C Hunger and appetite—hunger regulated by hypothalamus.
  D Thirst—regulated by hypothalamus.
5. General senses.
  A Pressure—end organs in deep tissues.
  B Temperature—heat and cold receptors separate. Adaptation (common to most other senses also).
  C Touch—receptors (tactile corpuscles). Close together in fingers, toes, tongue.
  D Pain—protective, no adaptation. Referred pain (from deeper organs but seemingly originating in nearby skin area. Areas mapped out for diagnostic purposes). Pain relief—application of cold, compression, analgesics, narcotics, anesthetics (local, general).
  E Position—receptors (proprioceptors in muscles, tendons, joints aided by semicircular canals).

Questions and Problems

1 Give a general definition of a sense and name 7 of the senses.

2 Name the main parts of the eye and trace the path of a light ray from the outside of the eye to the brain. Show the action of muscles.

3 Describe 3 eye infections and 4 eye defects. What are the main causes of blindness?

4 Outline the main parts of the ear and describe the process that ensues from the time that a sound wave activates the eardrum to the registration of the sound in the brain.

5 Name and describe 2 ear disorders and list some of the causes of deafness.

6 Name the 4 kinds of taste. Where are the taste receptors?

7 Describe the olfactory apparatus.

8 What is the difference between hunger and appetite?

9 What is the difference between a general and a special sense?

10 What does "adaptation" mean, with respect to the senses? Does this occur in the case of every sense?

11 Explain referred pain and give an example of its occurrence.

12 Name 3 categories of pain relieving drugs.

13 Where are the receptors for the senses of position and balance (equilibrium) located?

Chapter 13

The Blood

13

Glossary

Agglutination A process by which cells (bacteria, blood cells, others) collect in groups or clumps; clumping.

Antibody A specific substance produced in a person as a reaction to the presence of an exciting substance called antigen.

Antigen A substance that causes body cells to produce antibodies.

Coagulation The formation of a clot or mass.

Complement A system of protein enzymes that occurs in normal serum and interacts to combine with the antigen–antibody proteins.

Erythrocyte A red blood cell.

Hemocytometer An instrument used for counting blood cells.

Hemoglobin A protein occurring in the blood that contains iron.

Hemoglobinometer, hemometer An instrument used for measuring the amount of hemoglobin in the blood.

Hemolysis The disintegration of red blood cells which results in the appearance of hemoglobin in the surrounding fluid.

Hemorrhage Excessive bleeding which may be due to internal or external causes.

Leukocyte A white blood cell; any colorless ameboid cell mass.

Phagocytosis The engulfment of bacteria and other foreign particles by white blood cells.

Platelet, thrombocyte A fragment of a cell, essential in blood clotting.

Serum The clear liquid that separates from clotted blood. Whereas plasma contains clotting elements, serum contains none of them.

Transfusion Administration of blood from one person, the donor, into another person, the recipient.

We have noted that blood is sometimes classified as a tissue, since nearly half of it is made up of cells. However, it differs from other connective tissues because its cells are not fixed in position.

Blood is a viscous (thick) fluid that varies in color from bright scarlet to dark red, depending on how much oxygen it is carrying. The quantity of circulating blood differs with the size of the person; the average adult male, weighing 154 pounds, has about 5¼ quarts (5 liters) of blood in his body.

Blood is of fundamental importance in the maintenance of homeostasis.

Purposes of the Blood

The circulating blood serves the body in two ways: transportation and protection.

Transportation

1 The oxygen from the air that is breathed in diffuses into the blood through the thin lung membranes and is carried to all the tissues of the body. Carbon dioxide, a waste product of cell metabolism, is carried from the tissues to the lungs where it is breathed out.
2 The blood transports food and other needed substances to the cells. These materials may enter the blood from the digestive system or may be released from body stores.
3 The blood transports the waste products from the cells to the sites from which they are released. The kidney removes excess water, minerals, and urea from protein metabolism, and also maintains the acid–base balance of the blood. The liver removes bile pigments and drugs.
4 The blood transports heat that is generated in the muscles to other parts of the body, thus aiding in the regulation of body temperature.
5 The blood carries the secretions called hormones from their site of origin to the organs to be regulated.

Protection

1 The blood carries those substances that are among the body's defenders against pathogens. Other blood constituents are concerned with immunity to disease.
2 The blood also acts to maintain homeostasis (a stable internal environment).

Blood Constituents

The blood is composed of two prime elements:

1 The liquid element is called **plasma.**
2 The **formed elements** are cells and products

of cells (Fig. 13-1) The formed elements are also called **corpuscles** (kor'pus-ls) and are grouped as follows:

A **Erythrocytes** (e-rith'ro-sites) are the red blood cells ("erythro" means red).
B **Leukocytes** (loo'ko-sites) are the white blood cells ("leuko" means white). The spelling *leucocytes* may also be used.
C **Platelets** are cell fragments which initiate blood clotting. They are also called **thrombocytes** (throm'bo-sites).

Blood Plasma

Over one half of the total volume of blood is plasma. The plasma itself is 90% water with many different substances, dissolved or suspended in the water, making up the other 10%. The plasma content varies somewhat, since the blood carries substances to and from organs which use some of them and add others. However, the body tends to maintain a fairly constant level of the various substances. For example, the level of glucose, a simple sugar, is maintained at a remarkably constant level of about one tenth of 1% solution.

After water, the next largest percentage of material of which the plasma is composed is *protein.* Proteins are the principal constituents of protoplasm and are essential to the growth and the rebuilding of body tissues. The proteins include the following:

1 Albumin is the most abundant protein in plasma. It is manufactured in the liver.
2 The amino acids that have been absorbed by the capillaries of the intestinal villi. These are aptly described as the main building blocks of protein.
3 The antibodies that combat infection.
4 The blood clotting factors.
5 A system of enzymes made of several proteins, collectively known as *complement,* that assists antibodies in their fight against pathogens (see Chap. 23).

Nutrients are also found in the plasma. One group of nutrients has been given the collective name of *carbohydrates* (kor''bo-hi'drates). The principal form of carbohydrate found in the plasma is glucose, which is absorbed by the villus capillaries. Glucose is stored mainly in the liver and is released as needed to supply energy.

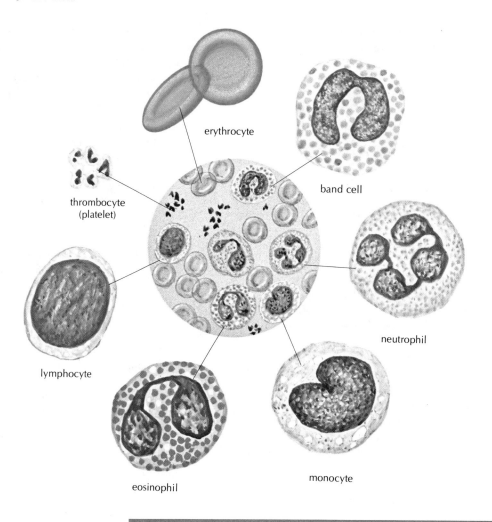

Fig. 13-1 *Blood cells.*

Lipids (lip'ids) constitute a small percentage of blood plasma. Lipids include fats. They may be stored as fat for reserve energy or carried to the cells as a source of energy.

The *mineral salts* in the plasma occur primarily as chloride, carbonate, or phosphate salts of sodium, potassium, calcium, and magnesium. These salts have a variety of functions including the formation of bone (calcium and phosphorus), the production of hormones by certain glands (iodine for the production of thyroid hormone), the transportation of the gases oxygen and carbon dioxide (iron), and the maintenance of acid–base balance (sodium and potassium carbonates and phosphates). Small amounts of other elements also help to maintain homeostasis. There are many other ma-terials such as waste products and hormones that are transported in the plasma.

The Formed Elements

Let us examine in more detail each of the formed elements: the erythrocytes, the leukocytes, and the platelets.

Erythrocytes

Erythrocytes, the red cells, are tiny disk-shaped bodies with a central area that is thinner than the edges. They are different from other cells in that the mature form found in the circulating blood does not have a nucleus. These cells live a much shorter time than most other cells of the body, some of which last a lifetime. One purpose of the red cells is to carry oxygen from the lungs to the tissues. This is accomplished by the *hemoglobin* (he-mo-glo'bin). Hemoglobin is a protein that contains iron. Hemoglobin combines with oxygen, and this gives the blood its characteristic red color. The more oxygen carried by the hemoglobin, the brighter the red color of the blood. Therefore, the blood that goes from the lungs, through the arteries, to the tissues is a brighter red because it carries a greater supply of oxygen. On the other hand, the blood that returns from the tissues, by way of the veins, and back to the lungs is a much darker red, since it has given up much of its oxygen. Hemoglobin that has given up its oxygen is able to carry hydrogen ions; in this way, hemoglobin plays an important role in acid–base balance (see Chap. 5). The red cells also carry a small amount of carbon dioxide from the tissues to the lungs for elimination when one exhales.

Carbon monoxide is a gas that can combine with hemoglobin to form a stable compound. It displaces the oxygen that is normally carried by the hemoglobin and reduces the oxygen-carrying ability of the blood.

Carbon monoxide may be produced by incomplete burning of various fuels such as gasoline, coal, wood, and other carbon-containing materials. It occurs also in automobile exhaust fumes and in cigarette smoke.

The erythrocytes are by far the most numerous of the corpuscles, averaging from 4.5 to 5 million per cubic millimeter of blood.

Leukocytes

The leukocytes, or white blood cells, are very different from the erythrocytes in appearance, quantity and function. They contain nuclei of varying shapes and sizes, and the cells themselves are shaped like balls. Leukocytes are outnumbered by red cells by 700 to 1, numbering but 5,000 to 10,000 per cubic millimeter of blood. Whereas the red cells have a definite color, the leukocytes tend to be colorless. The white cells are of many different kinds, but for the moment it is sufficient for us to know that the most important function of leukocytes is to destroy certain pathogens. At any time that pathogens enter the tissues, as through a wound, the white blood cells are attracted to that area. They leave the blood vessels and proceed by *ameboid* (ah-me'boid) or ameba-like motion to the area of infection. There they engulf the invaders by a process called *phagocytosis* (fag''o-si-to'sis) as shown in Fig. 13-2. If the patho-

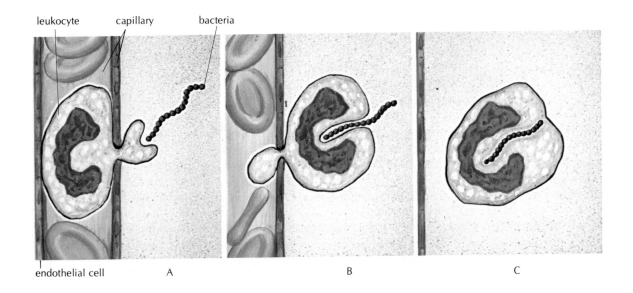

leukocyte   capillary   bacteria

endothelial cell   A   B   C

Fig. 13-2 (A) *A white blood cell squeezes through a capillary wall in the region of an infection.* (B and C) *The white cell engulfs the bacteria. This process, called phagocytosis, is a part of the body's mechanism for fighting infection.*

gens are extremely strong or numerous, they may destroy the leukocytes. A collection of dead and living bacteria, together with dead as well as living leukocytes, forms *pus.* A collection of pus localized in one area is known as an *abscess.*

Platelets or Thrombocytes

Of all the formed elements, the blood platelets (thrombocytes) are the smallest (see Fig. 13-1). These tiny structures are not cells in themselves, but fragments of cells. The number of platelets in the circulating blood has been estimated at 200,000 to 400,000 per cubic millimeter. If it were not for the platelets, we would not last very long; the slightest cut could prove to be fatal. We would bleed to death because the platelets are essential to coagulation (blood clotting). When blood is shed and comes in contact with any tissue other than that which normally carries blood, the platelets immediately disintegrate and release a chemical that reacts with a protein called *fibrinogen* (fi-brin′o-jen). Fibrinogen is manufactured in the liver and circulates in the plasma. The fibrinogen changes from a liquid to a solid mass called *fibrin,* which forms the clot.

Origin of the Corpuscles

The erythrocytes and most of the leukocytes are formed in red bone marrow, the connective tissue found in the numerous small spaces of the spongy part of all bones in children. In the adult, the red marrow is found only in the ends of the long bones and in the ribs, sternum, vertebrae, and the cranial and hip bones.

As has been noted, red cells as they normally appear in the bloodstream have no nuclei. However, when these cells were being formed in the red marrow, they did have nuclei. Thus, each red cell must lose its nucleus before it is considered to be mature and ready for release into the bloodstream. Therefore, if a routine blood examination is performed and some nucleated erythrocytes are seen, we know there is something wrong, and red cells are being released too soon. This may be a sign of a certain type of anemia, a disorder that is discussed later.

The life span of each type of corpuscle varies considerably. For example, after leaving the bone marrow, erythrocytes circulate in the bloodstream for approximately 120 days. On the other hand, the life span of the leukocytes within the circulating blood is usually a matter of hours. Blood platelets have a life span of about 5 to 9 days. In comparison with other tissue cells those in the blood are very short lived. Thus, the need for constant replacement of blood cells means that normal activity of the red bone marrow is absolutely essential to life.

The ancestors of blood cells are called *stem cells,* and they are all born in the red marrow. These stem cells continue their development to maturity within the red marrow except for one group of leukocytes, known as *lymphocytes* (lim′fo-sites). These develop not in the marrow but in the lymphoid tissues. (see Chap. 16)

When an invader enters the tissues, not only are the leukocytes in the blood attracted to the area, but the leukocyte-forming tissue goes into emergency war production, so to speak, with the result that the number of leukocytes in the blood is enormously increased. Therefore, if in the course of a blood examination an abnormally large number of white cells are seen to be present, this may be an indication of an infection somewhere. We shall also see that an abnormally small number of white cells is a characteristic sign of a different kind of disease.

The platelets are believed to originate in the red marrow as fragments of certain giant cells called *megakaryocytes* (meg″ah-kar′e-o-sites), which are formed in the red marrow.

Blood Clotting

Blood clotting, or coagulation, is a protective device that prevents blood loss when a blood vessel is ruptured by an injury. There are many substances involved in the clotting process; some, known as anticoagulants, prevent clotting, and others, called procoagulants, promote clotting. Whether blood will coagulate or not depends on the balance between these two groups of substances. Normally, the anticoagulant activity prevails, and blood does not clot. However, with injury to a blood vessel, the activity of the procoagulants becomes greater and a clot develops.

Basically, the clotting process occurs in these essential steps (Fig. 13-3):

1 The injured tissues release **thromboplastin** (throm-bo-plas'tin), a substance that triggers the clotting mechanism.

2 Thromboplastin reacts with certain protein factors and calcium ions to form **prothrombin activator**, which, in turn, reacts with calcium ions to convert the prothrombin to **thrombin.**

3 Thrombin, in turn, converts soluble fibrinogen into insoluble fibrin. **Fibrin** is a network of threads that entraps red blood cells and platelets to form a clot.

Several methods are in use to measure the body's ability to coagulate blood. These are described later in the chapter.

Blood Typing and Transfusions
Blood Groups

If for some reason the amount of blood in the body is severely reduced, through *hemorrhage* (hem'or-ij) (excessive bleeding) or through disease, the body cells suffer from lack of oxygen and food. The obvious measure to take in such an emergency is to inject blood from another person into the veins of the patient, a procedure called *transfusion.*

The plasma of one person may contain substances, called *antibodies,* that can damage the red cells of another person. The red cells of the donor's blood may become clumped or held together in

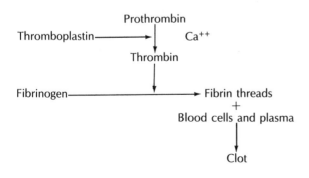

Fig. 13-3 Formation of a clot.

bunches, a process called *agglutination* (ah-gloo-ti-na'shun), by the antibodies in the patient's plasma. Sometimes the red blood cells may rupture and release their hemoglobin. Such cells are said to be *hemolyzed* (he'mo-lized), and this condition can be very dangerous.

These reactions are determined largely by the types of proteins, called *antigens* (an'ti-gens), on the red cell membranes. There are many types of these proteins, but only two groups are particularly likely to cause a transfusion reaction, the so-called A and B antigens and the Rh factor. Four blood types involving the A and B antigens have been recognized, A, B, AB, and O. These letters indicate the type of antigen present on the red cells, with O indicating that neither A nor B antigen is present. It is these antigens on the donor's red cells that react with the antibodies in the patient's plasma and cause the transfusion reaction.

Blood serum containing antibodies that can agglutinate and destroy red cells that have A antigen on the surface is called *anti-A serum,* while blood serum with antibodies that can destroy red cells with B antigen on the surface is called *anti-B serum.* These serums are used to determine blood type (Fig. 13-4).

Usually, a person can give blood safely to any person with the same blood type. However, because of other factors that may be present in the blood, determination of the blood type must be accompanied by further tests for incompatibility before a transfusion is given.

The RH Factor

About 85% of the population has another antigen called the *Rh factor.* Such individuals are said to be *Rh positive.* About 15% lack this protein and are said to be *Rh negative.* If Rh-positive blood is given to an Rh-negative person, he may become sensitized to the protein in the Rh-positive blood. The blood of this person may then produce antibodies to the "foreign" Rh-positive antigens and destroy the cells. A mother who is Rh negative may become sensitized by proteins from an Rh-positive baby (this factor having been inherited from the father), should these proteins enter the mother's circulation during childbirth. During a subsequent pregnancy with an Rh-positive fetus, some of the antibodies may pass from her blood

anti-B serum anti-A serum

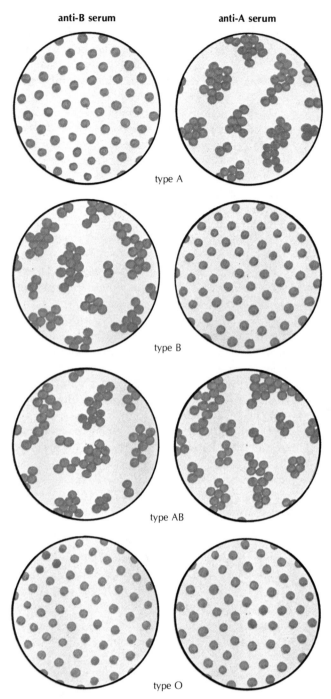

type A

type B

type AB

type O

Fig. 13-4 *Blood typing. Red cells in type A blood are agglutinated (clumped) by anti-A serum; those in type B blood are agglutinated by anti-B serum. Type AB blood cells are agglutinated by both serums; and type O blood is not agglutinated by either serum. Blood serum is the watery part of the blood that remains after the clot has been removed.*

into the blood of the fetus and there cause destruction of red cells. This results in the condition called *erythroblastosis fetalis* (e-rith''ro-blas-to'sis fe-ta'lis). The infant may be stillborn (born dead). If the infant is born alive, replacement transfusions with Rh-negative blood are begun at once.

Blood Banks

Blood can be packaged and kept in blood banks where it will be available for emergencies. In order to keep the blood from clotting, a citrate-phosphate-dextrose (CPD) solution is added. This blood may then be stored, usually for not more than 3 weeks. The supplies of blood in the bank are dated, and the date is noted before the transfusion is given to avoid giving blood in which red cells might have disintegrated. Blood banks usually have all types of blood available. However, it is important that a larger supply of type O, Rh-negative blood be maintained, since in an emergency this type can be used for all patients. The patient's blood must be tested for compatibility with the donor's blood before the transfusion is begun.

Typical Conditions Requiring Transfusion

The transfer of whole human blood from a healthy person to a patient is often a lifesaving process. Blood transfusions may be used for any condition in which there is insufficient blood or blood cells to perform the functions of the blood adequately. For example

1   In the treatment of hemorrhage from serious mechanical injuries, such as cuts or other wounds, or from disorders that may be accompanied by internal hemorrhage.
2   In the treatment of anemia from bleeding ulcers, tubercular lungs with blood loss, and other disorders in which there may be internal bleeding. "Anemia" here means "an insufficiency of blood."
3   In the treatment of *erythroblastosis fetalis.*
4   In cases of septic shock (blood poisoning), pneumonias, and nephritis (kidney disease).
5   For patients who are receiving chemotherapy for cancer and those who are on dialysis because of kidney failure.
6   As a preoperative procedure, or during an operation that causes considerable blood loss or that is performed on a patient in a weakened condition.
7   After operation as an aid in combating anemia and shock, and as an aid in the recovery process.

Uses of Blood Derivatives

Blood is capable of being broken down into its various components, and the substances derived

from it may be used for a number of purposes. One of the more common of these processes is to separate the blood plasma from the formed elements. This is accomplished by means of a *centrifuge* (sen′tre-fuge), which is a machine that spins a quantity of blood around in a circle at high speed. If you imagine a weight tied to the end of a string, and think of spinning the weight around in a circle, you will understand how a centrifuge works (Fig. 13-5). There is a force that tends to pull the weight outward. When the container of blood is spun rapidly, that same force will "pull" all the formed elements of the blood into a clump at the bottom of the container, separating them from the plasma, which can simply be drained off.

The blood plasma thus derived is a very useful substance. It may be given as an emergency measure to combat shock and to replace blood volume. The water can be removed, leaving the solids which can be stored in the dry state for a considerable length of time. Later, sterile distilled water may be added in order to reconstitute the plasma; it can then be given to treat an injured person, as, for example, in situations that do not make blood typing and the use of whole blood possible (on battlefields or in mass disasters). Since the red cells have been removed, there can be no incompatibility problems; plasma can be given to anyone. Plasma separated from the cellular elements can be further separated by either chemical means or by freezing. Plasma can be separated chemically into various components such as plasma protein, serum albumin, and gamma globulin.

Gamma globulin is a plasma protein that develops in certain tissues when they are attacked by harmful agents such as pathogenic bacteria and viruses; it is thought to be especially valuable as the first line of defense against these invaders (see Chap. 23). Gamma globulin is also prepared commercially to prevent or to reduce the severity of measles, hepatitis, and pertussis, especially in infants and in other persons who have been exposed to the disease and are in a debilitated (weakened) condition.

Fresh plasma may be frozen and saved. When frozen plasma is thawed, a white precipitate called *cryoprecipitate* (kri′o-pre-sip′i-tate) forms in the bottom of the container. Plasma frozen when it is less than 6 hours old and cryoprecipitate contain most of the factors needed for clotting, and may be given when there is a special need for these factors.

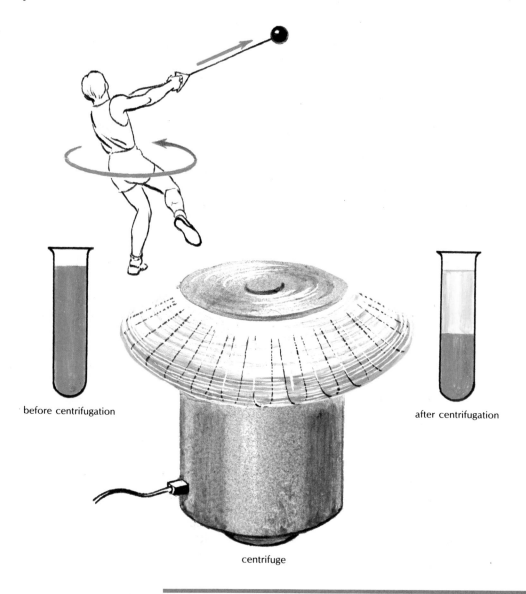

before centrifugation

after centrifugation

centrifuge

Fig. 13-5 Centrifugation.

Serum is another blood derivative. We all have observed that if a blood clot is removed (from a cut, for example) a watery fluid remains. This watery fluid is serum, and it is nothing more than plasma from which fibrinogen has been removed through the process of clotting. Serum may be derived from the blood of specially treated animals and then injected into humans in order to produce an immunity to certain diseases. Further discussion of this subject will be found in Chapter 23.

White blood cells may be separated from a donor's blood by a machine that removes the white blood cells and returns the plasma and red cells to the donor. This procedure is called *plasmapheresis* (plaz''mah-fe-re'sis). These white cells can be given to a patient who has bone marrow depression.

Blood Disorders

Abnormalities involving the blood depend on several factors and may be divided into three groups:

1 The **anemias.** The word anemia (ah-ne'me-ah) refers to a general condition in which there is a reduction in the hemoglobin or red blood

cell mass with impaired delivery of oxygen. Anemia may result from the following:

A **Excessive loss or destruction of red blood cells.** This may occur with hemorrhage or with conditions that cause hemolysis (hemol′i-sis), the rupture of red cells.

B **Impaired production of red cells or hemoglobin.** Both nutritional deficiencies and suppression of bone marrow may cause anemia.

2 **Neoplastic diseases** of the blood and blood-forming organs. A neoplasm is a new growth of abnormal cells or tissues, and neoplastic diseases may be cancerous. They include the **leukemias** (lu-ke′me-ah), a group of diseases characterized by an increase in the number of abnormal white blood cells.

3 **Hemorrhagic disorders.** These disorders are characterized by an abnormal tendency of the body to bleed which is caused by a breakdown in the body's clotting mechanism.

The Anemias

Anemia Due to Excessive Loss or Destruction of Red Cells

Excessive loss of red cells occurs with hemorrhage which may be sudden and acute or gradual and chronic.

As we know, the average adult has about 5¼ quarts of blood. If he loses as much as 2 quarts suddenly, death usually results. On the other hand, if the loss is gradual, over a period of days to weeks, the body can withstand the loss of as much as 4 or 5 quarts. If the cause of the chronic blood loss, such as bleeding ulcers, excessive menstrual flow, and bleeding hemorrhoids (piles) can be corrected, the body is usually able to restore the blood back to normal. This process can take as long as 6 months, and, until the blood returns to normal, anemia may be present.

Anemia caused by the excessive destruction of red cells is called *hemolytic* (he-mo-li′tik) anemia. Normally, an organ called the spleen destroys the older red blood cells. Occasionally, this destruction proceeds at too-rapid a pace so that an anemia is the result. More commonly, infections and infestations are the cause of blood cell loss. The action of the malarial organism is an interesting example of this. When a person is bitten by the mosquito, the malarial parasite is injected into the blood-stream. Each parasite enters a red cell, where it multiplies until the red cell bursts; that cell is now destroyed. The parasites, now freed, attack other red cells in the same manner. The result is an anemia. Certain bacteria, particularly streptococci, cause hemolysis and therefore a hemolytic anemia.

Certain inherited diseases that involve the production of abnormal hemoglobin may also result in hemolytic anemia. The hemoglobin in normal adult cells is of the A type and is designated HbA. In the inherited disease, *sickle cell anemia,* the hemoglobin in many of the red cells is abnormal so that the red cells may have a sickle shape (Fig. 13-6). These sickled cells are fragile and tend to break easily. Because of their odd shape, they also tend to become tangled in masses that may block smaller blood vessels. When this obstruction occurs, there may be severe joint swelling and pain, especially in the fingers and toes, and there may be abdominal pain. This development is referred to as sickle cell crisis.

This disease is seen almost exclusively in black persons. About 8% of American blacks have one of the genes for the abnormal hemoglobin and are said to have the *sickle cell trait.* It is only when the involved gene is transmitted from both parents that the clinical disease appears. About 1% of American blacks have two of these genes and thus have *sickle cell disease.*

Anemia Due to Impaired Production of Red Cells or Hemoglobin

Many factors can interfere with normal red cell production. Some are the result of the deficiency of some nutrient; they are referred to as nutritional anemias. The condition may arise from a deficiency of the specific nutrient in the diet, from the inability to absorb the nutrient, or from drugs that interfere with the body's use of the nutrient.

The most common nutritional anemia is *iron deficiency* anemia. Iron is an essential constituent of hemoglobin. The normal diet usually provides enough to meet the needs of the adult male but may be inadequate when there is an increased demand for iron. For example, children, women of childbearing age, pregnant women, and persons who lose iron because of chronic hemorrhage may need additional iron.

Pernicious (per-nish′us) anemia is characterized by a deficiency of vitamin B_{12}, a substance essential for the proper formation of red blood cells. The

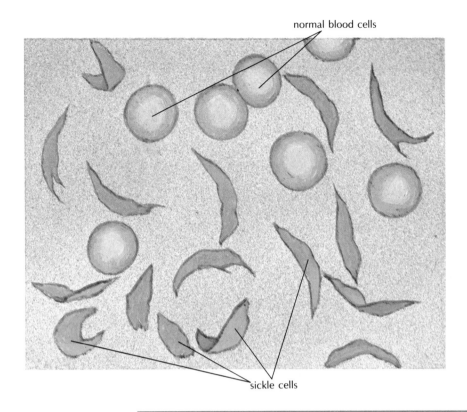

normal blood cells

sickle cells

Fig. 13-6 Sickling.

initial cause is a permanent deficiency of a factor in the gastric juice that is responsible for the absorption of vitamin B$_{12}$ from the intestine. Neglected cases of pernicious anemia can bring about conditions of deterioration in the nervous system, causing difficulty in walking, weakness and stiffness in the extremities, mental changes, and permanent damage to the spinal cord. Early treatment, including the intramuscular injection of vitamin B$_{12}$ and attention to a prescribed diet, now assures an excellent outlook. This treatment must be kept up for the rest of the patient's life if good health is to be maintained.

A decreased production of red blood cells may also be brought about by *bone marrow suppression* or failure. One type of bone marrow failure disease is *aplastic* (ay-plas′tick) anemia which may be caused by a variety of physical and chemical agents. Chemical substances that injure the bone marrow include benzene, arsenic, nitrogen mustard, gold compounds, and, in some persons, the antibiotic chloramphenicol. Physical agents that may injure the marrow include x-rays, atomic radiation, ra-

dium, and radioactive phosphorus. The damaged bone marrow fails to produce either red or white cells, so that the anemia is accompanied by leukopenia. Removal of the toxic agent followed by blood transfusions until the marrow is able to resume its activity may result in recovery.

Bone marrow may also fail to produce red blood cells when normal marrow cells are crowded out by abnormal cells such as cancer cells. In one type of leukemia, for example, the bone marrow is filled with abnormal blood cells that destroy the other cells in the marrow, resulting in a severe anemia.

Neoplastic Blood Disease

This group of diseases is characterized by an enormous increase in the number of white cells, owing to a cancer of the tissues that produce these cells. We noted that the white cells have two main sources: red marrow, also called myeloid tissue, and lymphoid tissue. If this wild proliferation of white cells stems from a tumor of the marrow, the condition is called *myelogenous* (mi-e-loj′e-nus) leukemia. When the cancer arises in the lymphoid tissue, so that the majority of abnormal cells are lymphocytes, the condition is called *lymphocytic* leukemia.

At the present time the cause of leukemia is unknown. Both inherent factors and various environmental agents have been implicated. Among the latter are chemicals such as benzene, excessive exposure to x-rays or to radioactive substances, and viruses.

The patient with leukemia exhibits the general symptoms of anemia. In addition, he has a tendency to bleed easily. The spleen is greatly enlarged, and several other organs may be increased in size because of the accumulation of white cells within them. X-ray treatments along with drugs are given in cases of leukemia; but because of the malignant character of the disease, it may be fatal. With new methods of chemotherapy, the outlook is improving, and many patients survive for years.

Hemorrhagic Disorders

A characteristic that these diseases have in common is a disruption of the coagulation process which brings about abnormal bleeding. A rare but interesting example of hemorrhagic disorder is a disease called *hemophilia* (he-mo-fil′e-ah). Hemophilia is the name given to a group of inherited disorders characterized by a deficiency in certain clotting factors so that any cut or bruise may cause serious abnormal bleeding. The deficient clotting factors are now available in concentrated form for treatment in case of injury, in preparation for surgery and for the painful bleeding into the joints that often occurs.

Another type of bleeding disease is *purpura* (pur′pu-rah) in which hemorrhages occur in the skin and mucous membranes. The abnormal bleeding in this disease may be due to a deficiency of platelets or to abnormalities of the blood vessel walls. There are probably a number of reasons for the deficiency of platelets. Suppression of bone marrow by drugs or cancer of the bone marrow may both lead to purpura.

A serious disorder of clotting in which there is excessive coagulation is called *disseminated intravascular coagulation* (DIC). It may occur in cases of tissue damage due to massive burns, trauma, certain acute infections, cancer, and some disorders of childbirth. During the progress of this disorder, platelets and various clotting factors are used up faster than they can be produced, and serious hemorrhaging may result.

Blood Studies

Many different kinds of studies may be made of the blood. Some of these have become a standard part of a routine physical examination. Machines have replaced many of the manual procedures, particularly in larger institutions.

The Hematocrit

The *hematocrit* (he-mat′o-krit) is the volume percentage of red blood cells in whole blood. It is also called the PCV, for *packed cell volume.* It is regarded as a more reliable indicator of red cell counts than either the manual counting, the use of a hemocytometer (he-mo-si-tom′e-ter), or the machine method. The hematocrit is determined by spinning a blood sample in a centrifuge for 30 minutes; in this way, the cellular elements are separated out from the plasma.

The hematocrit is expressed as volume of red cells per unit volume (100 ml) of whole blood. For example, if a laboratory report states "hematocrit, 38" that means that there are 38 ml of red cells per 100 ml of whole blood. In other words, 38% of the whole blood is red cells. For males, the normal range is 42 to 50 ml per 100 ml of blood, while for females the range is slightly lower, 36 to 40 ml per 100 ml of blood. These normal ranges, as with all normal ranges for humans, may vary depending on the method used and the interpretation of the results by an individual laboratory. Hematocrit values much below or much above these figures point to an abnormality requiring further study.

Blood Cell Counts

In most laboratories today, automatic counters such as the Coulter counter are used to count the blood cells. In very small laboratories, a hemocytometer may be used (Fig. 13-7). The normal count for red blood cells varies from 4.5 to 5.5 million cells per cubic millimeter of blood. The leukocyte count

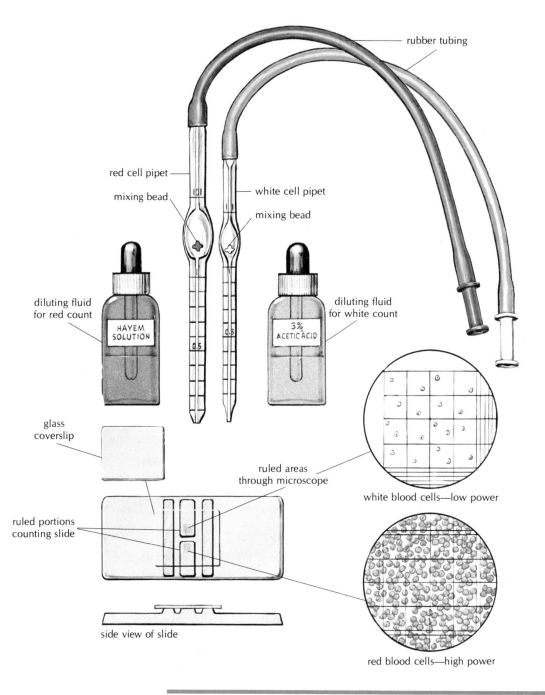

Fig. 13-7 Parts of a hemocytometer.

varies from 5,000 to 10,000 cells per cubic millimeter of blood.

In leukopenia the white count is below 5000. It is characteristic of a few infections such as malaria and measles, as well as certain disorders of the blood-forming organs.

Leukocytosis means that the white blood count is in excess of 10,000 per cubic millimeter. It is particularly characteristic of most infections. It may occur also after hemorrhage and in gout and uremia, a result of kidney disease.

The Blood Slide (or Smear)

A drop of blood is spread very thinly and carefully over a glass slide. A special stain is applied to differentiate the otherwise colorless white cells, and then this slide is studied under the microscope. Abnormal red cells that are characteristic of certain anemias may be noted, and malarial or other parasites may be found. Abnormalities in the white cells also are observed. In addition, the *differential white count* (*i.e.,* an estimation of the percentage of each type of white cell) is done using the same stained blood slide. Since each type of white blood cell has a specific function, changes in the amounts of the various types can be a valuable aid to the physician in making a diagnosis.

Amount of Hemoglobin

It is important to know that a person has an adequate amount of hemoglobin so that the tissues are assured a sufficient supply of oxygen. This is determined by means of a *hemometer* (he-mom'e-ter), also known as a *hemoglobinometer* (he-mo-glo-bi-nom'e-ter). These devices vary in design, but in general the principle is that a comparison is made between the blood and a standard color scale. The normal hemoglobin concentration ranges from 14 to 17 grams per 100 ml of blood for males, and, as with the hematocrit, the values are slightly lower for females, ranging from 12 to 15 grams per 100 ml of blood. A decrease in hemoglobin is a factor in anemia.

Blood Chemistry Tests

Batteries of tests on blood serum are often done by machine. One, the sequential multiple analyzer (SMA), provides for the running of some 12 or more tests per minute. Tests for electrolytes such as sodium, potassium, chloride, and bicarbonate, plus enzyme tests such as those for alkaline *phosphatase* (fos'fah-tase) and *transaminase* (trans-am'i-nase), may be included in this battery of tests. Others of importance include blood urea nitrogen (BUN), blood sugar, cholesterol, and triglyceride

evaluations. All of these may also be done manually using test tubes containing various chemicals that yield color changes or other kinds of determinants.

Many of these blood serum tests help in evaluating disorders that may involve such vital organs as the heart, kidneys, liver, and pancreas. For example, the presence of more than the normal amount of glucose (sugar) dissolved in the blood is called *hyperglycemia* (hi-per-gli-se'me-ah) and is found most frequently in unregulated diabetic persons. Sometimes several evaluations of sugar content are done following the administration of a known amount of glucose. This procedure is called the *glucose tolerance test* and usually is given along with another test which determines the amount of sugar in the urine. This combination of tests can indicate faulty cell metabolism.

Other Blood Tests
Clotting Time

Nature prevents excessive loss of blood from small vessels by the formation of a clot. Preceding surgery and under some other circumstances, it is important to know that the time required for coagulation to take place is not too long. Since clotting is a rather complex process involving many elements, a delay may be due to a number of different factors, including lack of certain hormone-like substances, calcium salts, and vitamin K.

The various clotting factors have each been designated by a Roman numeral, I through XIII. Factor I is fibrinogen, factor II is prothrombin, factor III is thromboplastin, and factor IV is assigned to calcium ions. The amounts of all thirteen factors may be determined and evaluated on a percentage basis, aiding in the diagnosis and treatment of some bleeding disorders.

Platelet Count

A count of the thrombocytes is done occasionally, but it is difficult to do accurately. Normal counts are said to vary from 200,000 to 400,000 per cubic millimeter. However, counts as low as 100,000 per cubic millimeter may not indicate an abnormality. In some severe hemorrhagic disorders, the counts have been known to go as low as 10,000 per cubic millimeter.

Bone Marrow Biopsy

A special needle is used to obtain a small sample of red marrow from the sternum, sacrum or iliac crest in a procedure called a bone marrow biopsy. If the marrow is taken from the sternum, the procedure may be referred to as a sternal puncture. Examination of the cells by a trained person will give valuable information that can be used to aid in the diagnosis of bone marrow disorders including leukemia and certain kinds of anemia.

Summary

1 General characteristics of blood.
   A Can be considered a connective tissue.
   B Thick fluid of varying red color.
   C Quantity—about 5¼ quarts in average adult male.
2 Main purposes of blood.
   A Transportation—gases, food, wastes, heat, and secretions.
   B Protection—internal environment, defense against disease.
3 Prime elements of blood.
   A Plasma (liquid element).
   B Formed elements (cell and cell-derived elements).
      (1) Erythrocytes (red cells).
      (2) Leukocytes (white cells).
      (3) Platelets (cellular fragments involved in clotting).
4 Plasma.
   A Ninety percent water.
   B Remainder—proteins, carbohydrates, lipids, salts, hormones, wastes.
5 Formed elements (corpuscles)—characteristics.
   A Erythrocytes—carry oxygen; main constituent is hemoglobin, which combines with gases; nonnucleated; most numerous of corpuscles.
   B Leukocytes—combat disease; nucleated; several different forms.
   C Platelets—fragments of cells; dissolve and combine with fibrinogen to form clot (fibrin).
6 Origin of corpuscles.
   A Erythrocytes—formed in red marrow; immature cells nucleated; mature cells lose nucleus before going to bloodstream.
   B Leukocytes—formed and mature mostly in red marrow; one form (lymphocytes) matures in lymphoid tissues.

   C Platelets—fragments of larger cells formed in red marrow.
7 Blood clotting.
   A Balance between anticoagulants and procoagulants prevents clotting.
   B Three essential steps—formation of thromboplastin; prothrombin converted to thrombin; fibrinogen converted to insoluble fibrin.
8 Blood groups.
   A Not all blood types compatible.
   B Blood types (A, B, AB, O).
   C Mixing of incompatible bloods may result in agglutination of red cells or hemolysis.
9 Rh factor.
   A Most people have special red cell protein (Rh factor); are Rh positive.
   B Minority lack it; are Rh negative.
   C Rh-negative mother may have Rh-positive baby (factor inherited from father); sensitized to Rh factor.
10 Blood banks—blood packaged and stored for emergencies; type O Rh-negative blood most commonly used.
11 Transfusions given in the following conditions—hemorrhage, anemia, erythroblastosis fetalis, treatment with chemotherapeutic drugs, shock, preoperatively and postoperatively.
12 Blood derivatives.
   A Plasma—separated, dried, stored, reactivated, used in emergencies to combat shock and to replace blood volume.
   B Fresh frozen plasma—rich in clotting factors.
   C Serum—provides for immunity; contains antibodies.
   D Others—plasma proteins; red blood cells; thrombocytes; leukocytes; gamma globulins.

13 Blood disorders.
  A Anemias.
    (1) Loss or destruction of red blood cells.
    (2) Impaired production of red cells or hemoglobin.
  B Neoplastic diseases—include leukemias.
  C Hemorrhagic diseases—characterized by faulty clotting.
14 Anemias.
  A Loss or destruction of red blood cells.
    (1) Hemorrhage—acute and chronic.
    (2) Hemolytic anemia—rupture of red blood cells; parasites or certain bacteria.
    (3) Sickle cell anemia—inherited disease; abnormal hemoglobin; red cells have sickle shape, are fragile and break; red cells tangle and obstruct small blood vessels; joint swelling and pain; abdominal pain; sickle cell crisis; seen primarily in black race.
  B Impaired production of red blood cells or hemoglobin.
    (1) Nutritional anemias—iron deficiency anemia; pernicious anemia due to lack of gastric juice factor, deficiency in vitamin B_{12} absorption, treatment with vitamin B_{12} and prescribed diet.
    (2) Bone marrow failure—aplastic anemia caused by poisonous agents; leukemic cells crowd out normal cells.
15 Neoplastic diseases.
  A Main group—leukemia (myelogenous and lymphocytic).
  B Caused by malignancy in white cell-producing tissue.
  C Characterized by greatly increased leukocyte count.
  D May be fatal; new treatment improving outlook.
16 Hemorrhagic disorders.
  A Characterized by disruption of clotting process.
  B Examples—hemophilia, purpura, DIC.
17 Blood studies.
  A Hematocrit, volume percent of red cells.
  B Total red and white blood counts.
    (1) Apparatus used called hemocytometer, or machine such as Coulter counter.
    (2) Too few white cells is called leukopenia.
    (3) More than normal number of white cells is known as leukocytosis.
  C Examine blood slide for parasites; used also for differential white count.
  D Differential white count.
  E Hemoglobin amount estimated, using hemometer.
18 Blood chemistry tests.
  A Machine such as SMA can perform 12 tests per minute.
  B Electrolytes and enzyme determinations.
  C Glucose, urea, others for status of organ function.
  D Glucose tolerance test.
19 Other blood tests.
  A Clotting time.
  B Clotting factors I through XIII.
  C Platelet count.
  D Bone marrow biopsy.

Questions and Problems

1 How does the color of blood vary with the amount of oxygenation?
2 Name the 2 main purposes of the blood.
3 Name the 2 prime elements of the blood.
4 Name and describe the 3 main groups of cellular structures in blood.
5 Name 4 main ingredients of blood plasma. What are their purposes?
6 What is the main function of erythrocytes? leukocytes? platelets? Where does each originate?
7 What are the names usually given to the 4 main blood groups? What are the factors that are the reason for the different groupings?
8 What is the Rh factor? What proportion of people possess this factor? In what situations is this factor of medical importance? Why?
9 Describe the three basic steps in the clotting process.
10 What are the advantages of blood banks? Are there any disadvantages? If so, what are they,

and is there a way of counteracting these disadvantages?

11 What are some of the conditions for which blood transfusions are useful?

12 What precautions should always be taken before a transfusion is given?

13 What substances obtained from the blood may be useful in the treatment of the sick, and in what way is each of these blood derivatives used?

14 Name the 3 general categories of blood disorders.

15 Differentiate between the types of anemia and give an example of each.

16 Name 2 kinds of leukemia. What is the chief symptom of leukemia, and what is the reason for it?

17 Name the main characteristics of hemorrhagic disorders and give an example of these.

18 What is the value of the hematocrit?

19 What are some of the conditions that are due to abnormal white counts?

20 What is determined by the blood smear?

21 What are some evaluations made by blood chemistry tests?

Chapter 14

The Heart and Heart Disease

14

Glossary

Arrhythmia Any variation from the normal rhythm of the heartbeat.

Atrium (pl. atria) A chamber (that affords entrance to another structure or organ).

Bradycardia A very slow heartbeat.

Catheter A tube that can be inserted into a body cavity through a canal to remove fluids, such as urine or blood.

Circulation The continuous one-way movement of blood.

Diastole The relaxing dilatation period of the heart muscle, especially the ventricles (adj. diastolic).

Echocardiograph An instrument for detecting abnormalities of the heart using high-frequency sound impulses.

Electrocardiograph An instrument used for making records of the heart's electric currents.

Endocardium The membrane that lines the heart chambers and assists in forming the heart valves.

Fluoroscope An instrument used to examine deep structures of the body by means of roentgen rays (x-rays).

Infarct An area that has been cut off from its blood supply.

Myocardium The middle, thick layer of the heart wall. It is composed of cardiac muscle.

Node A swelling.

Occlusion A closure.

Pericardium The serous membrane that lines the sac enclosing the heart, plus the reflection that attaches itself to the heart itself.

Septum A dividing wall or partition.

Stethoscope An instrument used for conveying sounds from the patient's body to the examiner's ears.

Systole The period of heart muscle contraction, especially that of the ventricles (adj systolic).

Tachycardia A very fast heartbeat.

Thrombus A blood clot.

Ultrasound Mechanical energy generated at a frequency beyond the range of sensitivity of the ear.

Circulation and the Heart

In the next two chapters we shall investigate the manner in which the blood acquires its food and oxygen to be delivered to the cells and disposes of the waste products of cell metabolism. This continuous one-way movement of the blood is known as its *circulation*. The fact that blood circulates throughout the body implies that there must be some sort of propelling mechanism. The prime mover in this case is the *heart;* and we shall have a look at the heart before going into the circulatory vessels in any detail.

The heart is a muscular pump that drives the blood through the blood vessels. This organ is slightly bigger than a fist and is located between the lungs in the center and a bit to the left of the midline of the body. The strokes (contractions) of this pump average about 72 per minute and are carried on unceasingly for the whole of a lifetime.

The importance of the heart has been recognized for centuries. The fact that its rate of beating is affected by the emotions may be responsible for the very frequent references to the heart in song and poetry. However, the vital functions of the heart and its disorders are of more practical importance to us at this time.

Structure of the Heart
Layers of the Heart Wall

The heart is a hollow organ the walls of which are formed of three different layers. Just as a warm coat might have a smooth lining, a thick and bulky interlining and an outer layer of a third fabric, so the heart wall has three tissue layers (Fig. 14-1).

1 **Endocardium** (en''do-kar'de-um) is a very smooth layer of cells that resembles squamous epithelium. This membrane lines the interior of the heart. The valves of the heart are formed by folds of this material with reinforcement.
2 **Myocardium** (mi''o-kar'de-um) is the muscle of the heart and is much the thickest layer.
3 **Pericardium** (per''i-kar'de-um) forms the outermost layer of the heart wall as well as serving as the lining of the pericardial sac that encloses the heart.

Two Hearts and a Partition

Physicians often refer to the right heart and the left heart. This is because the human heart is really a double pump. The two sides are completely separated from each other by a partition called the *septum*. The upper part of this partition is called the *interatrial* (in''ter-a'tre-al) *septum,* while the larger lower portion is called the *interventricular* (in''ter-ven-trik'u-lar) *septum.* This septum, as in the case of the heart wall, is largely myocardium.

Four Chambers

On either side of the heart there are two chambers, one of which is a receiving chamber and the other a pumping chamber:

1 The **right atrium** is a thin-walled chamber that receives the blood returning from the body tissues. This blood, which is low in oxygen is carried in the *veins,* which are the blood vessels leading *to* the heart from the body tissues.
2 The **right ventricle** pumps the venous blood received from the right atrium, and sends it to the lungs.
3 The **left atrium** receives blood high in oxygen content as it returns from the lungs.
4 The **left ventricle** has the thickest walls of all and it pumps oxygenated blood to all parts of the body. This blood goes through the *arteries,* which is the name for the vessels that take blood *from* the heart to the tissues.

Four Valves

Since the ventricles are the pumping chambers, the valves, which are all one-way, are located at the entrance and the exit of each ventricle (Fig. 14-2). The valves at the entrances are the *atrioventricular* (a''tre-o-ven-trik'u-lar) *valves,* while the exit valves are *semilunar* (sem''e-lu'nar) *valves.* "Semilunar" means "resembling a half-moon." Each valve has a specific name, as follows:

1 The **right atrioventricular valve** also is known as the **tricuspid** (tri-kus'pid) **valve,** since it has three cusps or flaps which open and close.

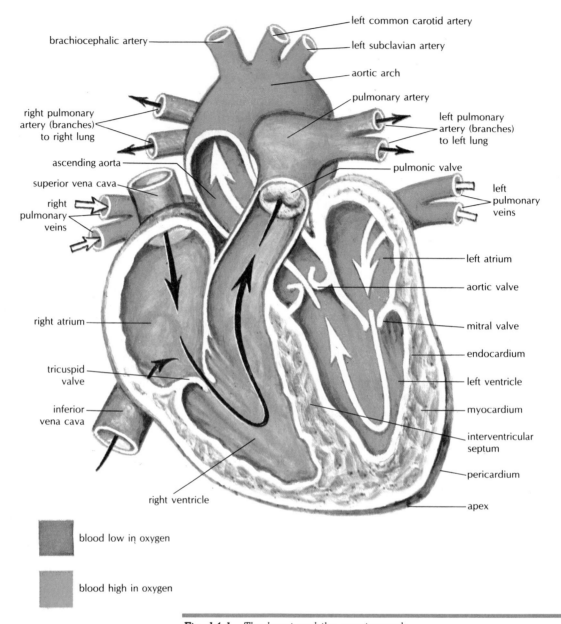

Fig. 14-1 *The heart and the great vessels.*

When this valve is open, blood flows freely from the right atrium into the right ventricle. However, when the right ventricle begins to contract, the valve closes so that blood cannot return to the right atrium; this ensures onward flow into the pulmonary artery.

2 The **pulmonary** (pul'mo-nar''e) **semilunar valve** is located between the right ventricle and the pulmonary artery which leads to the lungs. As soon as the right ventricle has finished emp-

tying itself, the valve closes in order to prevent blood on its way to the lungs from returning to the ventricle.

3 The **left atrioventricular valve** usually is referred to as the **mitral** (mi'tral) **valve**. It has two rather heavy flaps, or cusps, that permit blood to flow freely from the left atrium into the left ventricle. However, the flaps close when the left ventricle begins to contract; this prevents blood from returning to the left atrium

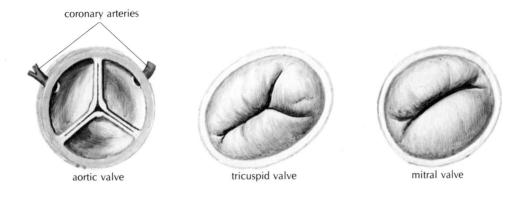

coronary arteries

aortic valve   tricuspid valve   mitral valve

Fig. 14-2 *Valves of the heart, seen from above, in the closed position.*

and ensures the onward flow of blood into the *aorta* (a-or'tah).

4   The **aortic** (a-or'tik) **semilunar** valve is located between the left ventricle and the aorta. Following contraction of the left ventricle, the aortic valve closes to prevent the flow of blood back from the aorta to the ventricle.

The appearance of the heart valves in the closed position is illustrated in Figure 14-2.

Blood Supply to the Myocardium

Although blood flows through the heart chambers, only the endocardium comes into contact with this vital fluid. Therefore, the myocardium must have its own blood vessels to provide oxygen and nourishment and to remove waste products. The arteries that supply blood to the muscle of the heart are called the right and left *coronary arteries,* so named because they encircle the heart like a crown (Fig. 14-3). These arteries are the first branches of the aorta. They arise just above the aortic semilunar valve (see Fig. 14-2). After passing through capillaries in the myocardium, blood drains into the cardiac veins and finally into the coronary venous sinus for the return trip to the right atrium.

Physiology of the Heart
The Work of the Heart

Although the right and the left sides of the heart are separated from each other, they work together.

The blood is squeezed through the chambers by a contraction of heart muscle beginning in the thin-walled upper chambers, the atria, and followed by a contraction of the thick muscle of the lower chambers, the ventricles. This active phase is called *systole* (sis'to-le), and in each case it is followed by a short resting period known as *diastole* (di-as'-to-le). The contraction of the walls of the atria is completed at the time the contraction of the ventricles begins. Thus, the resting phase (diastole) begins in the atria at the same time as the contraction (systole) begins in the ventricles. As soon as the ventricles have emptied, the atria (which meanwhile have been filling with blood) contract while the ventricles relax and again fill with blood. Then the ventricular systole begins (Fig. 14-4).

Cardiac muscle tissue has several unique properties. One of these is due to the interconnection of the muscle fibers (see Fig. 2-12). The fibers are interwoven so that the stimulation that causes the contraction of one fiber results in the contraction of the whole group. This plays an important role in the process of conduction and the working of the heart muscle.

Another property of heart muscle is its ability to adjust contraction strength to the amount of blood received. When the heart chamber is filled and the wall is stretched (within limits), the strength of the contraction is greater. When less blood enters the heart, the contraction is weaker. When more blood enters the heart, as occurs during exercise, it contracts with greater strength to push the larger volume of blood out into the blood vessels.

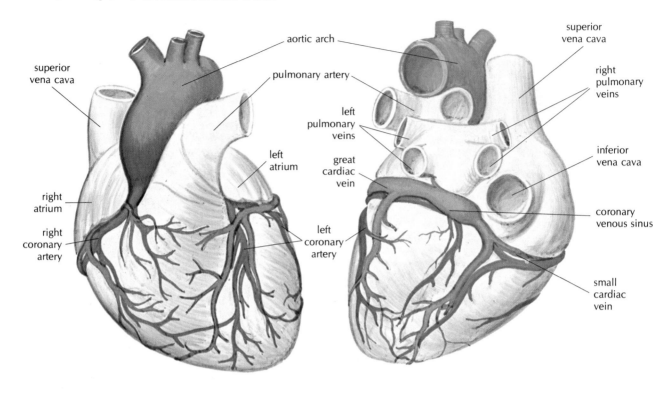

Fig. 14-3 *Coronary arteries and cardiac veins.* (Left) *Anterior view.* (Right) *Posterior view.*

Control of the Heartbeat

If the nerves that supply the voluntary muscles are cut, these muscles cease to function; that is, they are completely paralyzed. If the nerves that supply the heart are severed, however, the heart will continue to beat. The reason for this is that although the heart is under the control of the nervous system, heart muscle itself is capable of contracting rhythmically independently of outside control. Despite this, the impulses from the nervous system are required to cause a rapid enough beat to maintain circulation effectively. Without nerve connection, the heart rate might be less than 40 beats per minute instead of the usual 70 to 90 beats per minute.

The Conduction System of the Heart

Specialized masses of tissue in the heart wall form the conduction system of the heart, regulating the order of events. Two of these are called *nodes,* while the third is a branching structure called the *atrioventricular bundle.* The *sinoatrial node* is located in the upper wall of the right atrium and acts as a pacemaker. The second node is called the *atrioventricular node* and is located in the septum at the junction between the interatrial portion and the interventricular part. The atrioventricular bundle, which is also known as the *bundle of His,* is located in the interventricular septum with branches extending to all parts of the ventricle walls (Fig. 14-5). The order in which the impulses travel is as follows:

1   The beginning of the heartbeat is in the sinoatrial (S-A) node, the pacemaker.
2   The excitation (contraction) wave travels throughout the muscle of each atrium, causing it to contract.
3   The atrioventricular node is stimulated. The relatively slower conduction through this node allows the atrial contraction to fill the ventricle.

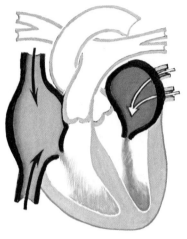

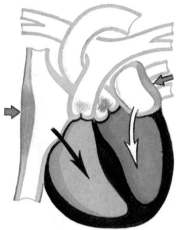

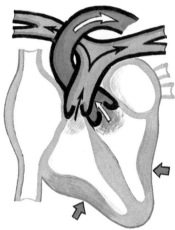

Diastole
Atria fill with blood which begins to flow into ventricles as soon as their walls relax.

Atrial Systole
Contraction of atria pumps blood into the ventricles.

Ventricular Systole
Contraction of ventricles pumps blood into aorta and pulmonary arteries.

Fig. 14-4 *Pumping cycle of the heart.*

4   The excitation wave travels rapidly through the bundle of His and throughout the ventricular walls. The entire musculature of the ventricles contracts practically all at once.

Heart Sounds and Murmurs

The normal heart sounds are usually described by the two syllables "lubb" and "dupp." The first is a longer and lower-pitched sound which occurs during the ventricular systole. It is probably caused by a combination of sounds including the closure of the atrioventricular valves. The second, or "dupp," sound is shorter and sharper. It occurs during the beginning of ventricular relaxation, and is due in large part to the sudden closure of the semilunar valves. Abnormal sounds are called *murmurs* and are usually due to faulty action of the valves. If, for example, the valves fail to close tightly and blood leaks back, a murmur is heard. Another condition giving rise to an abnormal sound is the narrowing (stenosis) of a valve orifice. The many conditions that can cause an abnormal heart sound may be due to congenital defects, to disease, or to physiologic variations. A murmur called a *functional* or *flow murmur* does not necessarily involve an abnormality but frequently is the result of the sounds produced during rapid filling of the ventricles. On the other hand, an abnormal sound caused by any structural change in the heart or the vessels connected with the heart is called an *organic murmur.*

Heart Rates

1   **Bradycardia** (brad''e-kar'de-ah) means the heart rate is relatively slow. During rest and sleep the heart may beat less than the normal 60 to 80 beats per minute, but usually not below 50 beats per minute.

2   **Tachycardia** (tak''e-kar'de-ah) refers to a heart rate over 100.

3   **Sinus arrhythmia** (ah-rith'me-ah) is a regular variation in rate due to changes in the rate and depth of breathing, a normal phenomenon.

4   **Premature beats,** also called extrasystoles, cause an arrhythmia that may occur in normal persons. These are beats that come in before the expected normal beats. They may be initiated by caffeine, nicotine or psychological stresses. They are also common in heart disease.

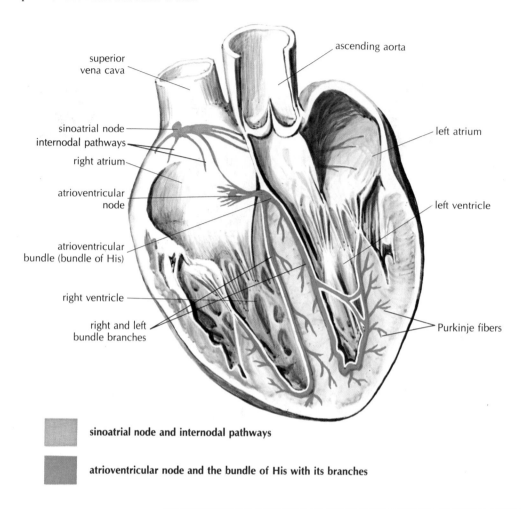

superior
vena cava

ascending aorta

sinoatrial node
internodal pathways
right atrium

left atrium

atrioventricular
node

left ventricle

atrioventricular
bundle (bundle of His)

right ventricle

right and left
bundle branches

Purkinje fibers

sinoatrial node and internodal pathways

atrioventricular node and the bundle of His with its branches

Fig. 14-5 *The conduction system of the heart.*

Heart Disease
Classification of Heart Disease

There are many ways of classifying heart disease. The three layers of the heart wall form the basis for one grouping of heart pathology.

1 **Endocarditis** (en''do-kar-di'tis) means "inflammation of the lining of the heart cavities," but it most commonly refers to valvular disease.
2 **Myocarditis** (mi''o-kar-di'tis) means inflammation of heart muscle.
3 **Pericarditis** (per''i-kar-di'tis) refers to disease of the serous membrane on the heart surface, as well as that lining the pericardial sac.

Another more generally used classification of heart disease is based on causative factors:

1 **Congenital** heart disease is present at birth.
2 **Rheumatic** heart disease begins with an attack of rheumatic fever in childhood or in youth.
3 **Coronary** (kor'o-na-re) heart disease involves the walls of the blood vessels that supply the muscle of the heart.
4 **Degenerative** heart disease is due to deterioration of the heart tissues, frequently the result of disorders of long duration such as high blood pressure.

Ischemic (is-kem'ik) heart disease is a term referring to coronary heart disease or degenerative heart disease in which there is a deficiency in blood supply to the heart muscle causing necrosis, or death, of the heart muscle.

Congenital Heart Disease

This category of heart disease includes certain abnormalities that have been present since birth, and which usually represent a failure of normal development.

The most common congenital heart defects are holes in the septum or partition between the left and right sides of the heart. Blood flow from one side of the heart to the other results in a mixture of venous and arterial blood being pumped to the tissues. This defect may be in either the atrial or ventricular septum.

The circulation of the fetus differs in several respects from that of the child after birth, one difference being that the lungs are not used until the child is born. Prior to birth the unused lungs are bypassed by a blood vessel that normally closes of its own accord once the lungs are in use. Sometimes, however, the vessel fails to close, with the result that much of the blood is detoured around the lungs instead of through them; and therefore the blood does not receive enough oxygen.

Another congenital heart defect is an obstruction or narrowing of the pulmonary artery which prevents the blood from passing in sufficient quantity from the right ventricle to the lungs.

In recent years many of these congenital defects have been remedied by heart surgery, one of the more spectacular advances in modern medicine.

Rheumatic Fever and the Heart

Streptococcal infections are indirectly responsible for rheumatic fever and rheumatic heart disease. The toxin produced by the streptococci causes an immune reaction that may be followed some 2 to 4 weeks later by rheumatic fever with marked swelling of the joints. Then the antibodies formed to combat the toxin attack the heart valves, producing a condition known as rheumatic endocarditis. The heart valves, particularly the mitral valve, become inflamed. The normally flexible valve cusps thicken and harden so that the opening becomes permanently narrowed (mitral stenosis). This con-

dition prevents an adequate flow of blood from the left atrium into the left ventricle, with a resulting pulmonary congestion, an important characteristic of mitral heart disease. The incidence of rheumatic fever and, hence, of rheumatic heart disease is being drastically reduced owing to the more prompt and effective antibiotic and other medical treatment of the streptococcal infections.

Coronary Heart Disease

The heart muscle receives its own blood supply through the coronary arteries. A common cause of sudden death, or at least disability, from heart disease is *coronary occlusion* (o-kloo′shun), that is, closure of one or more branches of the coronary arteries. Such interference with the blood supply will result in damage to the myocardium. The degree of injury sustained depends upon a number of factors, including the size of the artery that is involved and whether the occlusion is gradual or sudden.

Arteries of the heart as well as the rest of the body can undergo degenerative changes. It may happen that the lumen (space) inside the vessel narrows gradually owing to progressive thickening and hardening of the arteries. As a consequence of this, the volume of blood supplied to the heart muscle is reduced and the action of the heart is weakened. Degenerative changes of the artery wall may cause the inside surface to become roughened as well. This roughened artery wall is highly conducive to the formation of a *thrombus,* or blood clot. The thrombus may cause sudden closure of the vessel with complete obstruction of the blood flow. This life-threatening condition is known as *coronary thrombosis.* The area which has been cut off from its blood supply is called an *infarct* (in′farkt). The outcome of a myocardial infarction depends upon the extent of the damage and whether or not other branches of the artery can supply enough blood to maintain the heart's action. Death may occur swiftly if a large area of heart muscle is suddenly deprived of blood supply. If a smaller area is involved, the heart may continue to function. However, complete and prolonged lack of blood supply to any part of the myocardium results in death of tissue and weakening of the heart wall. In some cases, the weakened area may rupture, but in other cases there is a scar formed in the area of the infarct.

The person who suffers an acute coronary occlusion must be put on complete bed rest for a variable period of time, depending upon the severity of the attack and upon the time required for the damaged heart muscle to be replaced by scar tissue. During this period the most meticulous medical and nursing care is required.

Although myocardial infarction is one of the leading causes of death in the United States, prompt and effective treatment enables many individuals to survive a "heart attack," or "coronary." Despite the fact that the heart is damaged, it may be possible for the person to lead a fairly normal life so long as he moderates his activities, gets sufficient rest, follows a prescribed diet, and tries to minimize stressful situations.

When the blood flow to the heart muscle is inadequate, there results a characteristic agonizing pain, felt in the region of the heart and in the left arm and the shoulder, called *angina pectoris* (an-ji'nah pek'to-ris). Angina pectoris may be accompanied by a feeling of suffocation and a general sensation of forthcoming doom. Heart disease is a common cause of angina pectoris, although there are other causes as well.

Atrial and Ventricular Fibrillations

Fibrillations of the heart muscle begin as small local contractions of a few cells followed by convulsive movements of groups of cells within the muscle wall. They may affect the atria by themselves or they may involve the ventricles, a very serious cardiac disorder. There are rapid ineffective muscle contractions with symptoms of heart failure. First aid procedures include cardiopulmonary resuscitation (CPR) and then transfer by a paramedical unit to a hospital.

Degenerative Heart Disease

During a person's lifetime, many toxins, infections, and other kinds of injuries may cause weakening of the heart muscle. High blood pressure, known as *hypertension,* over a period of years may cause an enlargement of the heart, and finally heart failure. Malnutrition, chronic infections, and severe anemias may cause degeneration of heart muscle. Hyperthyroidism with its tendency to cause overactivity of all parts of the body, including the heart,

is another cause of heart failure. Although heredity may be responsible for an undue susceptibility to degenerative heart disease, it may also be a result of other diseases that cause damage to the heart.

Prevention of Heart Ailments

Although there may not be complete agreement on any set of rules for preventing or at least delaying the onset of heart disease, many authorities might concur on the following:

1 Proper nutrition, including all the basic food elements, will aid in maintaining all tissues, including those of the heart, in their optimum condition. The avoidance of eating more than is necessary, in order to prevent obesity, will be better for the heart.

2 Infections should be avoided as much as possible. Mild infections should be cared for to prevent serious complications from developing. Dental care should include the treatment of abscesses and the cleaning and filling of decayed teeth.

3 Temperate habits and adequate rest are desirable. People who wish to avoid heart disease need to avoid excesses in the use of tobacco, of alcohol, and of food. On the basis of numerous studies, it appears that the smoker is ten times more likely to die of coronary heart disease than is the nonsmoker. Emotional upsets and psychological upheavals are not conducive to maintaining a healthy heart. Playing too hard is just as damaging as working too hard.

4 Regular physical examinations may be useful, particularly in older persons and in those who have had symptoms that might suggest the presence of disease.

5 Appropriate exercise programs are an important part of prevention as well as of the treatment of heart disease. Regular exercise programs, with gradual increases in the length and difficulty of activity, have been found to be most helpful. To begin with, simple walking may be most effective, followed by such activities as swimming, bicycling, and jogging. Aerobic dancing or other vigorous exercises, in which the person increases the heart rate and

oxygen demand as well as getting recreation, are now used in some physical therapy programs.

Some Practical Aspects of Treatment
Instruments Used in Heart Studies

The *stethoscope* (steth'o-skope) is a relatively simple instrument used for conveying sounds from within the patient's body to the ear of the examiner. Experienced listeners can gain much information using this device. The *electrocardiograph* is used for making records of the changes in the electric currents produced by the contracting heart muscle. It is valuable in detecting certain myocardial injuries.

The *fluoroscope* (floo'o-ro-skop), which is an instrument for examining deep structures with x-rays, may be used to note heart action as well as for observing the size and relationships of some of the thoracic organs. It may be used in conjunction with *catheterization* (kath''e-ter-i-za'shun) of the heart. In this procedure, an extremely thin tube (a catheter) is passed through the veins of the right arm or the right groin, and then into the right side of the heart. During the passage of this tube the fluoroscope is used for observing the route taken by the catheter, and samples of blood are removed through the tube. Finally, the tube is passed all the way through the pulmonary valve and into the large lung arteries. Further samples of blood, removed for testing, are obtained along the way, pressure readings being taken meanwhile.

The *Swan-Ganz catheter* has several lumens and a terminal balloon that is filled with air during catheterization of the right heart. The air-inflated balloon allows the catheter to float through the right atrium, right ventricle and into the pulmonary artery. Used primarily in critically ill patients, it provides many valuable readings on heart function. This catheter is used to diagnose right and left ventricular failure, to monitor fluid replacement, and to regulate the administration of heart-stimulant drugs. The outlets of this tube may be connected to an impressive array of display screens and computers. This newer catheter accomplishes all the older types do and also provides additional information and more safety for the client.

Ultrasound is acoustic energy generated at a frequency above the range of sensitivity of the human ear. In *echocardiography* (ek''o-kar''de-og'rah-fe), also known as ultrasound cardiography, the high-frequency sound vibrations are sent into the heart through the chest wall, then recorded upon return. Cardiac structures return the echoes that are thus derived, giving information about the size and shape of the structures.

Movement of the echoes is traced on an electronic instrument called an oscilloscope, and recorded on film (the same principle is employed by submarines to detect ships).

Some Medicines Used for Heart Disease

The most important, one of the oldest, and still a very valuable drug for many heart patients is *digitalis* (dij''i-tal'is). Digitalis serves to slow and to strengthen contractions of the heart muscle. It is obtained from the leaf of the foxglove, a plant originally found growing wild in many parts of Europe. Foxglove is now being cultivated to ensure a steady supply of digitalis for medical purposes.

Anticoagulants (an''ti-ko-ag'u-lants) also are valuable drugs for heart patients. They may be used to prevent clot formation in persons with damage to heart valves or blood vessels, or following a myocardial infarction.

A potent group of drugs called *inotropins* are used to strengthen the contraction of the heart. These drugs increase the amount of blood pumped by the heart and improve blood flow in the coronary vessels. Dosage of these drugs is regulated by readings obtained by the Swan-Ganz catheter.

Pacemakers

Electric battery-operated pacemakers which supply impulses to regulate the heart beat have been implanted under the skin of many thousands of individuals, the site of implantation is usually in the left chest area. Electrode catheters attached to the pacemaker are then passed into the heart and anchored to the chest wall. The frequency of battery pack replacement varies with the type of pacemaker. Many people whose hearts cannot beat effectively alone have been saved by this rather simple device. In an emergency, a similar stimulus can be supplied to the heart muscle through electrodes placed externally on the chest wall.

Surgery Involving the Heart

The heart–lung machine has made it possible to perform many operations on the heart and other thoracic organs that could not otherwise be done. There are several types of machines in use, all of which serve as a temporary substitute for the patient's heart and lungs.

The machine siphons off the blood from the large vessels entering the heart on the right side so that no blood passes through the heart and lungs. While passing through the machine, the blood is oxygenated by means of an oxygen inlet, and carbon dioxide is removed by various chemical means. These are the processes that normally take place between the blood and the air in the lung tissue. While in the machine, the blood is also "defoamed" to be sure that all air bubbles are removed, since such bubbles could be fatal to the patient by obstructing blood vessels. An electric motor in the machine serves as a pump during the surgical procedure to return the processed blood to the general circulation by way of a large artery.

Coronary bypass surgery to relieve varying degrees of obstruction in the coronary arteries is a common and often successful treatment. The damaged coronary arteries are removed and replaced with healthy segments of blood vessels from the patient's body. Usually parts of the saphenous vein (a superficial vein in the leg) are used. Sometimes as many as six or seven segments are required to replace seriously damaged coronary vessels. The mortality rate in this operation is low. Some patients are able to return to a nearly normal lifestyle following recovery from the surgery.

Diseased valves may become deformed and scarred from endocarditis so that they are ineffective and often obstructive. In some cases a special small knife can be inserted into the heart chamber and the valve can be cut so that it no longer obstructs the blood flow. The valve may even become partially functional. In other cases there may be so much damage that replacement is the only resort. Substitute valves made of plastic materials have proved to be a lifesaving measure for many patients. Very thin butterfly valves made of Dacron or other synthetic material have also been successfully used.

Summary

1 Structure of the heart.
   A Three layers—endocardium, myocardium, and pericardium.
   B Two separate pumps, with an intervening septum.
   C Four chambers—left and right atria and the left and right ventricles.
   D Four valves—tricuspid, pulmonary, mitral, and aortic.
   E Blood supply to the myocardium—coronary arteries.
2 Physiology of the heart.
   A Cardiac cycle includes contraction (systole) and resting phase (diastole).
   B Properties of cardiac muscle—interconnection of muscle cells, variable contraction power.
   C Heart contractions self-sustaining, though nervous control essential for adequate circulation.
   D Events in heart action regulated by a conduction system of tissue—sinoatrial node, atrioventricular node, and bundle of His.
   E Heart sounds and murmurs.
      (1) First and second sounds—lubb, dupp.
      (2) Murmurs caused by faulty valve action—functional or organic.
   F Variations in heart rates.
3 Heart disorders.
   A One grouping according to layer of heart wall—endocarditis, myocarditis, and pericarditis.
   B Another grouping based on age and causation—congenital, rheumatic, coronary, and degenerative.
   C Congenital heart disease—some forms can be corrected by surgery.
   D Rheumatic fever—usually causes endocarditis, leaving scars and adhesions.
   E Coronary heart disease—damage to arteries leading to heart wall can cause sudden death.
   F Fibrillation—rapid, ineffective contractions.
   G Degenerative heart disease: weakening of

heart muscle because of prolonged effects of other diseases.

4 Prevention of heart ailments.
   A Proper nutrition.
   B Prevention and care of infections.
   C Temperate habits and adequate rest.
   D Regular evaluation of physical condition.
   E Avoidance of pollutants, especially tobacco smoke.
   F Regular exercise program.
5 Some practical aspects of diagnosis and treatment.
   A Instruments used in heart studies.
      (1) Stethoscope detects abnormal sounds.
      (2) Electrocardiograph records electric current changes in heart muscle.
      (3) Fluoroscope and catheterization of the heart are used together in visualization and evaluation of heart action and blood circulation.
      (4) Swan-Ganz catheter for diagnosis of heart failure.
      (5) Ultrasound cardiography is an important diagnostic tool.
   B Medications for heart patients include digitalis, anticoagulants, and inotropins.
   C Pacemakers to regulate the heartbeat.
   D Heart surgery.
      (1) Heart–lung machine.
      (2) Coronary bypass.
      (3) Artificial valves as replacements.

Questions and Problems

1 What are the 3 layers of the heart wall?
2 What are the 2 parts of the partition of the heart called? How do they differ from one another?
3 Name each of the chambers of the heart and tell what each does.
4 Name the valves of the heart. Explain the purpose of each valve.
5 Why does the myocardium need its own blood supply? Name these arteries.
6 Explain systole and diastole and tell how these phases are related to each other in the 4 chambers of the heart.
7 How does the heart's ability to contract differ from that of other muscles? What is required to maintain an effective rate of heartbeat?
8 What are the parts of the heart's conduction system called and where are these structures located? Outline the order in which the excitation waves travel.
9 What 2 syllables are used to indicate normal heart sounds, and at what time in the heart cycle can they be heard?
10 Distinguish between tachycardia and bradycardia.
11 Inflammation of the heart tissues is the basis for a classification of heart pathology. Give the 3 terms in this classification and explain each.
12 What is meant by congenital heart disease? Give an example.
13 What part does infection play in rheumatic heart disease?
14 What type of heart disease is the most frequent cause of sudden death?
15 What is the effect of a thrombus in an artery supplying the heart wall? What are some of the precautions that need to be taken by the person who is recovering from thrombosis?
16 What are some of the factors that aid in causing degenerative heart disease?
17 What are some rules that may at least delay the onset of heart ailments?
18 What is a fluoroscope and what is its purpose in heart studies?
19 Of what value is heart catheterization and how is this procedure carried out?
20 What is an electrocardiograph and what is its purpose?
21 How does echocardiography differ from electrocardiography?
22 How does digitalis help the person who has heart muscle damage?
23 What are artificial heart valves made of and how valuable are they?
24 What is the purpose of coronary bypass surgery?

Chapter 15

Blood Vessels and Blood Circulation

- A closed system
- Kinds of blood vessels
- Of what are blood vessels made?
- Names of arteries
- Names of larger veins
- How capillaries work
- Pulse and its meaning
- Blood pressure, normal and abnormal
- Arterial disease
- Hemorrhage and shock
- Disorders of veins

Glossary

Anastomosis A communication between 2 vessels, especially 2 arteries.

Aorta The largest artery.

Arteriole One of the smallest arteries.

Artery A vessel through which blood passes away from the heart to other parts of the body.

Capillary A minute vessel that connects the smallest arteries and the smallest veins.

Hypertension Abnormally high blood pressure.

Hypotension Abnormally low blood pressure.

Portal Pertaining to an entrance, especially to the liver.

Pulse The expansion and contraction of an artery.

Sinus A cavity or hollow space.

Sphygmomanometer An instrument for measuring blood pressure.

Vein A vessel through which blood passes from parts of the body back to the heart.

Venule One of the smallest veins.

Blood vessels, together with the four chambers of the heart, form a closed system for the flow of blood; only if there is an injury to some part of the wall of this system does any blood escape. The circulatory system will be easy to understand now that we know what the blood does and where it is supposed to go. If you keep one eye on the diagrams and the other on the text as the vessels are described, a picture of the system as a whole will gradually emerge.

Kinds of Blood Vessels
Functional Classification

On the basis of function, blood vessels may be divided into three groups: arteries, veins, and capillaries.

1 **Arteries** carry blood from the ventricles (pumping chambers) of the heart out to the capillaries in organs and other parts of the body.
2 **Veins** drain capillaries in the tissues and the organs, and return the blood to the heart.
3 **Capillaries** allow for exchanges between the blood and the body cells, or between the blood

and the air in the lung tissues. The capillaries connect the smallest arteries (arterioles) and the smallest veins (venules).

Arteries and veins both may be subdivided into two groups or circuits: pulmonary and systemic.

1 **Pulmonary** vessels are related to the lungs. They include the pulmonary artery and its branches to the capillaries in the lungs, and the veins that drain those capillaries. The pulmonary arteries carry blood low in oxygen from the right ventricle, while the pulmonary veins carry blood high in oxygen from the lungs into the left atrium (Fig. 15-1). This circuit concerns itself with eliminating carbon dioxide from the blood and replenishing its supply of oxygen.
2 **Systemic** (sis-tem'ik) arteries and veins are related to the rest of the body. This circuit is concerned with supplying food and oxygen to all the tissues of the body and carrying away waste materials from the tissues for disposal.

Structure of Blood Vessels

Artery Walls

The arteries have thick walls because they receive the pumping drive from the ventricles of the heart. There are three coats (tunics) which resemble the three tissue layers of the heart:

1 The innermost membrane of **endothelium** forms a smooth surface over which the blood may easily move.
2 The second, more bulky layer is made of **involuntary muscle** combined with elastic connective tissue.
3 An outer tunic is made of a supporting **connective tissue**.

The largest artery, the *aorta,* is about 1 inch in diameter and has the thickest wall because it receives blood under the highest pressure from the left ventricle. The smallest subdivisions of arteries, the *arterioles* (ar-te're-oles), have thinner walls in which there is very little connective tissue but relatively more smooth muscle.

Capillary Walls

The microscopic branches of these tiny connecting vessels have the thinnest walls of any vessels: one cell layer. The capillary walls are transparent and are made of smooth platelike cells that continue from the lining of the arteries. Because of the thinness of these walls, exchanges between the blood and the body cells are possible. The capillary boundaries are the most important center of activity for the entire circulatory system. Their function is explained later in this chapter.

Walls of Veins

The smallest veins, called *venules* (ven'ules), are formed by the union of capillaries. Their walls are only slightly thicker than those of the capillaries. As the veins become larger, the walls become thicker. However, veins have much thinner walls than those of comparable arteries because the blood within them is under much lower pressure. Although there are three layers of tissue in the walls of the larger veins, as in the artery walls, the middle tunic is relatively thin in vein walls. Therefore, veins are easily collapsed, and slight pressure on the vein by a tumor or some other mass may interfere with the return blood flow. Most veins are equipped with one-way valves which permit the blood to flow in only one direction. They are most numerous in the veins of the extremities (Fig. 15-2).

Names of Systemic Arteries

The Aorta and Its Parts

The aorta is by far the largest artery of the body. It extends upward and to the right from the left ventricle. Then it curves backward and to the left. It continues down behind the heart just in front of the vertebral column, through the diaphragm, and into the abdomen (Figs. 15-3 and 15-4). The aorta is one continuous artery that is divided into four sections:

1 The **ascending aorta** is near the heart and inside the pericardial sac.

(*Text continues on p. 210.*)

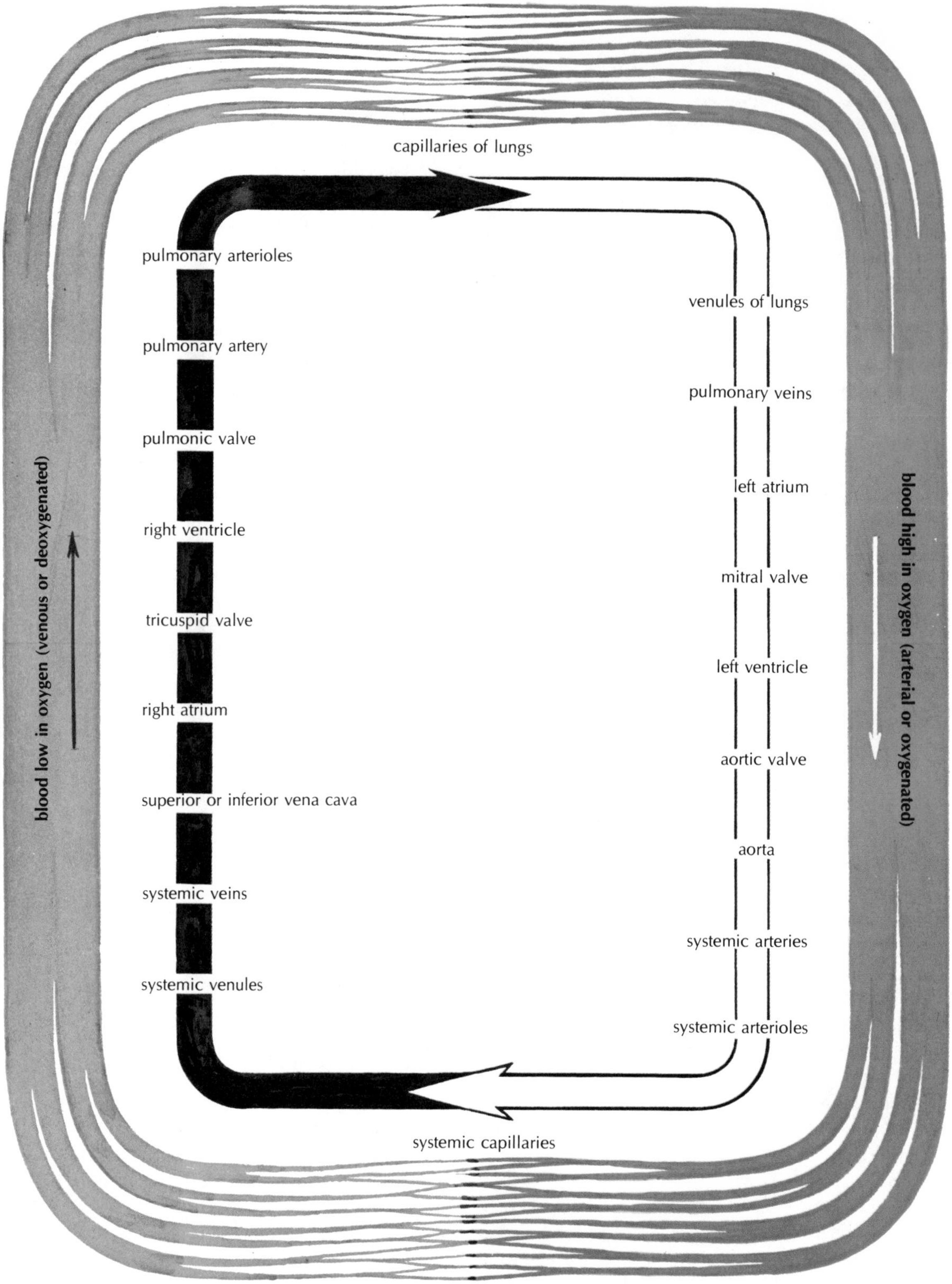

Fig. 15-1 *Blood vessels constitute a closed system for the flow of blood. Note that changes in oxygen content occur as the blood flows through capillaries.*

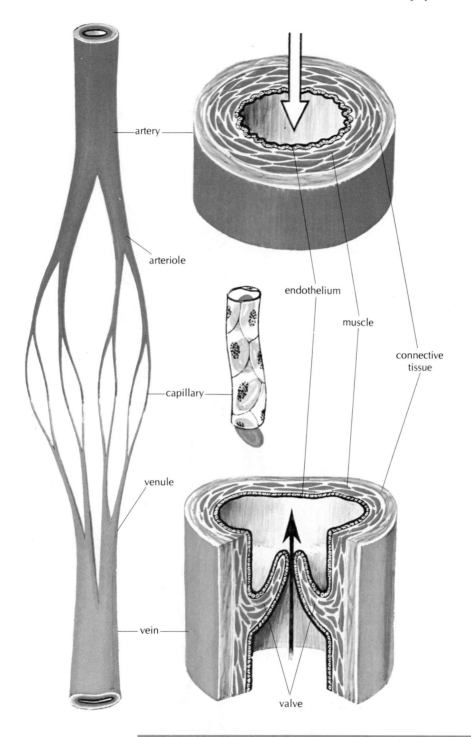

Fig. 15-2 *Sections of small blood vessels to show the thicker arterial walls and the thin walls of veins and capillaries. Venous valves also are shown. The arrows indicate the direction of blood flow.*

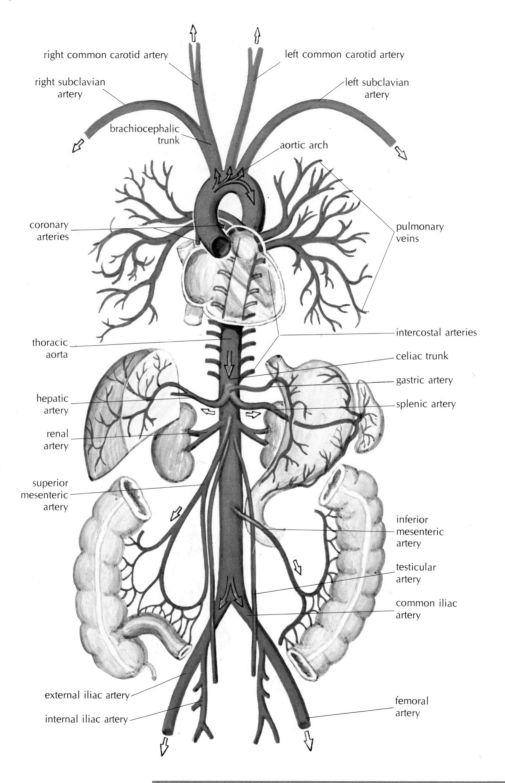

right common carotid artery

left common carotid artery

right subclavian artery

left subclavian artery

brachiocephalic trunk

aortic arch

coronary arteries

pulmonary veins

thoracic aorta

intercostal arteries

celiac trunk

gastric artery

hepatic artery

splenic artery

renal artery

superior mesenteric artery

inferior mesenteric artery

testicular artery

common iliac artery

external iliac artery

internal iliac artery

femoral artery

Fig. 15-3 *The aorta and its branches. The arrows indicate the flow of blood. The pulmonary veins carry oxygenated blood from the lungs to the left atrium of the heart.*

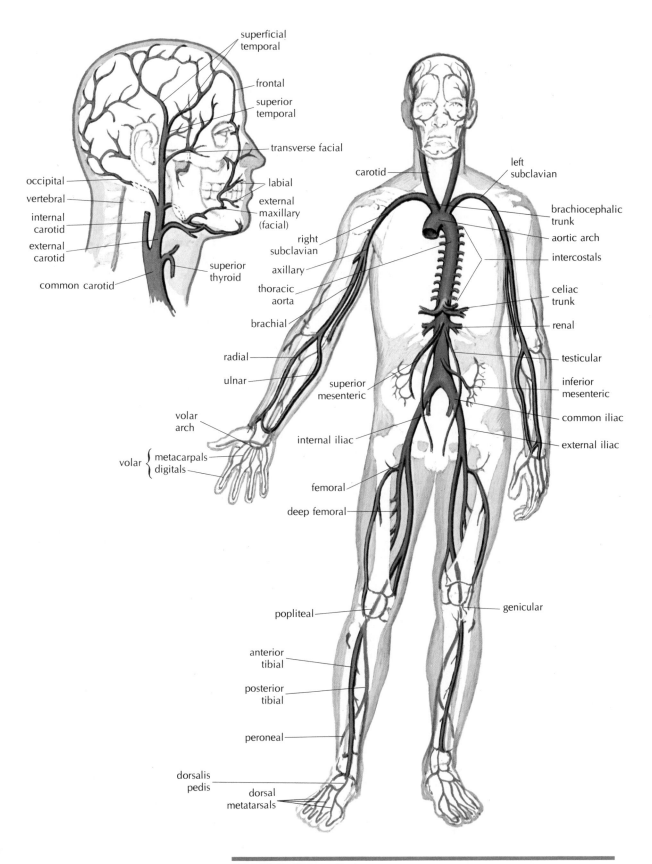

Fig. 15-4 Principal arteries.

2   The **aortic arch** curves from the right to the left, and also extends backward.

3   The **thoracic** (tho-ras′ik) **aorta** lies just in front of the vertebral column behind the heart and in the space behind the pleura.

4   The **abdominal aorta** is the longest section of the aorta, spanning the abdominal cavity.

Branches of the Ascending Aorta

The first, or ascending, part of the aorta has two branches called the left and right *coronary arteries,* which supply the heart muscle. These form a crown around the base of the heart and give off branches to all parts of the myocardium.

Branches of the Aortic Arch

The arch of the aorta, located immediately beyond the ascending aorta, gives off three large branches.

1   The **brachiocephalic** (brak″e-o-se-fal′ik) **trunk** is a short artery formerly called the innominate. After extending upward somewhat less than 2 inches (5 cm), it divides into the **right subclavian** (sub-kla′ve-an) **artery,** which supplies the right upper extremity (arm), and the **right common carotid** (kah-rot′id) **artery,** which supplies the right side of the head and the neck.

2   The **left common carotid artery** extends upward from the highest part of the aortic arch. It supplies the left side of the neck and the head.

3   The **left subclavian artery** extends under the left collar bone (clavicle) and supplies the left upper extremity. This is the last branch of the aortic arch.

Branches of the Thoracic Aorta

The third part of the aorta supplies branches to the chest wall, to the esophagus (e-sof′ah-gus), and to the bronchi (the treelike subdivisions of the trachea (windpipe) and their subdivisions in the lungs. There are usually nine to ten pairs of *intercostal* (in-ter-kos′tal) *arteries* that extend between the ribs, sending branches to the muscles and other structures of the chest wall.

Branches of the Abdominal Aorta

As in the case of the thoracic aorta, there are unpaired branches extending forward and paired arteries extending toward the side. The unpaired vessels are large arteries that supply the abdominal viscera. The most important of these visceral branches are listed below.

1   The **celiac** (se′le-ak) **trunk** is a short artery about ½ inch (1.25 cm) long that subdivides into three branches, namely, the *left gastric* to the stomach, the *splenic* (splen′ik) to the spleen, and the *hepatic* (he-pat′ik) *artery* which carries oxygenated blood to the liver.

2   The **superior mesenteric** (mes′en-ter′ik) **artery** is the largest of these branches, and carries blood to most of the small intestine as well as to the first half of the large intestine.

3   The much smaller **inferior mesenteric artery** is located below the superior mesenteric and near the end of the abdominal aorta, and supplies the last half of the large intestine.

The lateral (paired) branches of the abdominal aorta include the following right and left divisions:

1   The **phrenic** (fren′ik) **arteries** supply the diaphragm.

2   The **suprarenal** (su-prah-re′nal) **arteries** supply the adrenal (suprarenal) glands.

3   The **renal** (re′nal) **arteries,** largest in this group, carry blood to the kidneys.

4   The **ovarian arteries** in the female and **testicular** (tes-tik′u-lar) **arteries** in the male (formerly called the spermatic arteries), supply the sex glands.

5   Four pairs of **lumbar** (lum′bar) **arteries,** extend into the musculature of the abdominal wall.

Iliac Arteries and Their Subdivisions

The abdominal aorta finally divides into two common *iliac arteries.* Each of these vessels, about 2 inches (5 cm) long, extends into the pelvis, where each one subdivides into *internal* and *external* iliac arteries. The internal iliac vessels then send branches to the pelvic organs, including the urinary bladder, the rectum, and some of the reproductive organs. The external iliac arteries continue into the thigh, as the *femoral* (fem′or-al) *arteries*. These vessels give off branches in the thigh and then become the *popliteal* (pop-lit′e-al) *arteries* which subdivide below the knee. The subdivisions include the *tibial arteries* and the *dorsalis* (dor-sa′lis) *pedis* (pe′dis), which supply the leg and the foot.

Other Subdivisions of Systemic Arteries

Just as the larger branches of a tree give off limbs of varying sizes, so the arterial tree has a multitude of subdivisions. Hundreds of additional names might be included, but we shall mention only a few. For example, each common carotid artery gives off branches to the thyroid gland and other structures in the neck before dividing into *external* and *internal carotid arteries* that supply parts in the head. The hand receives blood that courses through the subclavian artery, which becomes the *axillary* (ak′si-lar-e) in the axilla (armpit). The longest part of this vessel, the *brachial* artery, is in the arm proper. It subdivides into two branches near the elbow. These are the *radial artery,* which continues down the thumb side of the forearm and wrist, and the *ulnar artery,* which extends along the medial or little finger side into the hand.

Anastomoses

A communication between two arteries is called an *anastomosis* (ah-nas-to-mo′sis). By this means, blood reaches vital organs by more than one route. Some examples of such unions of end arteries are described below.

1 The **circle of Willis** receives blood from the two internal carotid arteries as well as from the *basilar* (bas′i-lar) *artery,* which is formed by the union of two vertebral arteries. This arterial circle lies just under the center of the brain and sends branches to the **cerebrum** and to other parts of the brain.
2 The **volar** (vo′lar) **arch** is formed by the union of the radial and ulnar arteries in the hand. It sends branches to the hand and the fingers.
3 The **mesenteric arches** are made of communications between branches of the vessels that supply blood to the intestinal tract.

4 Arches are formed by the union of the tibial arteries in the foot, and similar anastomoses are found in various parts of the body.

Arteriovenous anastomoses are found in a few parts of the body including the external ears, the hands, and the feet. Vessels that have muscular walls connect arteries with veins and thus bypass the capillaries. This provides a more rapid flow and a greater volume of blood, thus protecting those exposed parts from freezing in cold weather.

Names of Systemic Veins
Superficial Veins

Whereas most arteries are located in protected and rather deep areas of the body, many veins are found near the surface. The most important of these superficial veins are in the extremities. These include the following:

1 The veins on the back of the hand and at the front of the elbow. Those at the elbow are often used for removing blood samples for test purposes, as well as for intravenous injections. The largest of this group of veins are the **cephalic** (se-fal′ik), the **basilic** (bah-sil′ik), and the **median cubital** (ku′be-tal) **veins.**
2 The **saphenous** (sah-fe′nus) **veins** of the lower extremities, which are the longest veins of the body. The great saphenous vein begins in the foot and extends up the medial side of the leg, the knee, and the thigh. It finally empties into the femoral vein near the groin.

Deep Veins

The deep veins tend to parallel arteries and usually have the same names as the corresponding arteries. Examples of these include the *femoral* and the *iliac* vessels of the lower part of the body and the *brachial,* the *axillary,* and the *subclavian* vessels of the upper extremities. However, exceptions are found in the veins of the head and the neck. The *jugular* (jug′u-lar) *veins* drain the areas supplied by the carotid arteries. Two *brachiocephalic* (innominate) *veins* are formed, one on each side, by the union of the subclavian and the jugular veins. (Remember, there is but one brachiocephalic artery.)

Superior Vena Cava

The veins of the head, the neck, the upper extremities, and the chest all drain into the *superior vena cava* (ve'nah ka'vah), which goes to the heart. It is formed by the union of the right and the left brachiocephalic veins which drain the head, the neck, and the upper extremities. The *azygos* (az'i-gos) *vein* drains the veins of the chest wall and empties into the superior vena cava just before the latter empties into the heart (Fig. 15-5).

Venous Sinuses

The word "sinus" means "a space" or "a hollow." The sinusoids (the word means "like a sinus") found in the liver, the spleen, the thyroid gland, and other structures are channels within the tissues of the organ. Larger channels that do not have the usual tubular structure of the veins also may drain deoxygenated blood. They are known as *venous sinuses*. An important example of a venous sinus is the *coronary sinus,* which receives most of the blood from the veins of the heart wall (see Fig. 14-3). It lies between the left atrium and left ventricle on the under (inferior) surface of the heart. It empties directly into the right atrium along with the two venae cavae.

Other important venous sinuses are located inside the skull. They are the *cranial venous sinuses* which drain the veins that come from all over the brain (Fig. 15-6). The largest of the cranial venous sinuses are described below.

1   The two **cavernous sinuses,** situated behind the eyeballs, serve to drain the *ophthalmic veins* of the eyes.
2   The **superior sagittal** (saj'i-tal) **sinus** is a single long space located in the midline above the brain and in the fissure between the two hemispheres of the cerebrum. It ends in an enlargement called the *confluence* (kon'floo-ens) of sinuses.
3   The two **transverse sinuses** which also are called the **lateral sinuses.** These sinuses are large spaces between the layers of the dura mater (a brain membrane) and extend toward each side after beginning posteriorly, in the region of the confluence of sinuses. As each sinus extends around the inside of the skull, it receives blood draining those parts not already drained by the superior sagittal and the other sinuses that join the back portions of the transverse sinuses. This means that nearly all the blood that comes from the veins of the brain eventually empties into one or the other of the transverse sinuses. On either side the sinus extends far enough forward to empty into an internal jugular vein, which then passes through a hole in the skull to continue downward in the neck.

Inferior Vena Cava

The *inferior vena cava* is much longer than the superior vena cava. The inferior vena cava returns the blood from the parts of the body below the diaphragm. It begins in the lower abdomen with the union of the two common iliac veins. It then ascends along the back wall of the abdomen, through a groove in the posterior part of the liver, through the diaphragm, and finally through the lower thorax to empty into the right atrium of the heart.

The drainage into the inferior vena cava is more complicated than drainage into the superior vena cava. We may divide the large veins below the diaphragm into two groups:

1   Those right and left veins that drain paired parts and organs. They include the *iliac veins* from near the groin; four pairs of *lumbar veins* from the dorsal part of the trunk and from the spinal cord; the veins from the testes of the male and the ovaries of the female called either the *testicular* (spermatic) *veins* or the *ovarian veins;* the *renal* and *suprarenal veins* from the kidneys and some glands near the kidneys; and finally the large *hepatic veins* from the liver. For the most part, these vessels empty directly into the inferior vena cava. The left testicular (spermatic) in the male and the left ovarian in the female empty into the left renal vein, which then takes this blood to the inferior vena cava; these veins thus constitute exceptions to the rule that the paired veins empty directly into the vena cava.
2   Unpaired veins which come from the spleen and from parts of the digestive tract (stomach and intestine) and empty into a vein called the portal vein. Unlike other veins, which empty into the inferior vena cava, the portal vein is part of a special system that enables blood to circulate through the liver before returning to the heart.

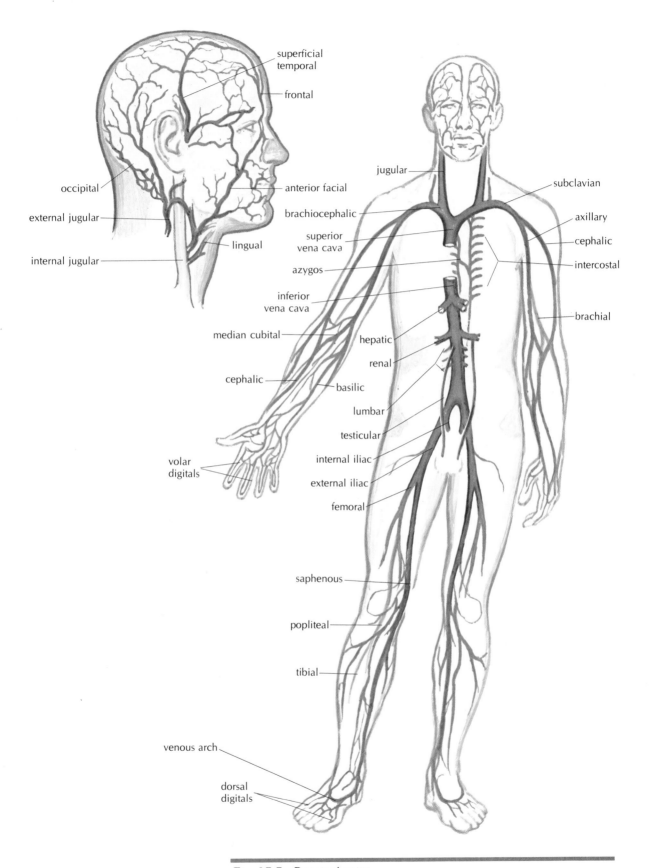

Fig. 15-5 *Principal veins.*

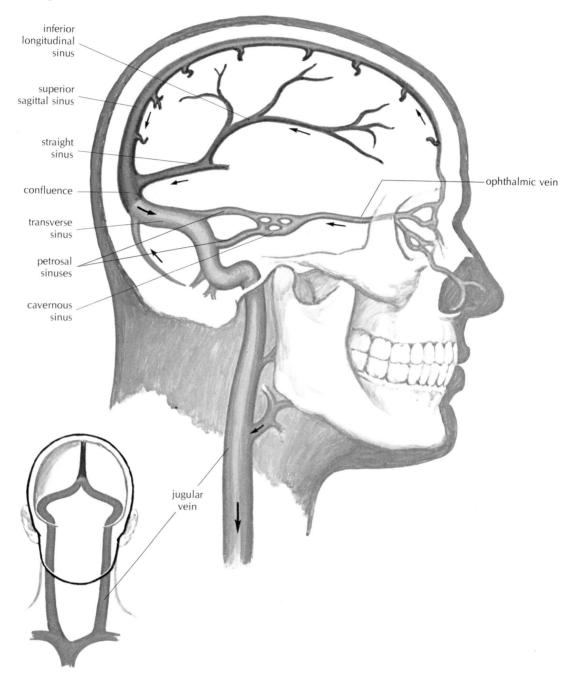

inferior longitudinal sinus

superior sagittal sinus

straight sinus

confluence

transverse sinus

petrosal sinuses

cavernous sinus

ophthalmic vein

jugular vein

Fig. 15-6 *Cranial venous sinuses. The paired transverse sinuses, which carry blood from the brain into the jugular veins, are shown in light blue in the inset.*

The Portal System

The portal system of veins includes those veins that drain blood from capillaries in the spleen, stomach, pancreas, and intestine. In general, these veins have the same names as the arteries that carry blood to the aforementioned organs. However, instead of emptying their blood directly into the inferior vena cava, they deliver it to the portal vein for a detour through the liver. The largest tributary of the portal vein is the *superior mesenteric vein.* It is joined by the *splenic vein* just under the liver. Other tributaries of the portal circulation are the *gastric,* the *pancreatic,* and the *inferior mesenteric veins.*

Upon entering the liver, the portal vein divides and subdivides into ever smaller branches. Eventually, the portal blood flows into a vast network of capillary-like vessels called *sinusoids* (si′nusoids). Since this portal blood has already passed through capillaries in other organs, its oxygen content is low. However, as noted earlier in this chapter, the hepatic artery is responsible for carrying oxygenated blood to the liver. After leaving the sinusoids, blood is finally collected by the hepatic veins which empty into the inferior vena cava (Fig. 15-7).

The purpose of the portal system of veins is to transport blood from the digestive organs and the spleen to the liver sinusoids so the liver cells can carry out their functions. For example, when food is digested, most of the end products are absorbed from the small intestine into the bloodstream and transported to the liver by the portal system. In the liver, these nutrients are processed, stored, and released as needed into the general circulation (see Chap. 18).

How Capillaries Work

In a general way, the circulating blood might be compared to a train that travels around the country, loading and unloading freight in each of the cities that it serves. For example, as blood flows through capillaries surrounding the air sacs in the lungs, it picks up oxygen and unloads carbon dioxide. Later, when this oxygenated blood is pumped to capillaries in other parts of the body, it unloads the oxygen and picks up the carbon dioxide (Fig.

15-8) as well as other substances resulting from cellular activities in the areas being served.

Although the heart, the arteries, and the veins all are essential parts of the circulatory system, the microscopic capillaries are of fundamental importance. It is only through these thin-walled vessels that the aforementioned exchanges can take place. However, one must not forget that all living cells are immersed in a slightly salty liquid called tissue fluid. Looking again at Figure 15-8, one can see how this fluid serves as a "middleman" between the capillary membrane and the neighboring cells. As water, oxygen, and other materials necessary for cellular activity pass through the capillary walls they enter the tissue fluid. Then these substances make their way (by diffusion) to the cells. At the same time, coming from the cells and moving in the opposite direction, are carbon dioxide and other end products of cell metabolism. These substances enter the capillary and are carried away in the bloodstream, to reach other organs or to be eliminated from the body.

The pressures within the capillaries vary considerably. In resting tissues, many of the capillaries are collapsed, while during activity an enormous amount of fluid moves across the capillary walls. The passage of fluids may occur through the tiny intervals between cells, or some fluids may pass through the endothelial cells. The movement of blood through the capillaries is relatively slow. This is due to the much larger cross-sectional area comprising the capillaries compared with that of the larger vessels from which capillaries branch. The slower progress through the capillaries allows more time for exchanges to occur.

Pulse and Blood Pressure
Meaning of the Pulse

The ventricles pump blood into the arteries regularly about 70 to 80 times a minute. The force of ventricular contraction starts a wave of increased pressure which begins at the heart and travels along the arteries. This wave is called the *pulse.* It can be felt in the arteries that are relatively close to the surface, particularly if the vessel can be pressed down against a bone. At the wrist the radial artery

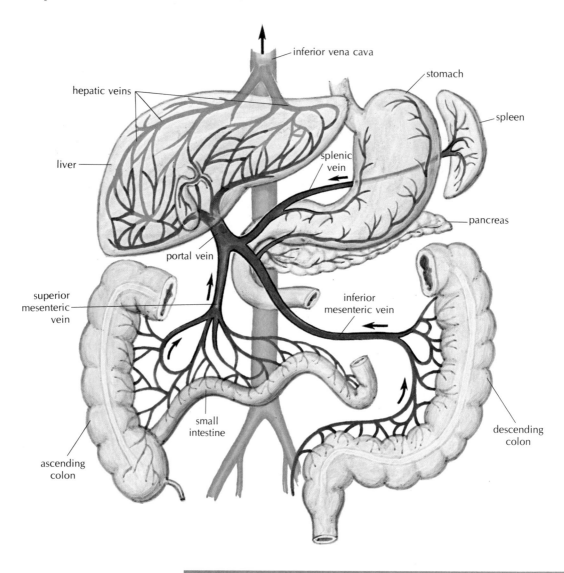

Fig. 15-7   *Portal circulation.*

passes over the bone on the thumb side of the forearm, and the pulse is most commonly obtained here. Other vessels sometimes used for obtaining the pulse include the carotid artery in the neck and the dorsalis pedis on the top of the foot.

Normally, the pulse rate is the same as the heart rate. Only if a heartbeat is abnormally weak, or if the artery is obstructed, may the beat not be detected as a pulse. In checking the pulse of another person, it is important to use the second or third fingers. If you use your thumb, you may find that you are getting your own pulse. When taking

a pulse, it is important to gauge the strength as well as the regularity and the rate.

Various factors may influence the pulse rate. We will enumerate just a few:

1   The pulse is somewhat faster in smaller people and usually is slightly faster in women than in men.

2   In a newborn infant the rate may be from 120 to 140 beats per minute. As the child grows, the rate tends to become slower.

3   Muscular activity influences the pulse rate. Dur-

ing sleep the pulse may slow down to 60 a minute, while during strenuous exercise the rate may go up to well over 100 a minute. If a person is in good condition, the pulse does not remain rapid despite a continuation of exercise.

4 Emotional disturbances may increase the pulse rate.

5 In many infections, the pulse rate increases with the increase in temperature.

6 An excessive amount of secretion from the thyroid gland may cause a rapid pulse. The pulse rate may serve as a partial guide for the person who must take thyroid extract.

Blood Pressure and Its Determination

Since the pressure inside the blood vessels varies with the condition of the heart and the arteries as well as with other factors, the measurement of blood pressure together with careful interpretation may prove a valuable guide in the care and evaluation of a person's health. The pressure decreases as the blood flows from arteries into capillaries and finally into veins. Ordinarily, measurements are made of arterial pressure only. The instrument used is called a *sphygmomanometer* (sfig''mo-mahnom'e-ter). The two measurements made are of

1 The **systolic pressure,** which occurs during heart muscle contraction and averages around 120, expressed in millimeters of mercury (mm Hg).

2 The **diastolic pressure,** which occurs during relaxation of the heart muscle and averages around 80 mm Hg.

The sphygmomanometer is essentially a graduated column of mercury connected to an inflatable

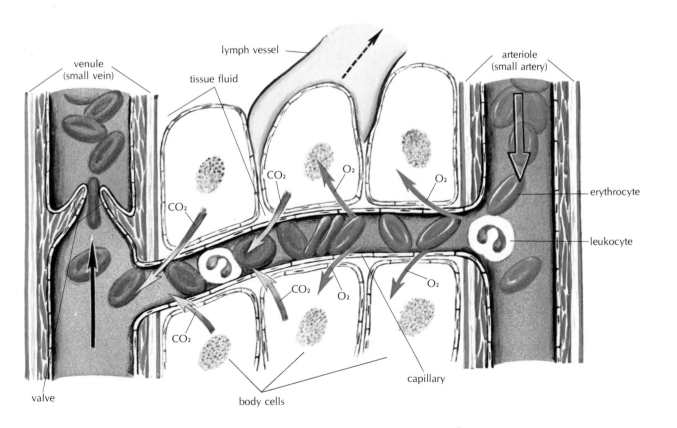

Fig. 15-8 *Diagram showing the connection between the small blood vessels through capillaries. Note the lymph capillary, a part of tissue drainage.*

cuff. The cuff is wrapped around the patient's upper arm and is inflated with air until the brachial artery is compressed and the blood flow cut off. Then, listening with a stethoscope, the doctor or nurse slowly lets air out of the cuff until the first pulsations are heard. At this point the pressure in the cuff is equal to the systolic pressure; and this pressure is read off the mercury column. Then, more air is let out until a characteristic muffled sound indicates the point at which the diastolic pressure is to be read. Considerable practice is required to insure an accurate reading.

Abnormal Blood Pressure

Lower-than-normal blood pressure is called *hypotension* (hi''po-ten'shun). However, there are individual variations in normal pressure levels, and what would be a low pressure for one person might be a normal or even a high pressure for someone else. For this reason, hypotension is best evaluated in terms of how well the body tissues are being supplied with blood. For example, a person whose systolic pressure is consistently below his normal range may experience episodes of fainting because of inadequate blood flow to the brain. The sudden lowering of blood pressure below a person's normal level is one symptom of shock. It may occur also in certain chronic diseases as well as in heart block.

Hypertension (hi''per-ten'shun), which is high blood pressure, has received a great deal of attention. Often it occurs temporarily as a result of excitement or exertion. It may be persistent in a number of conditions including the following:

1 Kidney disease and uremia or other toxic conditions.
2 Endocrine disorders such as hyperthyroidism and acromegaly.
3 Artery disease including the so-called hardening of the artery walls.
4 Tumors of the central portion of the adrenal (suprarenal) gland.

Hypertension that has no apparent medical cause is called *essential hypertension*. This condition is fairly common and is seen as a cause of strokes, heart failure, or kidney damage. Treatment is begun with young patients when the diastolic pressure is over 90 mm Hg. An excess of a hormone produced in the kidney, called renin (re'nin), seems to play a role in the severity of this kind of hypertension. Drugs may be given to block excessive renin production and to prevent fluid retention. General health measures such as weight control and avoidance of excessive alcohol and cigarette consumption plus adequate exercise are all beneficial.

Although stress has been placed on the systolic blood pressure, in many cases the diastolic pressure is even more important. The condition of small arteries may have more effect on the diastolic pressure. At any rate, the determination of what really constitutes hypertension depends on each person's normal range. As previously noted, a pressure that is normal for one individual may be abnormal for another.

Disorders Involving the Blood Vessels
Aneurysm of the Aorta

An *aneurysm* (an'u-rizm) is a bulging sac in the wall of an artery or a vein, owing to a localized weakness in that part of the vessel. The aorta is the vessel most commonly involved. The damage to the wall may be congenital, due to infections, or due to degenerative changes referred to as hardening of the arteries. Whatever the cause, the aneurysm continues to grow in size. Sometimes, as it swells, it may cause some derangement of other structures, in which case definite symptoms are manifested. Eventually, however, the walls of the weakened area yield to the pressure, and the aneurysm bursts like a balloon, usually causing immediate death. Some lives may be saved by surgical replacement of the damaged segment with a synthetic graft.

Arterial Degeneration

Changes in the walls of arteries frequently lead to loss of elasticity. This loss of elasticity is accompanied by irregular thickening of the artery wall at the expense of the lumen (space inside the vessel). Areas of yellow, fatlike material may replace the muscle and elastic connective tissue, leading to a disorder called *atherosclerosis* (ath''er-o''skle-ro'sis). Sometimes the lining of the artery is damaged,

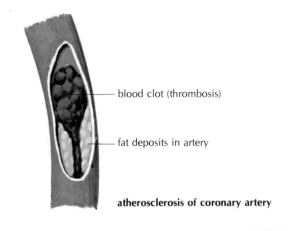

blood clot (thrombosis)

fat deposits in artery

atherosclerosis of coronary artery

Fig. 15-9 Development of coronary thrombosis.

and a blood clot (*thrombus*) may form at this point. Such a thrombus may more or less completely obstruct the vessel, as it sometimes does in coronary thrombosis (Fig. 15-9). In other cases calcium salts and scar tissue (fibrous connective tissue) may cause hardening of the arteries, known as *arteriosclerosis* (ar-te''re-o-skle-ro'sis).

Artery damage may be present for years without causing any noticeable symptoms. As the thickening of the wall continues and the diameter of the passage for blood flow is decreased, a variety of symptoms will appear. The nature of these disturbances will vary with the parts of the body affected and with the extent of the changes in the artery walls. Here are some examples:

1 Muscle cramps and sudden lameness while walking may be due to insufficient blood supply to the lower extremities as a result of artery wall damage.
2 Headaches, dizziness, and mental disorders may be the result of cerebral artery sclerosis.
3 Hypertension may be due to the decrease in size of the lumens within many arteries all over the body. Although hypertension may be present in many younger persons with no apparent artery damage, and arteriosclerosis may be present without causing hypertension, the two are more often found together in older people.
4 Palpitation, dyspnea, paleness, weakness, and other symptoms may be the result of arteriosclerosis of the coronary arteries. The severe pain of angina pectoris may follow the lack of

oxygen and myocardial damage associated with sclerosis of the vessels that supply the heart.
5 An increase in the amount of urine with the appearance of *albumin* (al-bu'min). Albumin is a normal body protein usually found in the urine only if there is kidney damage. Other symptoms referable to the kidneys may be due to damage to the renal arteries.

The gradual narrowing of the interior of the arteries, with a consequent reduction of the volume of blood that passes through them, gives rise to a general condition known as *ischemia* (is-ke'me-ah), which means literally "a suppression of blood." Those parts that are supplied by the damaged artery therefore will suffer from an inadequate blood supply, and the result is that certain vital cells of these organs will gradually die. The death of cells, for whatever cause, is called *necrosis* (ne-kro'sis).

Once these vital cells die, the organ loses its effectiveness. One example of necrosis due to ischemia is the death of certain cells of the brain, with mental disorders as a possible result. Another example of this is the chain of complications resulting from the gradual closure of the arteries of the leg or (rarely) of the arm. The circulation of blood in the toes or the fingers, never too brisk even at the best of times, may cease altogether. Necrosis occurs; the dead tissue is invaded by bacteria, and putrefaction sets in. This condition is called *gangrene* (gang'grene). Gangrene can result from a number of disorders that may injure the arteries, such as diabetes. Diabetic gangrene is a fairly common occurrence in elderly diabetic patients.

Hemorrhage and First Aid

A profuse escape of blood from the vessels is known as *hemorrhage,* a word that means "a bursting forth of blood." Such bleeding may be external or internal, may be from vessels of any size, and may involve any part of the body. Capillary oozing usually is stopped by the normal process of clot formation. Flow from larger vessels can be stopped by appropriate first-aid measures carried out at the scene. In most cases, pressure with a clean bandage directly on the wound will stop the bleeding effectively.

The loss of blood from a cut artery may be rapid and unpleasantly spectacular. Often it is rapidly fatal, and yet immediate appropriate action can be lifesaving. The Red Cross and other organizations that give instructions in first aid agree that excessive loss of blood can and should be prevented in all circumstances. Since hemorrhage is the number one problem in case of an accident, everyone should know that certain arteries can be pressed against a bone to stop hemorrhage. The most important of these "pressure points" are as follows:

1 The **facial artery,** which may be pressed against the lower jaw as the vessel extends along the side of the face, for hemorrhage around the nose, the mouth, and the cheek.
2 The **temporal artery,** which may be pressed against the side of the skull just in front of the ear, to stop hemorrhage on the side of the face and around the ear.
3 The **common carotid artery** in the neck, which may be pressed back against the spinal column, for bleeding in the neck and the head. Avoid prolonged compression which can result in lack of oxygen in the brain.
4 The **subclavian artery,** which may be pressed against the first rib by a downward push with the thumb, to stop bleeding from the shoulder or arm.
5 The **brachial artery,** which may be pressed against the humerus (arm bone), if one pushes inward along the natural groove between the two large muscles of the arm. This stops hand, wrist, and forearm hemorrhage.
6 The femoral artery (in the groin) which may be pressed in order to avoid serious hemorrhage of the lower extremity.

Shock

The word "shock" has a number of meanings. However, in terms of the circulating blood it refers to a life-threatening condition in which there is inadequate blood flow to the tissues of the body. The factor common to all cases of shock is an inadequate output by the heart. Shock can be instigated by a wide range of conditions that reduce the effective circulation. The exact cause of shock is often not known; however a widely used classification is based on causative factors. The most important of these include the following:

1 **Cardiogenic** (kar″de-o-jen′ik) **shock** is sometimes called pump failure. It is often a complication of heart muscle damage as is found in myocardial infarction. It is the leading cause of shock death.
2 **Septic shock** is second only to cardiogenic shock as a cause of shock death. It is usually due to an overwhelming bacterial infection.
3 **Hypovolemic** (hi″po-vo-le′mik) **shock** is due to a decrease in the volume of circulating blood, and may follow severe hemorrhage or burns.
4 **Anaphylactic** (an″ah-fi-lak′tik) **shock** is a severe allergic reaction to foreign substances to which the person has been sensitized.

In many cases the cause of shock is not known and so it is classified according to its severity.

In *mild shock* regulatory mechanisms act to relieve the circulatory deficit. Symptoms are often subtle changes in heart rate and blood pressure. Constriction of small blood vessels and the detouring of blood away from certain organs increase the effective circulation. Mild shock may develop into a severe, life-threatening circulatory failure.

Severe shock is characterized by poor circulation that causes further damage and deepening of the shock. Symptoms of late shock include clammy skin, anxiety, very low blood pressure, rapid pulse, and rapid, shallow breathing. Contractions of the heart are weakened owing to the decrease in blood supply to the heart muscle. The muscles in the blood vessel walls are also weakened so that they dilate. The capillaries become more permeable and lose fluid owing to the accumulation of metabolic wastes.

Treatment of the victim of shock includes first-aid measures such as placing him in a horizontal position and covering him with a blanket. Bleeding should be stopped if it is present. The head should be kept turned to the side to prevent aspiration (breathing in) of vomitus, an important cause of death in shock cases. Further treatment of shock depends largely on treating the causative factors. For example, shock due to fluid loss such as hemorrhage or burns is treated with blood products or plasma expanders. Shock due to heart failure is treated with drugs that will improve the contractions of the heart muscle. In any case, all measures are aimed at supporting the circulation and improving the output of the heart. Oxygen is frequently administered to improve the delivery of oxygen to the tissues.

Varicose Veins

Varicose veins is a condition in which superficial veins have become swollen, tortuous, and ineffective. It may be a problem in the esophagus or in the rectum, but the veins most commonly involved are the saphenous veins of the lower extremities (Fig. 15-10). This condition is found frequently in people who spend a great deal of time standing,

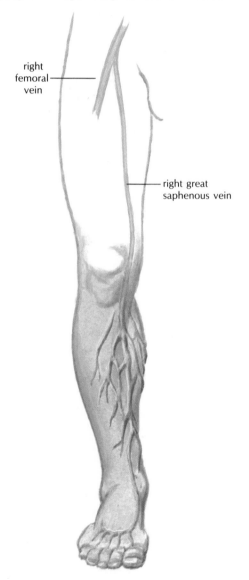

right femoral vein

right great saphenous vein

Fig. 15-10 Varicose veins.

salespeople, for instance. Also, pregnancy, with the accompanying pressure on the veins in the pelvis, may be a predisposing cause. Varicose veins in the rectum are called *hemorrhoids* (hem'o-roids), or *piles.* The general term for varicose veins is *varices* (var'i-sez), the singular form being *varix* (var'iks).

Phlebitis

Inflammation of a vein is called *phlebitis* (fle-bi'tis). There is marked pain, often considerable swelling, and involvement of the entire vein wall. A blood clot may form, causing the dangerous condition called *thrombophlebitis* (throm-bo-fle-bi'tis), with the possibility of a piece of the clot becoming loosened and floating in the blood as an *embolus* (em'bo-lus). If this embolus reaches the lungs, sudden death from *pulmonary embolism* (em'bo-lizm) may be the result. Prevention of infection, early activity to insure circulation following an injury or an operation, and the use of anticoagulant drugs when appropriate have greatly reduced the incidence of this complication.

Stasis Dermatitis and Ulcers

Stasis means a standing still or stoppage in normal blood flow. Often the valves in the veins of the lower extremity become incompetent and blood is not returned from the legs. The skin becomes inflamed and undergoes scaling, and fissures (cracks) form. This is followed by ulcer formation. Treatment of the causes as well as attention to the local lesions should be in the hands of a physician, and patient cooperation is most important.

Arterial Obstruction

When the lumen of an artery is completely blocked by arteriosclerosis, the condition is known as *arteriosclerosis obliterans* (o-blit'er-ans). The complete obstruction to blood flow causes intense pain; if the disease is allowed to progress and is not treated, the affected part or parts may become ulcerated or gangrenous. In such cases, it is often possible to treat the disease surgically.

In some cases, the obstruction is removed by making an incision into the artery after clamps are placed above and below the plug; then the plug is removed by a special instrument.

In other instances, the circulation can be restored by the use of vascular grafts. This is done by cutting out the diseased segment and suturing (sewing) a graft in its place. More often, however, grafts are implanted to bypass the obstructed segment. A vein from the patient's own body, usually the saphenous vein, may be used; or a synthetic vessel made of Dacron or Teflon may be chosen. Sometimes a patch graft is used to increase the lumen of small, narrowed areas of arteries. To accomplish this, the artery is clamped above and below the narrowed area and then incised in the long axis of the vessel. A patch of Teflon is sewn to the edges of the incision, thereby increasing its diameter.

Summary

1 Functional classification of blood vessels.
   A Arteries carry blood from the heart to other parts of the body. Smallest subdivisions are arterioles.
   B Veins drain tissues and return blood to the heart. Smallest subdivisions are venules.
   C Capillaries allow exchanges between blood and body cells. These take place through the tissue fluid.
2 Two circuits.
   A Pulmonary vessels—connected with the lungs.
   B Systemic vessels—form a network in all other parts of the body.
3 Structure of blood vessels.
   A Arteries have thick walls in 3 layers—endothelium, involuntary muscle, and connective tissue.
   B Capillaries are a single cell layer thick, a continuation of the endothelial lining of larger vessels.
   C Veins have 3-layer walls but are more easily collapsed than arteries because of their thinner walls, having less muscle and elastic connective tissue. Most have one-way valves.
4 Names of systemic arteries.
   A Parts of the aorta are the ascending aorta, aortic arch, thoracic aorta, and abdominal aorta.
   B Branches of the ascending aorta are the 2 coronary arteries that supply the heart muscle.
   C Three branches of the aortic arch.
      (1) Brachiocephalic trunk (formerly the innominate artery).
      (2) Left common carotid artery.
      (3) Left subclavian artery.

D Branches of the thoracic aorta.
   (1) Esophageal artery.
   (2) Bronchial arteries.
   (3) Intercostal arteries—9 or 10 pairs.
E Branches of the abdominal aorta.
   (1) Unpaired branches to the viscera.
      (a) Celiac artery to stomach, spleen, and liver.
      (b) Superior mesenteric to small intestine and first half of large intestine.
      (c) Inferior mesenteric artery to last half of large intestine.
   (2) Paired branches.
      (a) Phrenic arteries to the diaphragm.
      (b) Suprarenal arteries to the adrenal (suprarenal) glands.
      (c) Renal arteries to the kidneys.
      (d) Ovarian arteries or testicular (spermatic) arteries to the sex glands.
      (e) Lumbar arteries (4 pairs) to muscles of abdominal wall.
   (3) Iliac arteries.
      (a) Internal (hypogastric) arteries to pelvic organs.
      (b) External (femoral) arteries to thigh, which continue as the popliteal arteries. These subdivide below knee; latter group includes tibial arteries and dorsalis pedis.
F Other arteries and structures.
   (1) Common carotid divides into internal and external carotid arteries.
   (2) Subclavian becomes axillary and then brachial arteries.
   (3) Brachial artery subdivides into radial and ulnar arteries.

(4) Anastomoses are communications between arteries.
    (a) Circle of Willis to the brain.
    (b) Volar arch in the hand to supply fingers.
    (c) Mesenteric arches to the intestine.
    (d) Arches formed by the tibial arteries.
(5) Arteriovenous anastomoses bypass capillaries.

5 Names of systemic veins.
  A Superficial veins near the surface in extremities.
    (1) Cephalic, basilic, and the median cubital veins, all in the upper extremities.
    (2) Saphenous veins in lower extremities.
  B Deep veins accompany or parallel arteries and have the same names as the arteries.
    (1) Examples—femoral, iliac, brachial, axillary, subclavian.
    (2) Jugular veins from head and neck are important exceptions to the naming rule.
  C Superior vena cava receives all tributaries from above the diaphragm.
  D Venous sinuses.
    (1) Coronary sinus.
    (2) Cranial sinuses. Largest are 2 cavernous, a single superior sagittal, and 2 transverse (lateral) sinuses.
  E Inferior vena cava receives paired vessels from below diaphragm.
  F Portal system.
    (1) Portal vein receives unpaired veins from spleen, stomach, and intestine.
    (2) Portal vein subdivides in liver until sinusoids are formed.
    (3) Blood from sinusoids collected by hepatic veins empties into inferior vena cava.
    (4) System provides for detour of gastrointestinal and splenic blood through liver; important for liver functions.

6 Thin-walled capillaries provide place for exchanges of oxygen, nutrients, and metabolic waste products.
  A Tissue fluid serves as middleman between capillary and cell membranes.
  B Slow flow provides time for exchanges.

7 Pulse and blood pressure.

A Pulse is a wave in the arteries due to contraction of the heart muscle.
B Pulse varies with the size, sex, age, and activity of the healthy person.
C Pulse rate may be increased by emotional disturbances, fever, or excessive thyroid secretion.
D Blood pressure systolic during heart contraction, diastolic during relaxation of ventricles.
E Stethoscope and sphygmomanometer used for obtaining readings.
F Hypotension is an important symptom of shock.
G Hypertension may be temporary in cases of excitement and exertion.
H Hypertension is likely to be persistent in kidney, endocrine, and artery diseases.
I No known cause for essential hypertension.

8 Disorders involving the blood vessels.
  A Aneurysm is saclike enlargement of a vessel, commonly the aorta.
  B Arterial degeneration embraces many changes.
    (1) Atherosclerosis.
    (2) Arteriosclerosis.
    (3) Ischemia, necrosis, and gangrene can be complications of above.
  C Hemorrhage from arteries most serious emergency.
    (1) Direct pressure on wound often effective.
    (2) Use pressure points in certain cases.
  D Shock caused by factors that reduce circulatory effectiveness.
    (1) Decreased pumping capacity of damaged heart.
    (2) Inadequate venous return to the heart.
    (3) Treatment—whole blood, blood plasma, or drugs to improve circulation.
  E Varicose veins—swollen and ineffective. Common in legs and rectum (hemorrhoids).
  F Phlebitis—inflammation of a vein. Thrombophlebitis, a dangerous complication, may cause fatal pulmonary embolism.
  G Stasis dermatitis and ulcers.
  H Arterial obstruction.
    (1) Removal by surgery.
    (2) Vascular grafts or synthetic parts to replace damaged segments.

Questions and Problems

1 Name the 3 main groups of blood vessels and describe their functions. How has function affected structure?

2 Trace a drop of blood through the shortest possible route from the capillaries of the foot to the capillaries of the head.

3 What are the names and functions of some cranial venous sinuses? Where is the coronary venous sinus and what does it do?

4 What large vessels drain the blood low in oxygen from most of the body into the right atrium? What vessels carry blood high in oxygen into the left atrium?

5 Trace a drop of blood from capillaries in the wall of the small intestine to the right atrium. What is the purpose of going through the liver on this trip?

6 Why are capillaries of fundamental importance to the circulatory system?

7 What is meant by pulse? Where is it most often obtained? If a large part of the body were burned, leaving only the lower extremities accessible for obtaining the pulse, what vessel would you try to use?

8 What are some factors that cause an increase in the pulse rate?

9 What instrument is used for obtaining the blood pressure? What are the two values usually obtained called and what is the significance of each?

10 What are some examples of disorders that cause hypertension of a persistent kind? Of what importance is diastolic blood pressure?

11 What are some symptoms of arteriosclerosis and how are these produced?

12 What is the meaning of hemorrhage? What vessels cause the most serious bleeding if they should be cut? What are some of the most effective ways of stopping hemorrhage?

13 What is shock, and why is it so dangerous? Name some symptoms of shock.

14 In what organs are varicose veins found most commonly? In what situations are they given special names? Give examples.

15 What is the most serious complication of phlebitis of lower extremity veins?

Chapter 16

The Lymphatic System and Lymphoid Tissue

- What lymph is
- The lymphatic system and lymph circulation
- Lymphoid tissue
- Lymph nodes
- The reticuloendothelial system
- The tonsils, the thymus and the spleen
- Disorders of the lymphatic system and lymphoid tissue

Glossary

Duct A passage with defined walls, especially a tube for passage of excretions or secretions.

Hilus A depression at that part of an organ where vessels and nerves enter.

Lymph A yellowish, relatively clear, watery fluid found in the lymphatic vessels; a liquid containing cells, mostly lymphocytes, and, after a meal, fat globules; any clear, watery fluid resembling true lymph.

Reticuloendothelial Pertaining to tissues that have certain common characteristics and that work together to carry out certain functions related to body defense.

Spleen A large glandlike organ located in the upper part of the abdominal cavity.

Thymus An elongated mass of lymphatic tissue, usually consisting of 2 lobes, located in the upper chest cavity beneath the sternum. It is believed to play a part in the immunity responses of the body.

The Lymphatic System

It may be recalled, from the section called "How capillaries work" in the preceding chapter that the body cells live in tissue fluid, a liquid that is derived from the bloodstream. Water and dissolved substances, such as oxygen and nutrients, are constantly filtering through capillary walls into the spaces between cells, and constantly adding to the volume of tissue fluid. However, under normal conditions, there is also a constant removal of fluid so that it does not accumulate in the tissues. For example, part of this fluid simply returns (by diffusion) to the capillary bloodstream, taking with it some of the end products of cellular metabolism, including carbon dioxide and other substances. A second pathway for the drainage of tissue fluid involves the *lymphatic system*. In addition to the blood-carrying capillaries, there are microscopic vessels called *lymphatic capillaries*. These vessels drain away the excess tissue fluid that does not return to the blood capillaries (see Fig. 15-8). As soon as tissue fluid enters the lymphatic capillary, it is called *lymph*. The lymphatic capillaries join to form the larger lymphatic vessels, and these vessels (which we shall have a closer look at in a moment) eventually empty into the veins. However, before the lymph reaches the veins, it flows through a series of filters called *lymph nodes,* where bacteria and other foreign particles are trapped and destroyed. Thus, the lymph nodes may be compared in one way with the oil filter in an automobile.

Let us now have a closer look at the lymphatic capillaries, vessels, and nodes.

Lymphatic Capillaries

The lymphatic capillaries resemble the blood capillaries in that they are made of one layer of flattened cells to allow for easy passage of soluble materials and water through them. Unlike the capillaries of the blood stream, the lymphatic capillaries begin blindly; that is, they do not serve to bridge two larger vessels. Instead, one end simply lies within the lake of tissue fluid, while the other communicates with the larger lymphatic vessel.

In the intestine are some specialized lymphatic capillaries called *lacteals* (lak'te-als) which act as one pathway for the transfer of fats from digested food to the bloodstream. This process is covered in the chapter dealing with the digestive system. A lacteal is pictured in Fig. 18-4.

Lymphatic Vessels

The lymphatic vessels are thin-walled and delicate, and have a beaded appearance because of indentations at the regions at which valves are located. These valves prevent backflow in the same way as those that are found in some veins. Although there is no pumping mechanism comparable to the heart, compression of the lymphatic vessels by contraction of the skeletal muscles during exercise, and by changes in position of various parts of the body, help in maintaining the onward flow of lymph.

Lymphatic vessels include *superficial* and *deep* sets. The surface lymphatics are immediately below the skin, often continuing near the superficial veins. The deep vessels are usually larger and accompany the deep veins.

Lymphatic vessels are named according to their location. For example, those in the breast are called *mammary* lymphatic vessels, those in the thigh are called *femoral* lymphatic vessels, and those in the leg are called *tibial* lymphatic vessels. All the lym-

phatic vessels form networks, and at certain points they carry lymph into the regional nodes (the nodes that "service" a particular area). For example, nearly all of the lymph from the upper extremity and the breast passes through the *axillary* lymph nodes while that from the lower extremity passes through the *inguinal* nodes. Lymphatic vessels carrying lymph away from the regional nodes eventually drain into one of the two terminal vessels, the right lymphatic duct or the thoracic duct, which empty into the bloodstream.

The *right lymphatic duct* is a short vessel about ½ inch long (1.25 cm) which receives the lymph that comes from only the right side of the head, the neck, and the thorax, and also from the right upper extremity. It empties into the right subclavian vein. Its opening into this vein is guarded by two pocket-like semilunar valves to prevent blood from entering the duct. The rest of the body is drained by the *thoracic duct.*

The Thoracic Duct

The *thoracic duct* is much the larger of the two terminal vessels; it is about 16 inches (40 cm) in length. As shown in Figure 16-1, the thoracic duct receives lymph from all parts of the body except those above the diaphragm on the right side. This duct begins in the posterior part of the abdominal cavity, below the attachment of the diaphragm. The first part of this duct is enlarged to form a cistern or temporary storage pouch called the *cisterna chyli* (sis-ter'nah ki'li). *Chyle* (kile) is the milky-appearing fluid formed by the combination of fat globules and lymph, which comes from the intestinal lacteals. Chyle passes through the intestinal lymphatic vessels and the lymph nodes of the mesentery, finally entering the cisterna chyli. In addition to chyle, all the lymph from below the diaphragm empties into the cisterna chyli by way of the various clusters of lymph nodes and then is carried by the thoracic duct into the bloodstream.

The thoracic duct extends upward through the diaphragm and along the back wall of the thorax up into the root of the neck on the left side. Here it receives the left jugular lymphatic vessels from the head and the neck, the left subclavian vessels from the left upper extremity, and other lymphatic vessels from the thorax and its parts. In addition to the valves along the duct, there are two at its opening into the left subclavian vein to prevent the passage of blood into the duct.

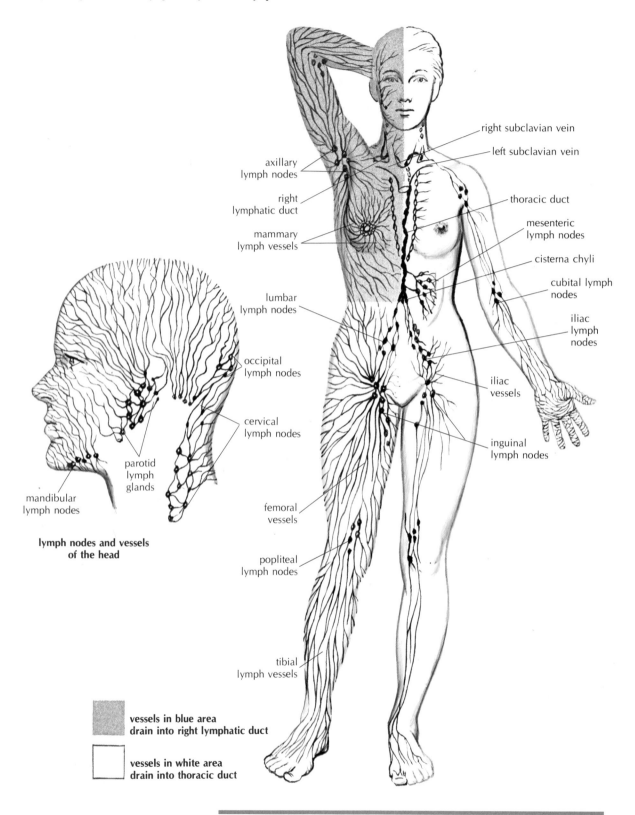

right subclavian vein

left subclavian vein

axillary
lymph nodes

right
lymphatic duct

thoracic duct

mesenteric
lymph nodes

mammary
lymph vessels

cisterna chyli

cubital lymph
nodes

lumbar
lymph nodes

iliac
lymph
nodes

occipital
lymph nodes

cervical
lymph nodes

iliac
vessels

parotid
lymph
glands

inguinal
lymph nodes

mandibular
lymph nodes

**lymph nodes and vessels
of the head**

femoral
vessels

popliteal
lymph nodes

tibial
lymph vessels

**vessels in blue area
drain into right lymphatic duct**

**vessels in white area
drain into thoracic duct**

Fig. 16-1 *The lymphatic system.*

Structures of Lymphoid Tissue

The foregoing section is a brief survey of the system of lymph vessels and lymph transport. The lymph nodes, or filters, have been mentioned repeatedly; but detailed discussion of them has been withheld until now. There has been a reason for this. The lymph nodes are made of a specialized tissue called *lymphoid* (lim'foid) *tissue.* A number of other organs also are made of lymphoid tissue, but some of them have nothing directly to do with the system of lymph transport itself.

Before looking at some typical organs of lymphoid tissue, let us first consider some properties of this kind of tissue and see what characteristics these organs have in common.

Functions of Lymphoid Tissue

Some of the general functions of lymphoid tissue include the following:

1 Removal of impurities such as carbon particles, cancer cells, pathogenic organisms, and dead blood cells.
2 Manufacture of lymphocytes, which make up 20% to 25% of the white blood cells.
3 Production of *antibodies,* which are chemical substances that aid in combatting infection. These will be discussed in a later chapter.

Lymph Nodes

The lymph nodes, as we have seen, are designed to filter the lymph once it is drained from the tissues. The lymph nodes are small rounded masses varying from pinhead size to as much as an inch in length (1 cm to 2.5 cm). Each node has a fibrous connective tissue capsule from which partitions extend into the substance of the organ. Inside the node are masses of lymphatic tissue, with spaces set aside for the production of lymphocytes. At various points in the surface of the node, lymphatic vessels pierce the capsule in order to carry lymph into the spaces inside the pulplike nodal tissue. An indented area called the *hilus* (hi'lus) serves as the exit for lymph vessels carrying lymph out of the node. At this region, other structures, including blood vessels and nerves, connect with the organ.

Lymph nodes seldom are isolated. As a rule, they are massed together in groups, the number in each group varying from 2 or 3 up to well over 100. Some of these groups are placed deeply, while others are superficial. Those of the most practical importance include the following:

1 **Cervical nodes,** located in the neck. They are divided into deep and superficial groups, which drain various parts of the head and the neck. They often become enlarged during upper respiratory infections as well as in certain chronic disorders.
2 **Axillary nodes,** located in the axillae (armpits). They may become enlarged following infections of the upper extremities and the breasts. Cancer cells from the breasts often metastasize (spread) to the axillary nodes.
3 **Tracheobronchial**   (tra-ke-o-brong'ke-al) **nodes,** found near the trachea and around the larger bronchial tubes. In persons living in highly polluted areas, these nodes become so filled with carbon particles that they are solid black masses resembling pieces of coal.
4 **Mesenteric** (mes-en-ter'ik) **nodes,** found between the two layers of peritoneum that form the mesentery. There are some 100 to 150 of these nodes.
5 **Inguinal nodes,** located in the groin region. They receive lymph drainage from the lower extremities and from the external genital organs. When they become enlarged, they are often referred to as *buboes* (bu'boes). The name for *bubonic plague,* which killed so many people during the Middle Ages, arose from the fact that the bacteria caused enlargement of various lymph nodes, especially those in the inguinal region.

This discussion of the lymph nodes completes our short outline of lymph drainage. The following organs of lymphoid tissue perform somewhat different functions, particularly with respect to the substances that they filter.

The Tonsils

There are other masses of lymphoid tissue that are designed to filter not lymph, but tissue fluid. These masses are found beneath certain areas of moist epithelium that are exposed to the outside, and hence to contamination. Such areas include parts of the digestive, the urinary, and the respiratory tracts. With this last-named system are associated those well-known masses of lymphoid tissue called the *tonsils.* The different tonsils include

1   The *palatine* (pal'ah-tin) **tonsils,** which are oval bodies located at each side of the soft palate. These are most commonly known as the tonsils.
2   The **pharyngeal** (fah-rin'je-al) **tonsil,** which, enlarged, is commonly referred to as **adenoids.** It is located behind the nose on the back wall of the upper pharynx.
3   The **lingual** (ling'gwal) **tonsils,** which are little mounds of lymphoid tissue at the back of the tongue.

Any or all of these tonsils may become so loaded with bacteria that the pathogens come to have the upper hand; removal then is advisable. A slight enlargement of any of them will not call for surgery. All lymphoid tissue masses tend to be larger in childhood, so that consideration must be made of the patient's age in determining whether or not these masses are enlarged abnormally.

The Thymus

Because of its appearance under the microscope, the *thymus* (thi'mus) has been considered a part of the lymphoid system. It is located in the upper thorax beneath the sternum. Recent studies point to its having a much more basic function than was originally thought. It now seems apparent that the thymus plays a key role in the formation of antibodies in the first few weeks of life and in the development of immunity. It manufactures lymphocytes and is essential to fetal growth. It seems that the factors that stimulate the formation of lymphocytes come from the thymus itself. Removal causes a decrease in the production of these cells, and a decrease in the size of the spleen and of lymph nodes throughout the body. The thymus is most active during early life. After puberty, the tissue undergoes changes and is replaced by adipose tissue.

The Spleen

The spleen is an organ that contains lymphoid tissue designed to filter blood. It is located in the upper left hypochondriac region of the abdomen and normally is protected by the lower part of the rib cage because it is high up under the dome of the diaphragm. The spleen is rather soft and of a purplish color. It is a somewhat flattened organ about 5 or 6 inches long (12.5 to 16 cm) and 2 or 3 inches wide (5 to 7.5 cm). The capsule of the spleen, as well as its framework, is more elastic than that of the lymph nodes. It contains involuntary muscle which enables the splenic capsule to contract as well as to withstand some swelling.

The spleen has an unusually large blood supply, considering its size. The organ is filled with a soft pulp, one of the functions of which is to filter out the worn-out red blood cells. The spleen also forms cells called phagocytes which engulf bacteria and other foreign particles. Prominent structures inside the spleen are round masses of lymphoid tissue, and it is because of these that the spleen often is classified with the other organs made of lymphoid tissue (although some other category might be better because of the other specialized functions of the spleen).

Some of the functions of the spleen include the following:

1   Destruction of old, worn-out red blood cells. As hemoglobin from the red cells is broken down, iron is salvaged and liberated into the bloodstream for reuse by the body.
2   Formation of certain white blood cells (lymphocytes and monocytes; see Fig. 13-1).
3   Production of antibodies which provide immunity to certain diseases.
4   Production of red blood cells before birth (this function is lost after birth).
5   A reservoir for blood which can be returned to the bloodstream in case of hemorrhage or other emergency.

Although the spleen is the largest unit of lymphoid tissue in the body, *splenectomy* (splen-nek'tome), the surgical removal of the spleen, usually is tolerated quite well since other lymphoid tissues can take over its functions. The human body has thousands of lymphoid units, and the loss of any one unit or group ordinarily is not a threat to life.

The Reticuloendothelial System

The *reticuloendothelial* (re-tik''u-lo-en''do-the'le-al) *system* consists of related cells, which are concerned with the destruction of worn-out blood cells, bacteria, cancer cells, and other foreign substances that are potentially harmful to the body. They include monocytes, which are relatively large white blood cells (see Fig. 13-1). Monocytes are formed in the bone marrow, then circulate in the bloodstream to various parts of the body, Upon entering the tissues, monocytes develop into *macrophages* (mak″ro-faj-es), a term that means "big eaters." Some of them are given special names, as for example, the *Kupffer's* (koop′ferz) cells which are located in the lining of the liver blood spaces (sinusoids). Other parts of the reticuloendothelial system are found in the spleen, bone marrow and in lymph nodes. Some macrophages are located in the lungs, where they are called 'dust cells' because they ingest solid particles that enter the lungs. Other macrophages are found in soft connective tissues all over the body, and are also considered to be part of this protective system.

Some Disorders of the Lymphatic System and Lymphoid Tissue

Lymphangitis

Inflammation of the lymphatic vessels is called *lymphangitis* (lim-fan-ji′tis). Red streaks can be seen to extend along an extremity, usually beginning in the region of an infected and neglected injury. Such inflamed vessels are a danger signal, since the lymph nodes may not be able to stop such a serious infection. The next step would be entrance of the pathogens into the bloodstream, causing *septicemia* (sep-ti-se′me-ah), or blood poisoning. Streptococci often are the invading organisms in such cases.

Elephantiasis

As was mentioned in Chapter 7, *elephantiasis* is a great enlargement of the lower extremities resulting from blockage of lymphatic vessels by small worms, called *filariae* (fi-la′re-e). These tiny parasites, carried by insects such as flies and mosquitoes, invade the tissues as embryos or immature forms. They grow in the lymph channels and thus obstruct the flow of lymph. The swelling of the legs or, as sometimes happens in men, the scrotum, may be so great that the victim becomes incapacitated. This disease is especially common in certain parts of Asia and in some of the Pacific islands. No cure is known.

Adenitis

The word *adenitis* (ad-eh-ni′tis) really means "inflammation of a gland," but is used most frequently to mean "enlarged, tender, and inflamed lymph nodes" (which are not truly glands). Such involvement of the lymph nodes reflects the body's attempt to combat an infection. Cervical adenitis occurs during measles, scarlet fever, septic sore throat, diphtheria, and, frequently, during the common cold. Chronic adenitis may be due to the tubercle bacillus. The so-called cold abscess may begin as a tuberculous adenitis. Lymph nodes in the thorax, especially the tracheobronchial nodes, are frequently involved in tuberculosis.

Splenomegaly

Enlargement of the spleen is known as *splenomegaly* (sple-no-meg′ah-le). Certain acute infectious diseases are accompanied by splenic enlargement. Among these are scarlet fever, typhus fever, typhoid fever, and syphilis. Many tropical parasitic diseases cause splenomegaly. A certain blood fluke (flatworm) which is fairly common among workers in Japan and other parts of Asia causes a marked splenic enlargement.

Splenic anemia is a disease in which enlargement of the spleen is one of a number of symptoms, others being hemorrhages from the stomach and accumulation of fluid in the abdomen. In this disease and others of the same nature, *splenectomy* (sple-nek′to-me), the surgical removal of the spleen, appears to constitute a cure.

Hodgkin's Disease

Hodgkin's disease is a chronic disorder characterized by enlargement of the lymph nodes. The nodes in the neck particularly, and often those in the armpit, thorax, and groin enlarge. The spleen also may enlarge. The condition is more common in young men. Chemotherapy and radiotherapy, either separately or in combination, have been used with good results, affording patients many years of life.

Lymphosarcoma

Lymphosarcoma (lim-fo-sar-ko′mah) is a malignant tumor of lymphoid tissue. It is likely to be a rapidly fatal disorder. Fortunately, it is not a common dis-ease. Early surgery together with appropriate ra-diotherapy offer the only possible cure at this time. (Note: a *lymphoma* is any tumor, benign or malig-nant, that occurs in lymphoid tissue.)

Summary

1 Lymph.
  A Tissue fluid that has entered lymphatic ves-sels.
  B Made of water and end products of cell me-tabolism.
  C Flows through lymphatic vessels, is filtered in lymph nodes, then enters the blood-stream.
2 Lymphatic capillaries.
  A Blind tubes lying in tissue fluid; called lac-teals in intestine.
  B Drain lymph from tissues.
3 Lymphatic vessels.
  A Receive lymph from capillaries.
  B Valves prevent backflow; muscular activity maintains onward flow of lymph.
  C Carry lymph to nodes for filtering, then to terminal ducts—right lymphatic and tho-racic.
  D Right lymphatic duct drains right side of the body above diaphragm. Empties into right subclavian vein.
  E Thoracic duct drains rest of body. Has cis-terna chyli, an enlargement at its beginning. Empties into left subclavian vein.
4 Lymphoid tissue.
  A Found in other structures than those in lymph conduction system.
  B Functions—removes bacteria and other for-eign particles, manufactures lymphocytes, produces antibodies.
  C Individual masses of tissue expendable.
5 Lymph nodes.
  A Act as lymph filters.
  B Main groups—cervical, axillary, tracheo-bronchial, mesenteric, inguinal.
6 Tonsils.
  A Are but 1 example of a group of lymphoid masses located beneath moist exposed ep-ithelium.
  B Forms—palatine, pharyngeal, lingual.
7 Thymus.
  A Most active during early life.
  B Plays role in development of immunity.
  C Manufactures lymphocytes.
8 Spleen.
  A In left hypochondriac region (upper abdo-men); designed to filter blood.
  B Functions—breakdown of old red blood cells; salvage of iron for reuse; destruction of bacteria and other foreign substances; formation of lymphocytes and monocytes; production of antibodies; formation of red blood cells in embryo; serves as reservoir for blood.
9 Reticuloendothelial system.
  A A system of cells derived from monocytes; concerned with destruction of foreign sub-stances and old cells.
  B Includes Kupffer's cells in liver and others in spleen, bone marrow, lymph nodes, and soft connective tissues.
10 Disorders of lymphatic system and lymphoid tissue.
  A Lymphangitis—infection of lymphatic ves-sels.
  B Elephantiasis—enlargement of lower ex-tremities caused by parasitic blockage of lymph vessels.
  C Adenitis—usually refers to lymph node in-flammation, enlargement, tenderness owing to disease.
  D Hodgkin's disease—a chronic disease occur-ring mostly in young men, characterized by enlargement of lymph nodes.
  E Lymphosarcoma—a malignant growth of lymphoid tissue.
  F Splenomegaly—enlargement of spleen. Splenectomy—removal of spleen.

Questions and Problems

1 What is lymph? Name some of its purposes.
2 Briefly describe the system of lymph circulation.
3 Describe the lymphatic vessels with respect to design, appearance, and depth of location.
4 Name the 2 main lymphatic ducts. What part of the body does each drain, and into what blood vessel does each empty?
5 What is the cisterna chyli and what are its purposes?
6 Name 3 functions of lymphoid tissue.
7 Describe the structure of a typical lymph node.
8 What are the neck nodes called and what are some of the causes of enlargement of these lymph nodes?
9 What parts of the body are drained by vessels entering the axillary nodes and what conditions cause enlargement of these nodes?
10. What parts of the body are drained by lymphatics that pass through the inguinal lymph nodes? What is the relationship of bubonic plague to these nodes?
11 What are the different tonsils called and where are they located? What is the purpose of these and related structures?
12 What is the function of the thymus?
13 Give the location of the spleen and name several of its functions.
14 What is lymphangitis?
15 Describe elephantiasis and its cause.
16 Describe Hodgkin's disease, lymphosarcoma.
17 What is splenomegaly and what can cause it?
18 Describe the reticuloendothelial system.

Chapter 17

Respiration

17

Glossary

Alveolus (pl. alveoli)   A small saclike dilatation.

Anoxia, hypoxia   A lack of oxygen supply to the tissues.

Apnea   A temporary cessation of breathing.

Asphyxia   An increase in carbon dioxide in the tissues, accompanied by an oxygen deficiency.

Bronchus   One of the larger air passageways of the lungs.

Chemoreceptor   A receptor that is stimulated by chemical substances or by a sense organ.

Cyanosis   Bluish color of the skin and mucous membranes resulting from insufficient oxygen in the blood.

Dyspnea   Difficult or labored breathing.

Glottis   Vocal apparatus of the larynx consisting of the vocal cords or folds and the opening between them.

Hyperpnea   An increase in depth and rate of respiration due to very rapid respiratory movements.

Larynx   The voice box.

Lung   The organ of respiration.

Mediastinum   The mass of tissue separating the lungs, and containing the heart and its great vessels, the trachea, esophagus, thymus, lymph nodes, and other structures.

Pharynx   The saclike tube extending from the nose and mouth above to the larynx and esophagus below; the "throat."

Respiration   The process by which cells take in oxygen and expel carbon dioxide.

Suffocation   A stoppage of respiration.

Surfactant   A secretion of certain lung cells that reduces surface tension and makes pulmonary tissue more elastic.

Trachea   A membranous and cartilaginous tube, commonly called the windpipe, extending from the larynx to its 2 branching bronchi.

Respiration

The word "respiration" means "to breathe again," and the fundamental purpose of the respiratory system is to supply oxygen to the individual tissue cells and to remove their gaseous waste product, carbon dioxide. Breathing refers to the inhaling and exhaling of air. Ventilation is the exchange of air between the lungs and the outside. Air is a mixture of oxygen, nitrogen, carbon dioxide, and other gases; the proportions of these gases varies depending upon the elevation above sea level and the amount of pollution in the specific locale. Respiration has two aspects; the first is that which takes place only in the lungs, where oxygen from the outside air enters the blood, and carbon dioxide is removed from the blood to be breathed into the outside air. This aspect is *external respiration* (Fig. 17-1). The second aspect is called *internal respiration*. Internal respiration refers to the gas exchanges between the blood and the body cells and within the cells. Oxygen leaves the blood and enters the cells at the same time that carbon dioxide leaves the cells and enters the blood. Internal respiration is also called *cellular respiration* (see Fig. 15-8).

The respiratory system is an intricate arrangement of spaces and passageways which serve to conduct air into the lungs. These spaces include the *nasal cavities;* the *pharynx* (far'inks) which is

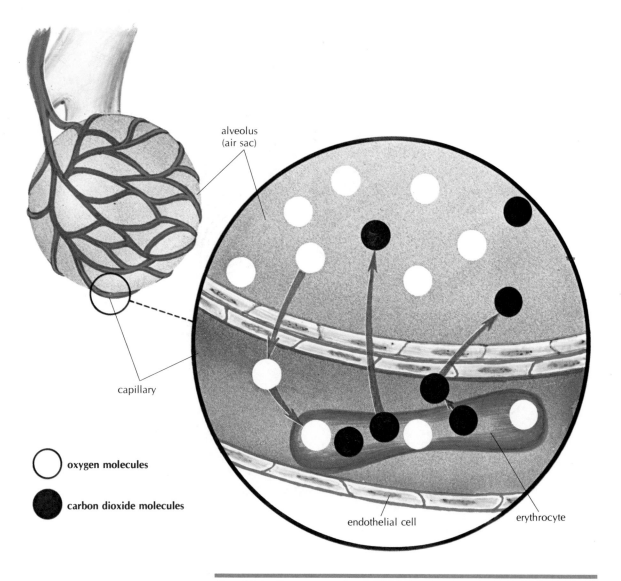

alveolus (air sac)

capillary

○ **oxygen molecules**

● **carbon dioxide molecules**

endothelial cell

erythrocyte

Fig. 17-1 Diagram to show diffusion of molecules through the cell membrane and throughout the air in the alveolus and the capillary blood.

common to the digestive and respiratory systems; the voice box, or *larynx* (lar'inks); the windpipe, or *trachea* (tra'ke-ah); and the *lungs* themselves, with their tubes and air sacs. The entire system might be thought of as a pathway for air between the atmosphere and the blood (Fig. 17-2).

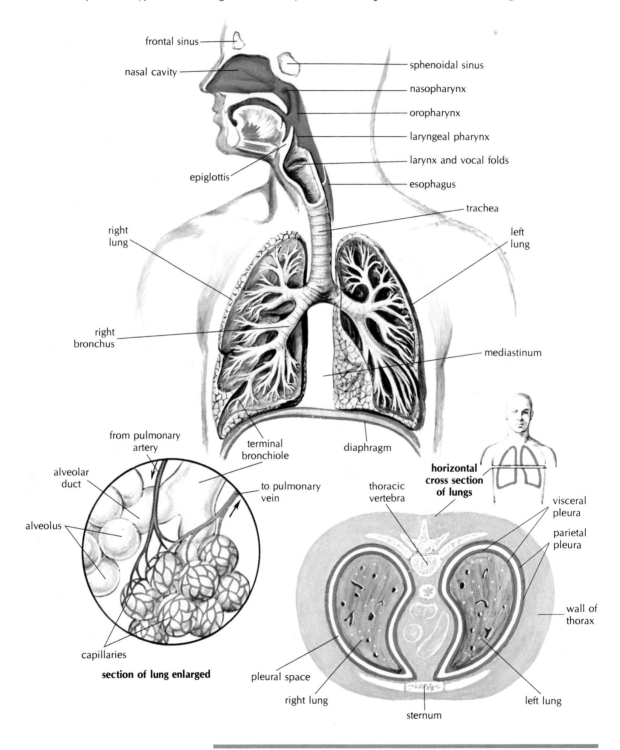

frontal sinus

nasal cavity

sphenoidal sinus

nasopharynx

oropharynx

laryngeal pharynx

larynx and vocal folds

esophagus

epiglottis

trachea

right lung

left lung

right bronchus

mediastinum

from pulmonary artery

terminal bronchiole

diaphragm

horizontal cross section of lungs

alveolar duct

to pulmonary vein

thoracic vertebra

visceral pleura

parietal pleura

alveolus

wall of thorax

capillaries

section of lung enlarged

pleural space

right lung

left lung

sternum

Fig. 17-2 The respiratory system.

The Respiratory System
Nasal Cavities

Air makes its initial entrance into the body through the openings in the nose called the **nostrils.** Immediately within are the two spaces known as the **nasal cavities,** located between the roof of the mouth and the cranium. These two spaces are separated from each other by a partition, the **nasal septum.** The septum and the walls of the nasal cavities are constructed of bone covered with mucous membrane. From the lateral (side) walls of each nasal cavity are three projections called the conchae. The conchae greatly increase the surface over which the air must travel on its way through the nasal cavities.

The lining of the nasal cavities contains many blood vessels; hence it is described as a *vascular membrane.* The blood brings heat and moisture to the mucosa. As much as a quart of liquid is secreted daily by this membrane. The advantages of breathing through the nasal cavities over breathing through the mouth are due to the various changes effected on the air as it comes in contact with the parts of the nose, particularly the lining. The following changes take place.

1 Foreign bodies, such as dust particles and pathogens, are removed by either being strained out by the hairs of the nostrils or being caught in the surface mucus.
2 Air is warmed by the blood in the vascular mucosa.
3 Air is moistened by the liquid secretion.

The sum of these changes amounts to a kind of air conditioning in a very real sense.

Also included in the discussion of the nasal cavities are the *sinuses,* which are small cavities, lined with mucous membrane, in the bones of the skull. The sinuses communicate with the nasal cavities, and they are highly susceptible to infection (see Chap. 7).

Another feature of the nasal cavities is a small duct communicating indirectly with the glands that produce tears. This is the *nasolacrimal* (na''zo-lak'ri-mal) *duct,* and its presence explains why the nose runs when tears flow freely.

The nasal cavities also contain the receptors for the sense of smell.

The Pharynx

The muscular pharynx serves as a passageway for air into the respiratory tract, and for foods and liquids into the digestive system. The upper portion located immediately behind the nasal cavity is called the *nasopharynx* (na''zo-far'inks). The middle section located behind the mouth is called the *oropharynx* (o''ro-far'inks); and finally the lowest portion is the *laryngeal* (lah-rin'je-al) *pharynx.* This last section opens into two spaces.

1 The air passageway into the larynx is toward the front.
2 The food path, toward the back, enters the esophagus.

The Larynx

The *larynx,* or voice box, is located between the pharynx and the trachea. It has a framework of cartilage which protrudes in the front of the neck and sometimes is referred to as the Adam's apple. The larynx is considerably larger in the male than in the female; hence, the Adam's apple is much more prominent in the male. At the upper end of the larynx are the *vocal folds.* These cordlike structures serve in the production of speech. They are set into vibration by the flow of air from the lung. It is the difference in the size of the larynx that accounts for the characteristic male and female voices. Because a man's larynx is larger than a woman's, his voice is lower in pitch. The nasal cavities, the sinuses and the pharynx all serve as resonating chambers for speech, just as the cabinet does for a radio speaker.

The space between these two vocal cords is called the *glottis* (glot'is), and the little leaf-shaped structure that closes this opening during swallowing is called the *epiglottis* (ep-e-glot'is). By the action of the epiglottis, food is kept out of the remainder of the respiratory tract. The epiglottis acts as a lid or a trapdoor. As the larynx moves upward and forward during swallowing, the epiglottis moves downward, closing the opening into the larynx. During breathing, the epiglottis rises to allow air to pass downward. Most of us are familiar with the choking sensation that occurs when we accidentally breathe and swallow at the same time.

The larynx is lined with ciliated mucous membrane. The cilia trap dust and other particles, moving them upward to the pharynx to be expelled, by coughing, sneezing, or blowing the nose.

The Windpipe, or Trachea

The *trachea* is a tube that extends from the lower edge of the voice box to the center of the chest behind the heart. It has a framework of cartilage to keep it open. These cartilages, shaped somewhat like a tiny horseshoe or the letter C, are placed near each other along the entire length of the trachea. All the open sections of these cartilages are at the back so that the esophagus can bulge into this region during swallowing. The purpose of the trachea is to conduct air between the larynx and the lungs.

The Bronchi

Near the center of the chest behind the heart, the trachea divides into two *bronchi* (brong'ki). These two main air passageways enter the lungs, one on each side. The right bronchus is considerably larger in diameter than the left and extends downward in a more vertical direction. Therefore, if a foreign body is inhaled, it is likely to enter the right lung. Each bronchus enters the lung at a notch or depression called the *hilus* (hi'lus) or *hilum* (hi'lum). In this same region the blood vessels and the nerves also connect with the lung.

The Lungs

The *lungs* are the organs in which external respiration takes place; that is, where blood and air meet through the medium of the extremely thin and delicate lung tissues. There are two lungs, set side by side in the thoracic cavity, and each of them is constructed in the following manner:

As soon as each bronchus enters the lung at the hilus, it immediately subdivides. These branches or subdivisions of the bronchi resemble the branches of a tree, hence the common name, *bronchial tree*. Each individual bronchus subdivides again and again, forming progressively smaller divisions. The smallest are called *bronchioles* (brong'ke-oles). The bronchi contain small bits of cartilage which give firmness to the walls and serve to hold the passageways open so that air can pass in and out easily. However, as the bronchi become

smaller, the cartilage decreases in amount until finally, in the most minute subdivisions—bronchioles—there is no cartilage at all.

At the end of each of the smallest subdivisions of the bronchial tree, called *terminal bronchioles,* there is a cluster of air sacs, resembling a bunch of grapes, known as *alveoli* (al-ve'o-li). Each alveolus is a single-cell layer of squamous (flat) epithelium. This very thin wall provides an easy passage for the gases entering and leaving the blood as it circulates through the millions of tiny capillaries of the alveoli. Certain cells in the alveolar wall produce *surfactant* (sur-fak'tant), a substance that prevents the alveoli from collapsing. There are millions of alveoli in the human lung. The resulting surface in contact with gases approximates 60 square meters, about three times as much lung tissue as is necessary for life. Surely nature has allowed an ample margin of safety! Because of the many air spaces, the lung is light in weight; and normally a piece of lung tissue dropped into a glassful of water will float.

It will be recalled that the pulmonary circuit brings the blood to and from the lungs. The blood passes through the capillaries of the alveoli, where the gas exchange takes place.

The Lung Cavities

The lungs occupy a considerable portion of the thoracic cavity, which is separated from the abdominal cavity by the muscular partition known as the *diaphragm.* Each lung is enveloped in a sac of serous membrane called the *pleura;* hence, there are two pleurae, one associated with each lung. As we noted in Chapter 3, the portion of the pleura that is attached to the chest wall is called *parietal pleura,* while that which is reflected onto the surface of the lung is called *visceral pleura.*

The pleural cavity around the lungs is an airtight space having a partial vacuum. The pressure in this space is less than the atmospheric pressure. The pressure inside the lungs is higher than in the surrounding pleural cavity.

The entire thoracic cavity is flexible, capable of expanding and contracting along with the lungs. Its interior is well sealed off from the outside by its layer of membrane; and, as we shall see, this is a feature of the mechanism of breathing.

Between the lungs is the *mediastinum* (me''de-as-ti'num), which contains the heart, great blood vessels, esophagus, and lymph nodes.

Physiology of Respiration
Pulmonary Ventilation

Ventilation is the movement of air into and out of the lungs. Breathing is the usual means of ventilating the lungs, but artificial respiration, as taught in first-aid classes, or various mechanical devices may be required to obtain adequate lung ventilation.

There are two phases of breathing (Fig. 17-3):

1 **Inhalation** is the drawing of air into the lungs.

2 **Exhalation** is the expulsion of air from the lungs.

Inhalation is the active phase of breathing, since it is then that the respiratory muscles contract to enlarge the thoracic cavity. The diaphragm is a strong dome-shaped muscle attached around the base of the rib cage. The contraction and flattening of the diaphragm causes a piston-like downward motion that results in an increase in the vertical dimension of the chest. The rib cage also moves upward and outward owing to the action of the diaphragm with the assistance of the external intercostals and other muscles. During quiet breathing, the movement of the diaphragm accounts for 75% of the increase in thoracic volume.

Exhalation is the passive phase of breathing, since the muscles of respiration then relax, allowing the lung and chest wall to return to their original

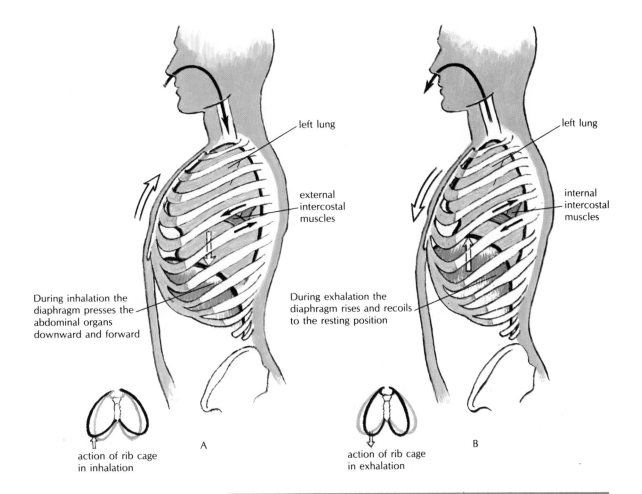

left lung

external intercostal muscles

During inhalation the diaphragm presses the abdominal organs downward and forward

action of rib cage in inhalation

A

left lung

internal intercostal muscles

During exhalation the diaphragm rises and recoils to the resting position

action of rib cage in exhalation

B

Fig. 17-3 (*A*) Inhalation and (*B*) exhalation.

position. The lung and chest wall tissues are elastic and recoil during exhalation. The abdominal viscera press upward, pushing air out of the lungs. During forced exhalation, the muscles of the abdominal wall contract, pulling the bottom of the rib cage in and down. There is also an increased push by the abdominal viscera against the diaphragm.

Air Movement

Air enters the respiratory passages and flows through the ever-dividing tubes of the bronchial tree. As the air traverses this passage it moves more and more slowly through the great number of bronchial tubes until there is virtually no forward flow as it reaches the alveoli. Here the air moves by diffusion which soon equalizes any differences in the amounts of gases present. Each breath causes relatively little change in the gas composition of the alveoli, but normal continuous breathing ensures the presence of adequate oxygen and the removal of carbon dioxide.

Gas Exchanges

The barrier that separates the air in the alveolus from the blood in the capillary is very thin and is ideally suited for the exchange of gases by diffusion. Normally, inspired air contains about 21% oxygen, while expired air has only 16% oxygen along with 3.5% carbon dioxide. A two-way diffusion takes place through the walls of the alveoli. Blood entering the lung capillaries is relatively lower in oxygen, which means that oxygen will diffuse from the alveolus, where its concentration is higher, into the blood. Carbon dioxide diffuses out of the blood into the air of the alveolus (see Fig. 17-1).

Gas Transport

The oxygen that has diffused into the lung capillary blood is bound to the hemoglobin of the red blood cell. The hemoglobin becomes a brighter red as it combines with larger amounts of oxygen, so oxygenated blood is a scarlet color, while deoxygenated blood is a dusky crimson red. The arterial blood (in systemic arteries and pulmonary veins) is 97% saturated with oxygen, while venous blood (in systemic veins and pulmonary arteries) contains about 70% oxygen saturation, a 27% difference. The bond between oxygen and hemoglobin is easily broken so oxygen can be readily released for use by the body cells.

The carbon dioxide produced in the tissues is transported to the lungs in three ways:

1 Most is transported as a compound, known as bicarbonate, which is formed by the union of the gas carbon dioxide with water.
2 Some is dissolved in the plasma.
3 Some is also combined with protein substances in the blood plasma.

The bicarbonate compound is formed slowly in the plasma but much more rapidly inside the red blood cells where an enzyme called carbonic anhydrase increases the speed of the reaction. These larger amounts of bicarbonate formed in the red blood cells are returned to the plasma and then carried to the lungs. The bicarbonate releases carbon dioxide in the lungs for diffusion into the alveoli and exhalation.

Regulation of Respiration

Regulation of respiration is a complex process which must keep pace with the moment-to-moment changes in cellular oxygen requirements and carbon dioxide production. Regulation depends primarily upon the respiratory control centers located in the medulla and pons of the brain stem. Nerve impulses from the medulla are modified by the pons. Respiration is regulated so that the levels of oxygen, carbon dioxide, and acid are kept within certain limits. The control centers regulate the rate, depth, and rhythm of respiration.

From the respiratory center in the medulla, motor nerve fibers extend into the spinal cord. From the cervical (neck) part of the cord, these nerve fibers continue through the *phrenic* (fren'ik) nerve to the diaphragm. Unlike the heart, the diaphragm does not continue to function if it is cut off from its nerve supply. The diaphragm and the other muscles of respiration are voluntary in the sense that they can be regulated by messages from the higher brain centers, notably the cortex. It is possible for a person deliberately to breathe more rapidly or more slowly, or to hold his breath and not breathe at all for a time. Usually, we breathe without thinking about it, while the respiratory centers in the medulla and pons do the controlling.

Of vital importance in the control of respiration are the *chemoreceptors* (ke''mo-re-sep'tors). These receptors are found in structures called the carotid and aortic bodies, as well as in the medulla of the brain stem. We have noted that carbon dioxide is carried in the form of a compound, bicarbonate. This compound releases acid, so that one of the effects of an increase in the production of carbon dioxide is an increase in acidity (*i.e.,* a lower pH). The carotid bodies are located near the bifurcation of the common carotid arteries, while the aortic bodies are located on or near the aortic arch. These bodies contain many small blood vessels and sensory neurons, which are sensitive to a decreased oxygen supply as well as to increases in carbon dioxide and acid. Impulses are sent to the brain from the receptors in the carotid and aortic bodies. The receptor cells in the medulla are affected by the concentrations of carbon dioxide and acid in the fluids related to it. This includes the capillary blood as well as the cerebrospinal fluid that circulates around it (see Fig. 11-10).

Respiratory Rates

Normal rates of breathing vary from 12 to 20 times per minute for adults. In children, rates may vary from 20 to 40 times a minute, depending on age and size. In infants, the respiratory rate may be more than 40 times per minute. To determine the respiratory rate, the health worker counts the client's breathing for at least 30 seconds, observing in such a way that the person is unaware that a count is being made. Changes in respiratory rates are important in various disorders and should be carefully recorded.

Abnormal Respiration

The following is a list of terms designating various abnormalities of respiration. They are symptoms, not diseases.

1 **Hyperpnea** (hi''perp-ne'ah) is overbreathing due to abnormally rapid respiratory movements. It refers to an increase in the depth as well as the rate of respiration.

2 **Apnea** (ap'ne-ah) is a temporary cessation of breathing.

3 **Dyspnea** (disp'ne-ah) is difficult or labored breathing.

4 **Cheyne-Stokes** (chan'stoks) respiration is a type of rhythmical variation in the depth of respiratory movements found in certain critically ill persons.

Situations that occur in relation to changes in respiration may include the following:

1 **Cyanosis** (si''ah-no'sis) is a bluish color of the skin and mucous membranes caused by an insufficient amount of oxygen in the blood.

2 **Hypoxia** (hi-pok'se-ah) and **anoxia** (ah-nok'se-ah) are often used interchangeably to mean reduced oxygen supply to the tissues.

3 **Suffocation** is the stoppage of respiration, often the result of a mechanical blockage of the respiratory passages. Suffocation can cause **asphyxia** (as-fik'se-ah), which is a lack of oxygen in the inspired air.

Disorders of the Respiratory System
Sinusitis and Nasal Polyps

"I have sinus" is an expression many people use to indicate disease of the sinuses. The sinuses are located close to the nasal cavities, and in one case near the ear. Infection may easily travel into these sinuses from the mouth, the nose and the throat along the mucous membrane lining, and the resulting inflammation is called *sinusitis.* Long-standing, or chronic, sinus infection may cause changes in the epithelial cells, resulting in tumor formation. Some of these growths have a grapelike appearance and cause obstruction of the air pathway. These tumors are called *polyps* (pol'ips).

Deviated Septum

The partition separating the two nasal spaces from each other is called the nasal septum. Since many of us have minor structural defects, it is not surprising that the nasal septum is rarely exactly in the midline. If it is markedly to one side, it is described as a *deviated septum.* In this condition one nasal space may be considerably smaller than the other. If such a person has an attack of hay fever or develops a cold with the accompanying swelling of the mucosa, this smaller nasal cavity may be completely closed. Sometimes the septum is curved in such a way that both nasal cavities are occluded, forcing the individual to breathe through the mouth. Such an occlusion may also prevent proper drainage from the sinuses and aggravate a case of sinusitis.

Nosebleed

The most common cause of nosebleed, also called *epistaxis* (ep-e-stak′sis), is an injury or a blow to the nose. Other causes include inflammation and ulceration such as may occur following a persistent discharge from a sinusitis. Growths including polyps can also be a cause of epistaxis. Rarely, an abnormally high blood pressure will cause the vessels in the nasal lining to break, resulting in varying degrees of hemorrhage. To stop the nosebleed, the victim should remain quiet with the head slightly elevated. Pressure applied to the nostril of the bleeding side, as well as cold compresses over the nose, is usually helpful. In some cases, it may be necessary to insert a plug into the bleeding side in order to encourage adequate clotting. If these methods fail, a physician should be consulted.

The Spread of Infection

The mucosa of the respiratory tract serves as one of the most important portals of entry for disease-producing organisms. This transfer of disease organisms from the respiratory system of one human being to another occurs much more rapidly in crowded places such as schools, auditoriums, theaters, churches, and prisons. Droplets from one sneeze may be loaded with many billions of disease-producing organisms. To a certain extent the mucous membranes can protect themselves by producing larger quantities of mucus. The runny nose, an unpleasant symptom of the common cold, is an attempt on the part of nature to wash away the pathogens and so protect the deeper tissues from further invasion by the infection. If the resistance of the mucous membrane is reduced, however, the membrane may act as a pathway for the spread of disease. The infection may travel along

the membrane into the nasal sinuses, into the middle ear, or down into the lung. Infections may also spread from the respiratory tract to the digestive system, or the reverse, because of the continuity of the mucosa.

Among the infections transmitted through the respiratory passageways, are the common cold, diphtheria, chickenpox, measles, influenza, pneumonia, and tuberculosis. Any infection that is confined to the nose, the throat, the larynx, or the trachea is called an *upper respiratory infection* (often called URI). In children's wards in hospitals the records show that the great majority of patients with these diseases had first developed symptoms of an upper respiratory infection. Very often, too, such an infection can precipitate the onset of such a serious disease as rheumatic fever.

The respiratory passageways may become infected one by one as the organisms travel along the lining membrane. The disorder is named according to the part involved as follows:

1 **Rhinitis** (ri-ni′tis) is inflammation of the nasal mucosa.
2 **Pharyngitis** (far-in-ji′tis) is inflammation of the pharynx, referred to also as sore throat.
3 **Laryngitis** (lar-in-ji′tis) is inflammation of the larynx, and is often characterized by hoarseness.
4 **Tracheitis** (tra-ke-i′tis) is inflammation of the trachea.
5 **Bronchitis** (brong-ki′tis) includes infection of the bronchi and their many subdivisions in the lungs.
6 **Pneumonia** is inflammation of the lungs in which the air spaces become filled with fluid.

The Common Cold

The common cold is the most widespread of all respiratory diseases—or any communicable disease, for that matter. The cause is a virus that is very easily spread; and one characteristic of the cold virus is that it may fail to produce an immunity, so that some persons suffer one cold after another. Medical science has yet to produce a method of preventing the common cold, although there are preventive inoculations that may be helpful for one person but ineffective for another.

The symptoms of the common cold are familiar: first the swollen and inflamed mucosa of the nose and the throat, then the copious discharge of watery fluid from the nose, and finally the thick and ropy discharge that occurs when the cold is subsiding. The scientific name for the common cold is *acute coryza* (ko-ri'zah); the word "coryza" can also simply mean "a nasal discharge."

A discharge from the nasal cavities may be a symptom not only of the common cold; it may also stem from sinusitis or be an important forerunner of a more serious disease.

The notion that all nasal mucus is undesirable is wrong. Normal mucous secretions are valuable and are required to keep the tissues moist as well as to help protect the cells against invasion by pathogens. The idea that excess secretion is caused by diets of eggs, milk, or any other food has no basis in fact.

Hay Fever and Asthma

Sensitivity to plant pollens, to dust, to certain foods, and to other allergens may lead to *hay fever* or *asthma* or both. Hay fever is characterized by a watery discharge from the eyes and nose, and about half of all hay fever attacks end in asthma. In asthma the symptoms are usually due to a spasm of the involuntary musculature of the bronchial tube walls. This spasm constricts the tubes so that the victim cannot exhale easily. He experiences a sense of suffocation and has labored breathing (*dyspnea*). Much has been written about the part that psychological factors play in the causation of asthma. It would seem advisable to leave the decision concerning the possible causes in the hands of the family physician or the specialist he may recommend. Individuals vary considerably, and most cases of asthma present a multiplicity of problems.

One great difficulty in the treatment of hay fever or asthma is to isolate the particular substance to which the patient is allergic. Usually a number of skin tests are given, but the results of these are far from conclusive in most cases.

Persons with asthma may benefit from treatment with a series of injections to reduce their sensitivity to specific substances.

Influenza

Influenza, or "flu," is an acute contagious disease characterized by an inflammatory condition of the upper respiratory tract accompanied by generalized aches and pains. It is caused by a virus and may spread to the sinuses as well as downward to the lungs. Inflammation of the trachea and the bronchi causes the characteristic cough of influenza, and the general infection brings about an extremely weakened condition of the victim. The great danger of influenza is its tendency to develop into a particularly severe form of pneumonia. At intervals in history there have been tremendous epidemics of influenza in which millions of people have died. Vaccines have been effective, though the immunity is of short duration.

Emphysema and Bronchitis

Chronic obstructive pulmonary disease (COPD) is the term used to describe several lung disorders including chronic bronchitis and emphysema. Most affected persons have symptoms and lung damage characteristic of both diseases. In chronic bronchitis the linings of the airways are chronically inflamed and produce excessive secretions. Emphysema is characterized by dilation and finally destruction of the alveoli.

In chronic obstructive pulmonary disease, respiratory function is impaired by obstruction to normal air flow, by air trapping and overinflation of parts of the lungs, and by reduced exchange of oxygen and carbon dioxide. In the early stages of these diseases, the small airways are involved, and several years may pass before symptoms become evident. Later, the person develops dyspnea, owing to the difficulty of exhaling air through the obstructed air passages.

The progressive character of these diseases may be reversed when they are detected early in their course and irritants to the respiratory system are eliminated. The major culprit is cigarette smoke, although industrial wastes and air pollution also play a large role. In the popular press the word emphysema is used to mean COPD.

Atelectasis

Atelectasis (at"e-lek'tah-sis) is the incomplete expansion of a lung or portion of a lung. This disorder may affect scattered groups of alveoli or an entire lobe, causing its collapse. The affected person will have hypoxia and dyspnea. Obstruction by mucus plugs in chronic obstructive lung disease, by foreign bodies or by lung cancer is a cause of this disorder. Another cause may be the insufficient production of surfactant as in hyaline membrane disease (seen in newborns) or adult respiratory distress syndrome. Atelectasis is also seen when there is external compression of the lung or interference with deep breathing, for example, with pain from fractured ribs.

Pneumonia

Pneumonia is an inflammation of the lungs in which the air spaces become filled with fluid. A variety of organisms including staphylococci, pneumococci, streptococci, *Legionella pneumophilla* (as in Legionnaire's disease), chlamydias, or viruses may be responsible. Many of these pathogens may be carried by a healthy person in the mucosa of the upper respiratory tract. If the person remains in good health, these pathogens may be carried for an indefinite period with no ill effect. However, if the individual's resistance to infection is lowered, the pathogens then may invade the tissues and cause disease. Exposure to inclement weather for long periods of time, alcoholism, malnutrition, a severe injury, or other debilitating (de-bil'i-ta-ting) or weakening conditions may cause a susceptibility to pneumonia.

There are two main kinds of pneumonia as determined by the method of lung involvement and other factors. These are

1 **Lobar pneumonia,** in which an entire lobe of the lung is infected at one time. The organism is usually a pneumococcus, although other pathogens also may cause this disease. The Legionella organism is the causative agent of a severe lobar pneumonia that occurs mostly in localized epidemics.
2 **Bronchopneumonia,** in which the disease process is scattered here and there throughout the lung. The cause may be a staphylococcus, a gram-negative proteus or colon bacillus (not normally pathogenic), or a virus. Bronchopneumonia most often is secondary to an infection or to some agent that has lowered the individual's resistance to disease. This is the more common form of pneumonia.

A characteristic of most types of pneumonia is the formation of a fluid, or *exudate,* in the infected alveoli; this fluid consists chiefly of serum and pus cells, products of infection. Some red blood cells may be present, as indicated by red streaks in the sputum. Sometimes so many air sacs become filled with fluid that the victim finds it hard to absorb enough oxygen to maintain life.

Tuberculosis

Tuberculosis is an inflammation caused by the bacillus *Mycobacterium tuberculosis.* Although the tubercle bacillus may invade any tissue in the body, the lung is the usual site. Tuberculosis remains a leading cause of death from communicable disease primarily because of the relatively large numbers of cases among recent immigrants and poor population groups in metropolitan areas.

The lungs, with the pleuras, are the organs affected most often by tuberculosis. The bacillus can be spread in a number of ways, chiefly by inhalation. The sputum deposited by a person who carries the organism dries out; and the bacilli, which are extremely hardy, are carried about for long periods of time in the dust of the air from which they are inhaled by another individual. This organism withstands exposure to many disinfectants, but it is vulnerable to sunlight. Therefore, we might expect to find the greatest frequency of tuberculosis to be among the poorer inhabitants of the large cities, where disease and malnutrition are common and where there is a maximum of crowding and a minimum of fresh air and sunlight.

In addition to the lungs, many other organs may become infected by tubercle organisms. The lymph nodes in the thorax, especially those surrounding the trachea and the bronchi, frequently are involved. Tuberculous pleurisy (inflammation of the pleura) with fluid formation is fairly common. The fluid may collect in the pleural cavity, and such a collection is called an *effusion* (e-fu' zhun). The fluid presses against the pleura and compresses the lung. The fluid may be absorbed over a period of time, if it is not removed artificially to relieve pressure against the lung. Chronic hoarseness may be due to tuberculosis (or cancer) of the larynx. Other organs which may be infected by tubercle organisms include the kidneys, certain tubes of the reproductive system, and, particularly in children, the bones of the vertebral column. Occasionally, vast numbers of the organisms may enter the bloodstream and cause a rapidly fatal tuberculosis.

Drugs are used quite successfully in many cases of tuberculosis. However, this *chemotherapy* may have the undesirable effect of producing resistant strains of bacteria. These resistant organisms can be transmitted to additional victims, who then cannot be treated effectively with these particular medications. Best results have been obtained by the use of a combination of several drugs, along with prompt, intensive, and uninterrupted treatment once such a program is begun. Such therapy is usually continued for a minimum of 12 to 18 months, therefore close supervision by the health-care practitioner is important. Adverse drug reactions are rather common, necessitating changes in the drug combinations.

Lung Cancer

The death rate due to cancer of the lungs has increased more than 25 times in males and has more than doubled in females in the last 45 years. It is considerably higher in industrial areas. By far the most important cause of lung cancer is cigarette smoking. Additionally, it has been found that smokers who are exposed to toxic chemicals or particles in the air have an even higher rate of lung cancer. Smoking has also been linked with an increase in chronic obstructive pulmonary disease and cancers of respiratory passages.

Early lung cancer has few symptoms. However, it may be discovered during a routine chest x-ray examination. Too often, emphasis upon the danger of exposure to radiation from x-ray machines can frighten people away from routine chest x-ray examination and thus prevent an early diagnosis of lung cancer. Early detection is absolutely essential if any possibility of a cure is to be maintained. Modern x-ray machines in competent hands pose such slight danger, at least to those over 40 years of age, that this would be much more than offset by the advantages of discovering a tumor while it is still small enough to be completely removed.

A common form of lung cancer is *bronchogenic* (brong-ko-jen′ik) *carcinoma*, so-called because the malignancy originates in a bronchus. The tumor may grow until the bronchus is blocked, cutting off the supply of air to that lung. The lung then collapses, and the secretions trapped in the lung spaces become infected, with a resulting pneumonia or the formation of a lung abscess. Such a lung cancer can also spread to cause secondary growths in the lymph nodes of the chest and neck as well as in the brain and other parts of the body. The only treatment that offers a possibility of cure, before secondary growths have had time to form, is to remove the lung completely. This operation is called a *pneumonectomy* (nu-mo-nek′to-me).

Malignant tumors of the stomach, the breast, the prostate gland, and other organs may spread to the lungs, causing secondary growths.

Pleurisy

Pleurisy (ploor′i-se) is inflammation of the pleura, and it usually accompanies a lung infection—particularly pneumonia and tuberculosis. This condition can be quite painful, because the inflammation produces a sticky exudate which roughens the pleura of both the lung and the chest wall; when the two surfaces rub together during respiration, the roughness causes acute irritation. If the two surfaces stick together, this condition is called an *adhesion* (ad-he′zhun). Infection of the pleura also causes an abnormal flow of pleural fluid. This may accumulate in the pleural cavity in such large amounts that the lung will be compressed, and the patient cannot obtain enough air. Withdrawal of the fluid by chest tube or syringe may be necessary.

Pneumothorax is an accumulation of air in the pleural cavity. The lung on the affected side collapses and the person has great difficulty in breathing. Pneumothorax may be caused by a wound in the chest wall or by rupture of lung air spaces. In a pneumothorax caused by a penetrating wound in the chest wall, an airtight cover over the opening will prevent further air from entering. The remaining lung will function and owing to the increased blood flow received by that lung the person can obtain adequate amounts of oxygen for the body tissues.

Hyperventilation is deep, rapid respiration that occurs during anxiety attacks. The oxygen level in the blood increases, and the carbon dioxide level drops. After an episode of several minutes of hyperventilation, there often occurs a period of apnea (cessation of breathing). The respiratory center responds to the abnormal oxygen and carbon dioxide levels by not sending impulses to the diaphragm. Gradually, these levels return to normal, and a regular breathing pattern is resumed.

Some Practical Aspects of Ventilation

People usually devote a great deal of thought to the food that they take into their bodies but very little to the air that they breathe. Consideration of the latter will go a long way toward the maintenance of health. So many ideas concerning ventilation are erroneous. There are fresh-air fiends who open windows at night, allowing cold air to chill their bodies unduly. This habit may be a carryover from the days when wood stoves or gas heaters had no vent to the outside, and it was important to prevent an accumulation of deadly carbon monoxide and other gases in the room. On the other hand, there are others who seemingly are not happy outside of an unbearably stuffy, unventilated, and overheated room. Scientific studies have shown that the factors that make air healthy and comfortable are

1 Enough coolness to remove some body heat without chilling.
2 Avoidance of drafts, which have been shown to create disturbances within the body that cause a predisposition to colds and other infections.
3 Enough circulation of air to remove unpleasant odors or other pollutants.

Various mechanisms for modifying or conditioning the air have been devised. Most of their emphasis has been on the alteration of temperature, the air being heated if the outside temperature is low and cooled if the outside air is too warm. Modern heaters are vented so that noxious gases do not enter the living quarters, and in many areas laws have been passed prohibiting the installation of unvented heaters. Nevertheless, deaths from the escape of poisonous gases from heaters still are all too common. The general public should be better informed about the whole field of ventilation and air conditioning.

Desirable modification of air includes more than merely heating or cooling it. The humidity should be maintained at the proper level, and some effective means of filtering the air should be provided. Air filters, needless to say, should be cleaned regularly; otherwise, they are worse than useless. An acceptable air conditioner should be able to maintain adequate air circulation without blowing a gale and chilling everyone within its range.

Special Equipment for Respiratory Tract Treatments

The *bronchoscope* (brong'ko-skope) is a tubular instrument containing tiny mirrors so arranged that the doctor can inspect the bronchi and the larger bronchial tubes. The bronchoscope is passed into the respiratory tract by way of the mouth and the pharynx. It may be used to remove foreign bodies or to inspect the tubes for tumors or other evidence of disease. Children inhale a variety of objects such as pins, beans, pieces of nuts, and small coins, all of which are removed with the aid of a bronchoscope. If such things are left in the lung, an abscess or other serious complication may cause death.

Oxygen therapy is employed to sustain life when some condition interferes with adequate oxygen supply to the tissues. Oxygen must first have moisture added by bubbling it through room temperature or heated water. Oxygen may be delivered to the person by mask, catheter or nasal prongs. Since there is danger of fire when oxygen is being administered, the individual and his visitors must not smoke.

Intermittent positive pressure breathing (IPPB) apparatus delivers oxygen or medicines into the lungs. These devices exert pressure during inhalation to deliver the desired treatment to larger areas of the lung. This makes exhalation easy. For the person who is unable to regulate his own respirations, these devices may be automatically set. In other cases, the individual's respiratory effort triggers the machine.

Suction apparatus for removing mucus or other substances from the respiratory tract also may be required. Usually, the device takes the form of a drainage bottle, with one tube from it leading to the area to be drained, and another tube from the bottle leading to a suction machine. When the suction is applied, the drainage flows from the patient's respiratory tract into the bottle.

A *tracheostomy* (tra''ke-os'to-me) tube is used if the pharynx or the larynx is obstructed. It is a small metal or plastic tube which is inserted through a cut made in the trachea, and it acts as an artificial airway for ventilation. The procedure for the insertion of such a tube is a tracheostomy. The word *tracheotomy* (tra''ke-ot'o-me) refers to the incision in the trachea for the purpose of removing a growth or a foreign body, or for obtaining a specimen for a biopsy. Very often emergency tracheotomies are performed on children who have inhaled something large enough to block the respiratory passages; otherwise they would die in a very short time.

Artificial respiration is resorted to in cases in which an individual has temporarily lost the capacity to perform the normal motions of respiration. Such emergencies include smoke asphyxiation, electric shock, and drowning.

Classes are offered by many public agencies in the techniques of mouth-to-mouth respiration as well as cardiac massage to revive persons experiencing respiratory or cardiac arrest. This technique is known as cardiopulmonary resuscitation, or CPR.

Summary

1 Respiration.
  A Purpose—supply oxygen to tissues, remove carbon dioxide.
  B Aspects.
     (1) External—gas exchange in lungs.
     (2) Internal—gas exchange in tissues.
2 Respiratory system as a whole.
  A Nasal cavities—include sinuses, nasolacrimal duct.
  B Pharynx (throat)—passageway for both air and food.
  C Larynx (voice box).
  D Trachea (windpipe—conducts air to bronchi, lungs.
  E Bronchi—2 tubes branching at end of trachea; each to a lung at hilus. (Primary bronchi.)
  F Bronchial tubes—subdivisions of bronchi in lungs. (Also called secondary bronchi.)
  G Bronchioles—smallest subdivisions of bronchial tree.
  H Alveoli—air sacs where gas exchange occurs. Connected to terminal bronchioles. Contain capillaries of pulmonary circulation.
3 Lung cavities. Lungs occupy most of thoracic cavity. Both lungs covered by, and thoracic cavity lined with, pleura. Diaphragm separates thoracic and abdominal cavities. Space between lungs is mediastinum, containing heart and other organs.
4 Physiology of respiration.
  A Phases of breathing—inhalation, exhalation.
  B Air movement.
  C Gas exchange.
  D Gas transport.
     (1) Oxygen bound to hemoglobin.
     (2) Carbon dioxide as bicarbonate compound.
  E Regulation of respiration.
     (1) Respiratory control centers.
     (2) Phrenic nerve to diaphragm.
     (3) Chemoreceptors—carotid and aortic bodies, medulla.
  F Respiratory rates.
5 Abnormal respiration—hypernea, apnea, dyspnea and Cheyne-Stokes; situations—cyanosis, hypoxia, and suffocation.
6 Disorders of respiratory system.
  A Sinusitis—inflammation of membrane lining of sinuses; may cause obstructing tumors (polyps).
  B Deviated septum—may cause closure of a nasal cavity in infection; aggravate sinusitis.
  C Epistaxis (nosebleed)—many causes. Failure to stop of own accord may indicate more serious disorder.

D Spread of infection—upper respiratory infection can spread down mucosa, develop into more serious diseases. Progression of inflammation—rhinitis, pharyngitis, laryngitis, tracheitis, bronchitis, pneumonia.

E Common cold—caused by a virus; no sure prevention.

F Hay fever and asthma—latter may follow the former. Difficult to identify allergen.

G Influenza—caused by virus. Can develop into pneumonia.

H Bronchitis and emphysema—chronic obstructive pulmonary disease; serious, often fatal.

I Atelectasis—incomplete lung expansion.

J Pneumonia—inflammation of lungs.

K Tuberculosis.
   (1) Cause—bacillus *Mycobacterium tuberculosis*.
   (2) Inhalation main method of transmission.
   (3) Treatment—drugs and rest.

L Lung cancer.
   (1) Common form—bronchogenic carcinoma.
   (2) Pneumonectomy may halt progress if done early.

M Pleurisy—inflammation of pleura. Adhesions, fluid accumulation.

N Pneumothorax.

O Hyperventilation.

7 Ventilation. Good ventilation includes coolness without chilling, avoidance of drafts, adequate air circulation.

8 Special equipment—bronchoscope, oxygen equipment, suction apparatus, tracheostomy tube.

9 Artificial respiration—CPR.

Questions and Problems

1 What is the purpose of respiration and what are its 2 aspects?

2 Trace the pathway of air from the outside into the blood.

3 What are the advantages of breathing through the nose?

4 What are some causes of mouth breathing and what should be done about them?

5 Describe the lung cavities.

6 Describe normal breathing, including 2 phases, respiratory rates, mechanism of breathing, and nerve control.

7 Describe the method of exchange and transport of oxygen and carbon dioxide.

8 Name and describe 4 types of abnormal respiration.

9 What are sinusitis, polyps, deviated septum? What is the effect of each?

10 What are some causes of nosebleed?

11 Describe some possible developments and complications of upper respiratory infections. Trace the course of infection along the respiratory tract and give the name for the inflammation of each area.

12 Describe the common cold and influenza.

13 What changes occur in the lungs in chronic obstructive lung disease?

14 What are the symptoms of atelectasis?

15 What do hay fever and asthma have in common?

16 What are some possible causes of lung cancer?

17 What is pleurisy? Its complications?

18 Describe pneumothorax. What first aid measure can be used?

19 Describe hyperventilation. Is apnea associated with it?

20 Name 3 characteristics of ideal ventilation.

21 Name and describe 3 devices used in treatments of the respiratory tract.

Chapter 18

Digestion and Indigestion

18

Glossary

Absorption   The taking up of fluids or other substances by the mucous surfaces.

Deciduous   Relating to anything that is cast off at maturity, as for example, the first set of teeth.

Digestion   The process of conversion of food materials to a state in which they can be taken into the cells.

Esophagus   The gullet (the tubular passage extending from the pharynx to the stomach).

Intestine   The portion of the alimentary canal that extends from the pylorus of the stomach to the anus.

Peristalsis   A rhythmic wavelike motion of the muscle tissue of the alimentary canal which moves the food through the digestive tube.

Saliva   The clear, somewhat sticky secretion from the mucous glands of the oral cavity.

Sphincter   A ringlike band of muscle fibers that constricts a passage or closes a body orifice.

Ulcer   A loss of the substance on a skin or mucous surface, causing breakdown and death of the tissue.

Uvula   A soft, fleshy, V-shaped mass which hangs from the soft palate.

What the Digestive System Does

In this chapter we shall study the mechanism by which the food that we eat nourishes the cells of every part of the body. This process is not so simple as it might seem. A solitary cell would be baffled if a fragment of food, in the state that is familiar to us, appeared across the lake of tissue fluid and sought admission. Food must be converted to a state in which it is capable of being taken into the cells. This conversion process is known as digestion. Once the food is digested, however, it must be transferred to the blood or lymphatic vessels, and the process by which this transfer occurs is called *absorption*. Digestion and absorption are the two chief functions of the digestive system (Fig. 18-1).

For purposes of study, the digestive system may be divided into two groups of organs as follows:

1 The **alimentary canal** is a continuous passageway beginning at the mouth, where food is

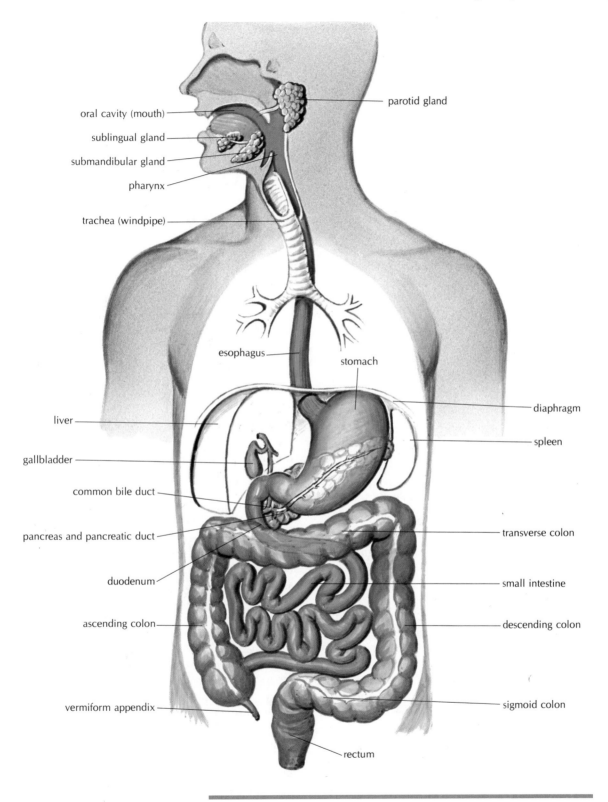

oral cavity (mouth)

sublingual gland

submandibular gland

pharynx

trachea (windpipe)

esophagus

liver

gallbladder

common bile duct

pancreas and pancreatic duct

duodenum

ascending colon

vermiform appendix

parotid gland

stomach

diaphragm

spleen

transverse colon

small intestine

descending colon

sigmoid colon

rectum

Fig. 18-1 *The digestive system.*

taken in, and terminating at the anus, where the solid waste products of digestion are expelled from the body.

2 The **accessory organs,** while vitally necessary for the digestive process, do not happen to be part of the alimentary canal.

The Alimentary Canal

The *alimentary* (al-e-men′tar-e) *canal* is a muscular digestive tube extending through the body. It is composed of several parts: the *mouth,* the *pharynx,* the *esophagus,* the *stomach,* the *small intestine,* and the *large intestine,* all of which will be defined and described as we encounter them. In this chapter, there will be a separate section devoted to the accessory organs, although we shall be familiar with at least the main functions of all of them by the time we have finished our survey of the alimentary canal.

The word "aliment" comes from a Latin word which means "food" or "nutrients." Those foods that undergo changes and are absorbed into the blood leave the tube from the region of the small intestine. Indigestible substances such as the cellulose in food pass the whole distance through the alimentary canal and are expelled from the body.

The Mouth, or Oral Cavity

The mouth is also called the oral cavity. A digestible substance begins the tour of the alimentary canal in this cavern. The oral cavity has three purposes:

1 To receive food.
2 To prepare food initially for the digestive process.
3 To aid in the accomplishment of speech.

Into this space there projects a muscular organ, the tongue, an accessory organ for digestion. The tongue is an aid to chewing and swallowing, and, in addition, is one of the principal organs of speech. The tongue has on its surface a number of special organs called *taste buds,* by means of which taste sensations (bitter, sweet, sour, or salty) can be differentiated.

Other accessory organs within this cavity are the teeth. There are 20 teeth in a child between 2 and 6 years of age. The adult with a complete set has 32 teeth. The cutting teeth, or *incisors* (in-si′zers), occupy the front part of the oral cavity, while the larger grinding teeth, called the *molars,* are in the back portion.

Deciduous, or Baby, Teeth

The first eight *deciduous* (de-sid′u-us) *teeth* to make their appearance through the gums are the incisors. Later the *canines* (eyeteeth) and molars appear. Usually, the 20 baby teeth have all made their appearance by the time the infant has passed his second birthday. During this time, the permanent teeth continue development within the jawbones. The first permanent tooth to make its appearance is the very important 6-year molar. This permanent tooth comes in before the baby incisors are lost, and a parent may not realize that a key permanent tooth has appeared. Decay and infection of the adjacent deciduous molars may spread to and involve the new permanent molar tooth. Deciduous teeth need proper care in order to help preserve the six-year molars and other permanent teeth.

Permanent Teeth

Although the buds for the second set of teeth are present at birth, the first permanent tooth does not usually make its appearance until the child is about 6 years old. At that time, the first molar, the keystone for the future grinding surfaces, appears in the space now present behind the baby molars. As the child grows, the jawbones grow also; therefore, there is space for more teeth than are in the first set. After the first permanent molar has made its appearance, the baby incisors loosen and are replaced by *permanent incisors.* Then the baby canines (cuspids) are replaced by *permanent canines,* and finally the baby molars are replaced by the bicuspids (premolars) of the permanent set. Now the larger jawbones are ready for the appearance of the 12-year or second permanent molar teeth. Somewhat later, the third molars, or so-called *wisdom teeth,* appear. In some cases, the jaw is not large enough, or there are other abnormalities, so that these teeth may have to be removed early in life.

Diseases of the Mouth and the Teeth

Infection of the gum is called *gingivitis* (jin-je-vi-tis), while infection of the rest of the mucous lining of the mouth is called *stomatitis* (sto-mah-ti′tis).

Stomatitis has become a problem for people who use antibiotic types of lozenges. These medicated wafers may encourage fungous infections of the mouth and the tongue. *Vincent's angina* (trench mouth) is a kind of gingivitis, causing redness and ulceration of the mucous membrane of the mouth and gums. It is contagious and is caused by a spirochete. *Pyorrhea* is an inflammation involving the tooth socket or *alveolus* (al-ve'o-lus). It is accompanied by discharge of pus, so the name is really pyorrhea alveolaris (pi-o-re'ah al-ve-o-la'ris).

Tooth decay or dental *caries* (ka're-ez), which means "rottenness," has a number of causes. Among persons who injest high quantities of sugar, it is a particularly prevalent disease. In addition to diet, such factors, as heredity, mechanical problems and endocrine disorders are believed to play a part. Since a baby's teeth begin to develop before birth, the diet of the mother during pregnancy also is very important in insuring the formation of healthy teeth in her baby.

The Salivary Glands

Another contribution to the digestive mechanism furnished by the oral cavity is the production of *saliva*. The purpose of saliva is to dissolve the food and to facilitate the processes of *mastication* (chewing) and *deglutition* (swallowing). Saliva also coats the food with mucus, allowing it to "go down" more easily. The chemical function of saliva will be discussed later in this chapter.

Saliva is manufactured by three pairs of glands which are also accessory organs.

1 The **parotid** (pah-rot'id) glands, the largest of the group are located near the ear.
2 The **submandibular** (sub-man-dib'u-lar), or **submaxillary** (sub-mak'si-ler-e), glands are located near the body of the lower jaw.
3 The **sublingual** glands are under the tongue.

The parotid salivary glands are infected in the contagious disease commonly called mumps. The infecting agent is a virus. *Parotitis* (par''o-ti'tis), inflammation of the parotid glands, may lead to inflammation of the testicles by the same virus. Males affected after puberty are at risk for permanent damage to these sex organs, resulting in sterility. Another complication that may occur in 10% of cases is meningitis. As is true of many contagious diseases, mumps is now preventable by the use of a vaccine routinely given to children early in life.

The Walls of the Alimentary Canal

Beyond the oral cavity and the throat, the walls of the alimentary canal from the esophagus to the anus are all similar in structure, but modified to perform particular functions. Beneath the mucosa is a layer of connective tissue containing blood vessels and nerves. Next come layers of involuntary muscle tissue with a most interesting function. When food reaches the first part of the canal (the esophagus) this muscle tissue is stimulated to produce a rhythmic, wavelike motion known as *peristalsis* (per''i-stal'sis), as a result of which food is transported the entire length of the alimentary canal and mixed with digestive juices *en route*.

The involuntary muscle layers include an outer longitudinal one whose fibers run lengthwise, and an inner circular layer that reduces the size of the lumen during contraction. In some areas the circular layer is markedly thickened to form valves that close openings. These muscular valves are called *sphincters* (sfingk'ters).

The final layer of the alimentary canal is fibrous connective tissue—except for those parts that extend into the abdominal cavity, which have an additional layer called peritoneum—and are discussed later in this chapter (See Fig. 3-1).

The Esophagus and the Pharynx

The *pharynx* (far'inks) is often referred to as the *throat*. Food is pushed by the tongue into the pharynx. The tongue and the walls of the pharynx are voluntary muscle with a lining of mucosa. The tonsils may be seen at either side of the pharynx. The *soft palate* is muscular tissue that forms the back of the roof of the oral cavity. From it hangs a soft, fleshy, V-shaped mass called the *uvula* (u'vulah) (Fig. 18-2). The soft palate guards the opening to the nasal cavity from the upper pharynx, preventing foods and liquids from entering the nasal cavities. During the process of swallowing, the muscles of the pharynx contract and so constrict the space. At this time, the openings into the air spaces both above and below the mouth are closed

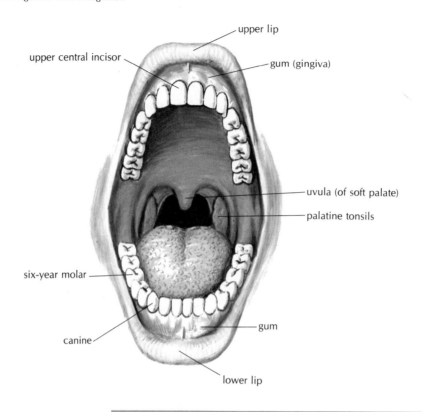

upper lip

upper central incisor

gum (gingiva)

uvula (of soft palate)

palatine tonsils

six-year molar

gum

canine

lower lip

Fig. 18-2 *The mouth, showing the teeth and the tonsils.*

off by the soft palate above and by the *epiglottis* (ep''i-glot'is), a leaf-shaped lid, below.

The *esophagus* (e-sof'ah-gus), or *gullet,* receives the contents of the contracting pharynx and forces them on by peristalsis. The esophagus, about 22.5 cm long, extends through the neck and the thorax. After passing through the diaphragm, the esophagus reaches the abdominal cavity. There it empties into a saclike structure, the stomach.

The Stomach

The stomach is actually an enlarged (dilated) section of the alimentary tube. It is shaped somewhat like a gourd, and both ends of it are guarded by sphincters that permit the passage of substances in only one direction. The first of these is the *lower esophageal* (e-sof''ah-je'al) *sphincter* (sfink'ter), located between the esophagus and the stomach. We frequently are aware of the existence of this sphincter; sometimes it does not relax as it should, and then there is a feeling of having a place one can't swallow past. At the distal or far end of the stom-

ach, connecting it with the small intestine, is the other valve called the *pyloric* (pi-lor'ik) *sphincter.* This valve is especially important in that it plays a role in determining how long food remains in the stomach (Fig. 18-3).

The stomach is a combination storage pouch and churn. If the stomach is empty, there will be many folds in the lining. These folds are called *rugae* (ru'ge), and they disappear as the stomach dilates (it may be stretched so that it holds a half gallon of food and liquid). When the stomach is filled, the pyloric sphincter closes and retains the contents until the food has been mixed with digestive juices collectively called *gastric juice.* These juices are secreted by many glands in the stomach wall. The mixture of gastric juice and food is known as *chyme* (kime).

The gastric juice itself has two main components: *hydrochloric acid* and *enzymes.*

Stomach Acid

The hydrochloric acid in the stomach juice has three important functions:

1 It softens the connective tissues in meat.
2 It kills bacteria and thus destroys many potential disease-producing agents.
3 It activates at least one of the stomach enzymes, which are chemicals that begin the digestion of food.

An abnormally low production of stomach acid may cause digestive disturbances which are greatly aggravated by the soda or other alkaline substances contained in many patent medicines purporting to relieve indigestion. Such substances neutralize the valuable normal functions of the stomach acid, and, in many cases, grave harm is done by such self-medication. Occasionally, hydrochloric acid is pro-

duced in excess, and its presence can be determined by an analysis of the stomach contents. This condition is called hyperacidity and may be associated with ulcer disease.

Heartburn, Vomiting, and Related Disorders

A burning sensation in the region of the esophagus and stomach is popularly known as *heartburn*. It may be caused by the sudden intake of a large amount of fluid or food resulting in excessive stretching of the lower esophagus. This interferes with the functioning of the lower esophageal sphincter, allowing gastric acid to enter the esophagus. Heartburn is not due to hyperacidity of the

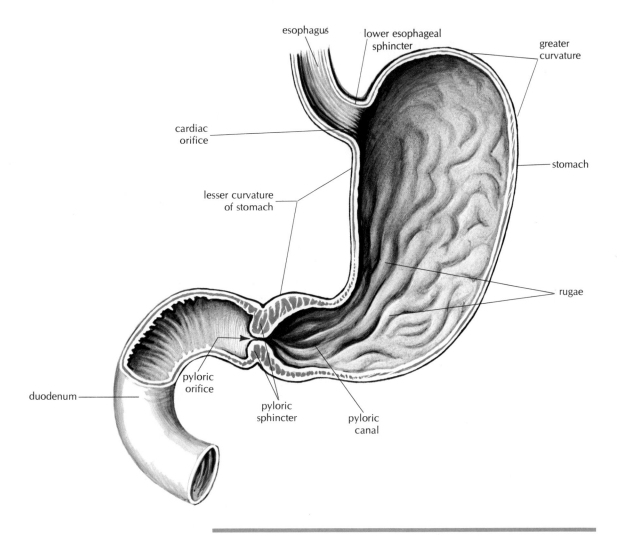

Fig. 18-3 *Longitudinal section of stomach and a portion of the duodenum, showing interior.*

stomach contents. *Nausea* is an unpleasant sensation that may follow distention or irritation of the lower esophagus or of the stomach as the result of various nervous and mechanical factors. It may be a symptom of interference with the normal forward peristaltic motion of the stomach and intestine and thus may be followed by vomiting. *Vomiting* is the expulsion of stomach (and sometimes bowel) contents through the mouth by reverse peristalsis. The contraction of the abdominal wall muscles forcibly empties the stomach. Vomiting is frequently caused by overeating or by inflammation of the stomach lining, a condition called *gastritis* (gas-tri′tis). Gastritis results from irritation of the mucosa by certain drugs, foods, or drinks. For example, long-term use of aspirin, highly spiced foods, or alcohol can lead to gastritis. Likewise, the nicotine in cigarettes can cause gastritis.

Flatus (fla′tus) usually refers to excessive amounts of air (gas) in the stomach or intestine. The resulting condition is referred to as *flatulence* (flat′u-lens). In some cases it may be necessary to insert a tube into the stomach or rectum to aid the patient in expelling flatus.

Stomach Cancer

While stomach cancer is common in many parts of the world, it has become infrequent in the United States. Nevertheless, it is an important disorder owing to the high death rate associated with it. Males are more susceptible than females. The tumor nearly always develops from the epithelial or mucosal lining of the stomach and is often of the type called adenocarcinoma (ad″e-no-kar″si-no′mah). Sometimes the victim has suffered from long-standing indigestion but has failed to consult a physician until the cancer has spread to other organs, such as the liver, in which there may be several metastases. Persistent indigestion is one of the important warning signs of cancer of the stomach.

Peptic Ulcer

An ulcer is an area of the skin or mucous membrane in which the tissues are gradually disintegrating. Peptic ulcer occurs in the mucous membrane of the esophagus, the stomach, or the duodenum (du″o-de′num), the first part of the small intestine. Peptic ulcers in the stomach are gastric ulcers; those in the duodenum are duodenal (du″o-de′nal) ulcers. An ulcer may be the result of the acid action

of the gastric juice. Peptic ulcers are found most frequently in people between the ages of 30 and 45. Duodenal ulcers are much more common in males. Emphasis is now being placed on mental and emotional factors as a contributing cause of ulcers. The person suffering from peptic ulcer needs the best medical and nursing care, and most certainly should not depend on patent medicines such as antacids.

More about the Pyloric Sphincter

The pyloric sphincter is a ringlike muscle surrounding the end of the stomach. Normally, the stomach contents escape through this muscular ring in about 2 to 6 hours after eating. This action may be delayed by a spasm of the muscle (pylorospasm). In some infants, more often males, there may be a congenital obstruction called *pyloric stenosis* (ste-no′sis). Usually, surgery is required to modify the muscle so food can pass from the stomach into the duodenum.

The Small Intestine

The small intestine is the longest part of the alimentary canal. It is known as the small intestine because its diameter is smaller than that of the large intestine. The small intestine is about 6 m (20 feet) long compared with 1.2 m to 1.5 m (4 or 5 feet) for the large intestine. In addition, the mucosal surface of the small intestine has a greatly increased surface area, owing to the presence of tiny, finger-like projections called *villi* (vil′li) (Fig. 18-4). The first 25 cm to 27 cm (10 to 12 inches) of the small intestine is called the duodenum. In the duodenum is an opening into which lead two ducts, carrying digestive juices from two accessory organs of digestion, the *pancreas* and the *liver*. Pancreatic juice arrives in the duodenum by way of the pancreatic duct, while bile from the liver and gallbladder is carried by the *common bile duct*. Bile contains no enzymes, but it is important in the digestion of fats. The small intestine secretes its own intestinal juice. Thus, as the chyme passes into the duodenum, it is exposed to several digestive juices.

Beyond the duodenum, there are two more divisions of the small intestine: the *jejunum* (je-joo′num), which forms the next two fifths of the small intestine; and finally the *ileum* (il′e-um), constituting the remaining portion of the small intes-

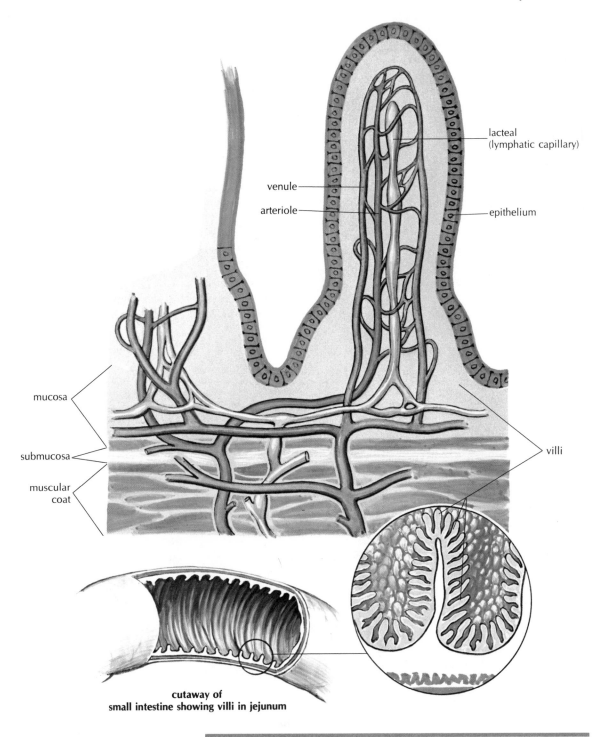

lacteal
(lymphatic capillary)

venule

arteriole

epithelium

mucosa

villi

submucosa

muscular
coat

cutaway of
small intestine showing villi in jejunum

Fig. 18-4   *Structure of a villus.*

tine. The ileum joins the large intestine through a muscular ring called the ileocecal (il''e-o-se'kal) *valve.*

The food in the stomach is partially digested by the gastric juices, but the small intestine is the organ in which most of the digestive and absorptive processes occur. We shall have a closer look at these two processes.

The Process of Digestion

In Chapter 13, The Blood, it was pointed out that the blood plasma contains the water, the food substances, and the mineral salts which together are necessary for the life and growth of the cells. Ingested foods must be converted to simple substances before they can nourish the cells. This conversion process is called digestion.

Let us review once more these basic materials that the cells need, and that are found in foods.

1 **Carbohydrates** include starches and sugars, and contain the elements carbon, hydrogen, and oxygen.
2 **Fats** are more concentrated in fuel value than carbohydrates, and are important for the absorption of certain vitamins.
3 **Proteins** form the stuff of which, besides water, protoplasm is made.
4 **Mineral salts** include a large variety of somewhat simpler compounds than those mentioned above. Salts maintain the proper conditions for osmosis in the cells, form a part of the body structure (as in bone), and play an important part in such life processes as muscle contraction, nerve responses, and blood clotting (Table 18-1).
5 **Vitamins** help to regulate cell metabolism. They are food substances which are essential for good health (Table 18-2).

Table 18-1 Mineral salts.

Mineral	Functions	Sources	Deficiencies
Potassium (K)	Nerve and muscle activity	Fruits and other foods	Muscular and neurologic disorders
Sodium (Na)	Body fluid balance	Most foods and table salt	Weakness, cramps, diarrhea, dehydration
Calcium (Ca)	Formation of bones and teeth, blood clotting, nerve conduction	Dairy products, eggs	Rickets, tetany, bone demineralization
Phosphorus (P)	Formation of bones and teeth required for processes that need energy	Beef, egg yolk, dairy products	Bone demineralization, abnormal metabolism
Iron (Fe)	Oxygen carrier (hemoglobin)	Meat, eggs, spinach, prunes	Anemia, dry skin, indigestion
Iodine (I)	Thyroid hormones	Seafood, iodized salt	Hypothyroidism, goiter
Magnesium (Mg)	Catalyst for enzyme reactions, carbohydrate metabolism	Green vegetables	Spasticity, arrhythmia, vasodilation
Manganese (Mn)	Catalyst in the actions of calcium and phosphorus	Legumes, nuts, cereals, green leafy vegetables	Possible reproductive disorders
Copper (Cu)	Necessary for absorption and oxidation of vitamin C & iron and in formation of hemoglobin	Liver, fish, oysters, legumes, nuts	Anemia
Cobalt (Co)	Part of vitamin B_{12}, involved in blood cell production and in synthesis of insulin	Animal products	Pernicious anemia
Zinc (Zn)	Promotes carbon dioxide metabolism, aids in the breakdown of proteins	Many foods	Alopecia, (baldness) possibly related to diabetes
Fluorine (F)	Prevents tooth decay	Water and many foods	Dental caries

Table 18-2 Vitamins.*

Vitamin	Functions	Sources	
Retinol (A)	Required for healthy epithelial tissues and for eye pigments	Yellow vegetables, fish-liver oils	Night blindness, dry scaly skin
Thiamin (B$_1$)	Required for some enzyme systems involved in converting food into energy	Pork, cereal grains	Beriberi, a disease of nerves (neuritis)
Riboflavin (B$_2$) (also called G)	Needed for enzyme systems that aid oxidation of sugars and amino acids (proteins)	Milk, eggs, kidney, liver	Skin and tongue disorders
Niacin (nicotinic acid) or PP or B$_5$	Involved in oxidation of carbohydrates	Yeast, lean meat, liver	Pellagra with dermatitis, diarrhea, mental disorders
Pyridoxine (B$_6$)	Involved in metabolism of various food substances, transport of amino acids	Liver, rice, milk, cereals	Skin disorders, anemia, lack of growth
Pantothenic acid	Essential for normal growth	Yeast, liver, eggs	Skin lesions, gray hair
Cyanocobalamin (B$_{12}$)	Production of blood cells (hemopoiesis)	Meat, liver, milk, eggs	Pernicious anemia
Biotin	Involved in carbon dioxide and fat metabolism	Peanuts, liver, tomatoes, eggs	Lack of coordination, dermatitis
Folic acid and folates	Required for synthesis of amino acids in DNA	Vegetables, liver	Anemia, digestive disorders
Ascorbic acid (C)	Maintains healthy skin and mucous membranes synthesis of collagen	Citrus fruits, green vegetables	Scurvy, poor bone and wound healing
Calciferol (D)	Aids in absorption of calcium from intestinal tract, and prevents rickets	Fish liver oils, sun on skin oils	Rickets, bone deformities

* Vitamin E has been omitted because its role in normal nutrition is not established. It is widely distributed in common foods.

6 **Water** constitutes about 66% of an adult's entire body composition. Eighty percent or more of many fruits and vegetables, and from fifty percent to seventy-five percent of meats and fish is water.

The digestive juices, by their chemical action, extract these materials so that they can be absorbed. Most of the digestive juices contain the chemicals known as *enzymes,* which speed up the chemical reactions that make possible the breakdown of food. It should be pointed out that although the enzymes enable the chemical reaction to take place, the enzymes themselves do not enter into the reaction. For example, an enzyme may assist a basic protein to separate itself from the rest of the food, but the enzyme itself does not become a part of the protein. There are several different enzymes, and each acts on a specific food compound and no other. For example, some enzymes act only on fats, others act only on starches, and so forth. But let us see what happens to a mass of food from the time it is taken into the mouth to the moment that it is ready to be absorbed.

In the mouth, the food is chewed, and saliva, the first of the digestive juices, acts on it, softening it so that it can be swallowed easily. Saliva contains the enzyme *salivary amylase* or *ptyalin* (ti'ah-lin), which initiates the process of digestion by changing some of the starches into sugars. Recall at this point that carbohydrates are found in the blood plasma in the form of simple sugar—glucose—and thus we should begin to understand where this blood sugar comes from.

When the food reaches the stomach, it is acted upon by the gastric juice, which contains hydrochloric acid and certain enzymes. The most important functions of the gastric juice are those related to the actions of the hydrochloric acid (as previously outlined) and the liquefying of the food. In addition, there is some action, particularly on proteins, by the enzyme *pepsin.* Although secreted by the cells of the gastric lining in an inactive form, the presence of hydrochloric acid in the stomach activates pepsin in order that it may aid in the digestion of protein. Nearly every type of protein in the diet begins to be digested by the action of pepsin. Two other enzymes are secreted by the stomach, but they are of minor importance. Due to the churning action of the stomach, food, gastric juice and mucus, secreted by cells of the stomach wall, are mixed until the semiliquid substance, chyme, is formed. From the stomach chyme proceeds to the small intestine for more chemical treatment.

In the duodenum, the chyme is mixed with the greenish yellow bile delivered from the liver and the gallbladder through the common bile duct. The bile does not contain enzymes; its action is purely mechanical. It works on fat, acting as a sort of liquid crowbar that splits the bits of fat into ever smaller particles so that the next digestive juice, the powerful secretion from the pancreas, can act more efficiently. The pancreatic juice contains a number of enzymes including the following:

1   **Lipase.** Following the physical division of fats into tiny particles by the action of bile, the powerful pancreatic lipase actually does almost all the digesting of fats. In this process, fats are usually broken down into two simpler compounds, glycerol and fatty acids, which are more readily absorbable. If pancreatic lipase is absent, fats are expelled with the feces in undigested form.
2   **Amylase** (am'i-lase). This changes starch to sugar.
3   **Trypsin** (trip'sin). This splits proteins into *amino* (am'e-no) acids, which are the form in which proteins enter the blood stream.

The intestinal juice contains a number of enzymes including three that act on complex sugars to transform them into the simpler form in which they are absorbed. These are *maltase, sucrase,* and *lactase.* It must be emphasized that most of the chemical changes in foods occur in the intestinal tract because of the pancreatic juice, which could probably adequately digest all foods even if no other digestive juice were produced. If pancreatic juice is absent, serious digestive disturbances always occur.

This, in a nutshell, is the process of digestion. It should be noted that the food materials that the enzymes break down to absorbable forms are carbohydrates (*i.e.,* sugars and starches), fats, and proteins. The mineral salts are dissolved in the water, and this solution is absorbed as it is. The vitamins behave a bit differently according to their type. Some are incorporated in fats and are absorbed along with the fats. Other vitamins are dissolved in water and are absorbed in much the same way that mineral salts are. Still other vitamins (such as vitamin K) are produced by the action of bacteria in the colon and are absorbed from the large intestine (see Table 18-3).

Absorption in the Small Intestine

The means by which the digested food reaches the bloodstream is known as *absorption.*

The small intestine is the chief organ of absorption. This process takes place through the mucosa by means of its countless minute projections known as villi. The villi are so small and so numerous that they give a velvety appearance to the lining of the small intestine. Each villus is epithelium underlaid with connective tissue. Within each villus is a system of miniature arteries and veins, bridged with capillaries. All the basic food materials, including water and salts, but with the exception of most fats, are absorbed into the bloodstream through the capillary walls in the villi. From here, they pass by way of the portal system to the liver, to be stored or released and used as needed.

Fats have an alternative method of reaching the bloodstream. As noted, some fat is absorbed by way of the blood capillaries of the villi. However, most fats also are absorbed by way of the lymphatic capillaries of the villi, which are called lacteals. The word "lacteal" means "like milk," an apt description of the appearance of the mixture of lymph and fat globules that is drained from the small intestine after a quantity of fat has been digested. This mixture of fat and lymph, called *chyle,* collects in the cisterna chyli and eventually reaches the bloodstream.

Table 18-3 *Digestive juices and enzymes.*

Juices and Glands	Place of Action	Enzymes	Changes in Foods
Saliva from 3 pairs of salivary glands	Oral cavity	Salivary amylase (ptyalin)	Begins starch digestion
Gastric juice from the stomach wall	Stomach	Pepsin	Begins protein digestion
Pancreatic juice from the pancreas	Small intestine	Amylase Trypsin Lipase	Acts on starches Acts on proteins Acts on fats
Intestinal juice from the small intestine (tubular glands)	Small intestine	Lactase Maltase Sucrase	Breaks down complex sugars into simpler forms
Bile from the liver	Small intestine	None	Breaks down fats physically so that lipase can digest them

In summary, the products of the digestive process, namely simple sugars, amino acids, fatty acids, and glycerol are absorbed into the capillaries of the villi.

The Large Intestine

Once the processes of digestion and absorption have taken place in the stomach and small intestine, all that remains is water and those parts of the food that are of no use to the body. These materials and anything else that may be indigestible will pass out of the body through the large intestine.

The materials to be eliminated continue through the ileocecal valve from the small intestine and enter the small pouch at the beginning (proximal) part of the large intestine. This pouch is called the *cecum* (se'kum) and is located in the lower iliac region of the abdomen. To the cecum is attached a small blind tube called the *vermiform* (ver'me-form) *appendix*. "Vermiform" means wormlike.

The next part of the large intestine is called the *colon*. The colon comprises four subdivisions: the *ascending colon* extends upward from the cecum along the right side toward the liver. There it bends, extending across the abdomen to the left side, forming the *transverse colon*. At this point, the colon bends sharply and extends downward on the left side of the abdomen into the pelvis. This part is called the *descending colon*. The lower part of the colon bends posteriorly in an S shape and con-

tinues downward, forming the *sigmoid colon*. The sigmoid colon empties into the *rectum,* a portion about 15 cm to 20 cm long. The rectum serves as a temporary storage area for the indigestible and unabsorbable food residue (see Fig. 18-1). A narrow portion of the distal part of the large intestine is called the *anal canal,* which leads to the outside of the body through an opening called the *anus* (a'nus).

No enzymes are secreted by the large intestine. Its walls are lined with mucous membrane and contain layers of involuntary muscle which move the solid waste products, called *fecal matter,* toward the rectum. Absorption of large amounts of water takes place through the walls of the large intestine. The action of bacteria within the large intestine aids in the production of vitamin K and some of the B-complex vitamins.

Intestinal Disorders
Inflammation

Difficulties with digestion or absorption may be due to *enteritis* (en''ter-i'tis), an intestinal inflammation. When both the stomach and the small intestine are involved, the illness is called *gastroenteritis* (gas''tro-en-ter-i'tis). The symptoms include nausea, vomiting, and diarrhea as well as acute abdominal pain or colic. Gastroenteritis may be caused by a variety of pathogenic organisms including viruses, bacteria, and protozoa. Chemical irritants such as alcohol, spray residues on fruits and vegetables, and other toxins have been known to cause this disorder.

Appendicitis is inflammation of the vermiform appendix. It may result from infection of the appendix mucosa by organisms causing enteritis or from obstruction by accumulated, hardened fecal material or occasionally by pinworms.

Diarrhea and Dysentery

Diarrhea is a symptom characterized by abnormally frequent watery bowel movements. *Dysentery* usually refers to an inflammation of the mucosal lining, although deeper tissues also may be affected. The two main types of dysentery are as follows:

1   **Bacillary** (bas'e-la-re) dysentery, which is caused by rod-shaped bacteria that are transferred to food and water primarily by human carriers.
2   **Amebic** dysentery, which is due to an infestation by a one-celled animal called *Entamoeba histolyica.* See Chapter 7, Figure 7-4.

Bacillary dysentery may be prevented by a combination of water chlorination, milk pasteurization and observation of all sanitary measures in the handling of food. Restaurant workers should receive periodic examinations and should observe ordinary precautions such as frequent hand washing, particularly after every trip to the toilet. Amebic dysentery is especially prevalent in areas in which food is grown in fields where human waste is used for fertilizer. When traveling in countries in which this is the custom, one should avoid the use of raw food and unboiled or unsterilized water. The traveler should carry chemical tablets to kill contaminants in water if he is unable to boil it.

Diarrhea is a symptom found in many conditions in addition to the dysenteries. Some of these disorders include the following:

1   Epidemic diarrhea, or diarrhea of the newborn, which is somewhat more common in the premature infant. This symptom may be due to poor handwashing techniques by those who care for newborn infants, resulting in the transfer of pathogens between infants.
2   Bacterial infection of the intestinal wall, due to ingested pathogens such as staphylococci, common in food poisoning, or to the spread of pathogens from other infected sites, such as the respiratory tract.
3   Ptomaine poisoning which is sometimes confused with the bacterial food poisoning caused by staphylococci but is actually due to putrid meat. It is now rather rare.
4   Nutritional deficiency diseases such as pellagra (pel-lag'rah) or sprue.
5   Acute emotional disturbances, such as those sometimes experienced by students just before and during an important test ("State Board" diarrhea).
6   Ulcerative colitis, a chronic inflammatory disease with ulceration of the intestinal wall frequently causing bleeding.
7   Cancer, in which constipation may alternate with diarrhea.

In order to determine the cause of the diarrhea, an examination of the intestinal excretions may be required. Various terms are used to refer to this bowel waste including *feces* (fe'sez), fecal material, excrement, and most commonly, the word "stool." A stool examination may reveal the presence of amebae, bacteria, the ova of worms, or blood.

Constipation

Millions of dollars are spent each year in an effort to remedy a condition called constipation. What is constipation? Many people erroneously think of themselves as constipated if they have days during which there are no bowel movements. Actually, normal people vary greatly, so that one person may be perfectly well although he has a bowel movement only once in two or three days, while another may be equally well with more than one movement daily.

On the basis of its onset, constipation may be classified as acute or chronic. Acute constipation occurs suddenly and may be due to an intestinal obstruction such as a tumor associated with cancer or an inflammation of the saclike bulges (diverticula of the intestinal wall as seen in *diverticulitis* (di''ver-tik''u-li'tis). Laxatives and enemas should be avoided and a physician should be consulted at once. Chronic constipation, on the other hand, has a more gradual onset and may be divided into two groups:

1   **Spastic** constipation in which the intestinal musculature is overstimulated, so that the canal

becomes narrowed and the space (lumen) inside the intestine is not large enough to permit the passage of fecal material.

2 **Flaccid** (flak'sid) constipation which is characterized by a lazy or *atonic* (ah-ton'ik) intestinal muscle. Elderly persons and those on bed rest are particularly susceptible to this condition.

The overactive spastic type of constipation is probably much more common than the atonic lazy kind. Nervous tensions, excessive amounts of bulky foods, and the use of laxatives increase the muscle tone of the intestine. The person who has sluggish intestinal muscles may be helped by moderate exercise, an increase in vegetables and other bulky foods in the diet, and an increase in fluid intake.

The use of enemas and so-called colonic flushings is unnecessary and should be discouraged for most persons. The lining of the intestine may be injured by streams of water that remove the normal protective mucus. In addition to this, those who have piles (hemorrhoids) will aggravate this condition by enemas. Enemas should be done on the order of a physician, and sparingly.

Cancer of the Colon and Rectum

Tumors of the colon and rectum are among the most common types of cancer in the United States. These tumors usually arise from the mucosal lining and are called adenocarcinomas. The occurrence of cancer of the colon is evenly divided between the sexes, but malignant tumors of the rectum are more common in men. Tumors may be detected by examination of the rectum and lower colon with an instrument called a *sigmoidoscope* (sig-moi'do-scope). Early detection and treatment is a key to increasing survival rates.

The Accessory Structures
The Liver

The liver, or *hepar* (he'par), is the largest of the glandular organs of the body. It is located under the dome of the diaphragm so that, if of normal size, it cannot be felt through the abdominal wall. The human liver is the same brownish red color as the animal livers seen in the market. It has a large right lobe and a somewhat smaller left lobe, as well as two other lesser lobes. The liver has a double blood supply: the portal vein and the hepatic artery. These two vessels deliver about 1½ quarts of blood to the liver every minute. The hepatic artery carries oxygenated blood, while the portal system of veins carries blood that is rich in the end products of digestion as well as in other raw materials required for metabolic activities in the liver. This most remarkable organ has so many functions that only some of its major activities can be listed here:

1 The storage of glucose (simple sugar) in the form of *glycogen* (gli'ko-jen), an animal starch. When the blood sugar level falls below normal, the liver cells convert glycogen to glucose and release it into the bloodstream; this serves to restore the normal concentration of blood sugar.

2 The formation of albumin, fibrinogen, and certain other blood plasma proteins.

3 The synthesis of *urea* (u-re'ah), a waste product of protein metabolism. Urea is released into the bloodstream for transport to the kidneys for elimination.

4 The modification of fats so that they can be more efficiently used by cells all over the body.

5 The manufacture of bile. Liver cells synthesize bile salts, the substances that aid in the digestion of fats. *Bilirubin* (bil''e-roo'bin), a pigment released during red blood cell destruction in the spleen, is extracted from the bloodstream and eliminated in the bile.

6 The detoxification (de-tok''si-fi-ka'shun) (removal of poisonous properties) of harmful substances such as alcohol and certain drugs. The end products resulting from these activities are eliminated in the bile.

7 The manufacture of heparin (hep'ah-rin), a substance that prevents clotting of blood.

Diseases of the Liver

Inflammation of the liver is called *hepatitis* (hep-ah-ti'tis). Epidemic hepatitis is caused by a virus. Outbreaks of this disease, which are more common in the fall and winter, occur in military establishments and in other populous institutions as epidemics. It varies in severity from cases that are so mild as to be scarcely recognizable to serious infections in which the liver may become permanently damaged. A more prevalent type of virus infection is called serum hepatitis. The infection is transmitted by administration of infected blood, plasma or blood products, or by improperly sterilized needles and syringes (as used by drug addicts). (See Table 3 of the Appendix.) Because of the fact that the blood from the intestinal tract passes through the liver, any toxins or microorganisms that may get into the intestinal (mesenteric) veins enter the liver. The most important of these organisms is the *Entamoeba histolytica* which causes amebic colitis at first. If it is carried into the liver, it causes the same destruction of tissue that it does in the colon. However, since the liver is not open to the outside as the colon is, the softened and liquid area becomes an abscess. This condition is very hard to treat.

Cirrhosis (si-ro′sis) of the liver is a chronic disease in which the active liver cells are replaced by inactive scar tissue (connective tissue). The most usual type is *portal cirrhosis,* which is fairly common in alcoholics. Many believe that the cause is related to poor nutrition. Destruction of the liver cells curtails the portal circulation, causing blood to accumulate in the spleen and the gastrointestinal tract, and fluid in the peritoneal cavity. This fluid may have to be removed periodically by puncture, or *paracentesis* (par-ah-sen-te′sis).

Cancer of the liver also is common in cases that begin as a cancer in one of the organs of the abdominal cavity. The tumor cells are carried from the intestine or another organ through the veins that go to the liver. Secondary growths or metastases in the liver therefore are fairly common. With new surgical techniques, large sections of diseased liver can be removed. Also, liver transplantation is a successful treatment for some persons with liver disease.

The Gallbladder

The gallbladder is a muscular sac that serves as a storage pouch for bile. While the liver may manufacture bile continuously, the need for it is likely to arise only a few times a day. Consequently, bile from the liver flows into the liver ducts and then up through the duct connected with the gallbladder. When the chyme enters the duodenum, the gallbladder contracts, squeezing bile into a duct leading to the duodenum.

The gallbladder may become infected, a condi-

tion called *cholecystitis* (ko-le-sis-ti′tis), while the presence of stones in the gallbladder is called *cholelithiasis* (ko-le-le-thi′ah-sis). Sometimes a chronic gallbladder infection may lead to stone formation. If a stone finds its way into the tube from the gallbladder, the person may suffer from *biliary* (bil′e-a-re) *colic* (i.e., acute pain) because of the muscle spasm in the wall of the duct.

The Pancreas

The pancreas produces the pancreatic juice. Pancreatic juice is extremely powerful because of the presence of digestive enzymes. Since it is usually confined to its proper channels, the action of the pancreatic enzymes will not damage body tissues. However, it may happen that the pancreatic duct becomes blocked, with the result that these enzymes become backed up in tissues that are not supposed to receive them. Also, in some cases of gallbladder disease the infection of that organ may extend into the duct connected with the pancreas and cause an abnormal activation of the pancreatic enzymes. In either circumstance, the pancreas will suffer destruction by its own juice, and the outcome can be fatal. This condition is known as *acute pancreatitis.* Additional disorders that may involve the pancreas include cancer and other tumors.

Also, the pancreas manufactures a substance called *insulin* which is released directly into the blood and has the function of regulating the amount of sugar that is "burned" in the tissues.

The Peritoneum

The *peritoneum* is a serous membrane that covers the surface of most of the abdominal organs to form the visceral serosa and lines the abdominal wall to form the parietal layer. In addition to these parts of the peritoneum, there are more complex double layers of membrane that separate the abdomen into areas and spaces, and in some cases aid in supporting the organs and holding them in place. (See Fig. 3-1.)

The *mesentery* (mes′en-ter-e) is a double-layered peritoneal structure shaped somewhat like a fan, with the handle portion attached to the back wall. The expanded long edge is attached to the small intestine. Between the two layers of membrane that form the mesentery are the blood vessels, nerves, and other structures that supply the intestine.

Another double-layered peritoneal structure, called the *greater omentum* (o-men'tum), hangs downward from the lower border (greater curvature) of the stomach. This double layer of peritoneum extends into the pelvic part of the abdomen and then loops back and up to the transverse colon. It has been aptly described as an apron inside the abdomen. It may, in some cases, serve to prevent the spread of infection inside the abdominal cavity. There is also a peritoneal structure called the *lesser omentum,* which extends between the stomach and the liver.

Disorders Involving the Peritoneum

Peritonitis

Peritonitis is inflammation of the peritoneum. It is a serious complication following infection of one of the organs that the peritoneum covers—often the appendix. The frequency of peritonitis has been greatly reduced by the use of antibiotic drugs. However, it still occurs and can be very dangerous. If the infection is kept in one area, it is said to be a *localized* peritonitis. A *generalized* peritonitis may cause so much absorption of disease organisms and their toxins that the outcome will be fatal. A ruptured appendix or ulcer may pour such masses of bacteria into the abdominal cavity that the resulting peritonitis could overwhelm the individual. Immediate surgery to repair the rupture, together with meticulous nursing care, will be needed to save the person's life.

Since many of the infections of such epithelial membranes have their origins in relatively mild disorders such as tonsillitis, appendicitis, sinusitis, and related infections, careful attention to the general health, as well as nursing care directed toward the prevention of the extension of lesser infections, is the best way to forestall these serious complications.

Ascites

An accumulation of fluid in the peritoneal cavity is called *ascites* (ah-si'tez). The abdomen becomes greatly enlarged and the pressure on the organs may require removal of liquid by paracentesis. Obstruction of the portal flow, which may occur in cirrhosis of the liver, is one important cause of ascites.

Some Practical Aspects of Nutrition

Good nutrition is absolutely essential for the maintenance of health. This means basically that all the fundamental food materials necessary for the life and growth of the body cells must be continuously provided, in adequate quantity, in the food that is eaten. If one or more of these vital materials are not supplied, the body will suffer in a number of ways, the effect being *malnutrition.* One commonly thinks of a malnourished person as one who does not have enough to eat; but malnutrition can occur just as easily from eating too much of the wrong foods. The normal manner by which malnutrition is avoided is to adhere to a balanced diet; that is, to ensure that most of what is eaten includes adequate quantities of the basic nutrients.

In order that homemakers and others who plan meals may understand more easily how to provide a balanced diet, food groupings have been publicized. One grouping arranges foods as follows.

1 **Protective** foods are those especially high in vitamins and mineral salts. These include citrus and other fruits plus a variety of vegetables, particularly leafy green and yellow ones (Tables 18-2 and 18-3). Protective foods are especially valuable in staving off disease.
2 **Protein** foods are required for growth and repair of tissues. Since they cannot be stored, they should be included daily.
3 **Energy** foods contain fats and carbohydrates. They are needed in larger amounts by those who are especially active physically.

Many assertions about food combinations, such as the common one that cherries and ice cream (or fish and milk) are poisonous mixtures, are not based on the laws of nature; nor can any scientific basis be found for such ideas. For the normal, healthy person, a balanced diet including a variety of fruits, vegetables, and cereals, together with adequate amounts of such protein foods as milk and milk products, eggs, and meats, will maintain nutritional health.

Infants may need supplements of certain vitamins, but normal, healthy children and adults should be able to obtain adequate amounts of all the different vitamins from a well-balanced diet. When required, vitamin supplements should be selected by a physician to fit the particular needs of the individual. The so-called megavitamin dosages now fashionable in some quarters may cause unpleasant reactions and in some cases are hazardous. Vitamins A and D have both been found to cause serious toxic effects, and a relatively small excess of vitamin D may result in the appearance of dangerous symptoms.

A few people develop severe allergic (hypersensitive) manifestations if they eat certain foods. Some find that strawberries cause such a response. In others, shellfish cause a reaction resembling poisoning. However, the great majority of people can eat any food. The most common causes of temporary digestive disturbances are overeating, bacterial contamination, and virus infections.

Summary

1 Digestive system as a whole.
  A Functions—digestion and absorption.
  B Components—alimentary canal, accessory organs.
2 Alimentary canal.
  A Mouth, or oral cavity.
    (1) Structures.
      (a) Tongue.
      (b) Teeth—deciduous and permanent.
      (c) Salivary glands—parotid, submandibular (submaxillary), sublingual.
    (2) Diseases—gingivitis, stomatitis, pyorrhea, caries, mumps.
  B Swallowing tubes and their accessories.
    (1) Pharynx (throat).
    (2) Uvula.
    (3) Epiglottis.
    (4) Esophagus ("gullet"). Has peristaltic action.
    (5) From swallowing tubes to anus, alimentary canal is lined with mucous membrane; has involuntary muscle for peristaltic action.
  C Stomach.
    (1) Characteristics and accessory structures.
      (a) Lower esophageal sphincter (guards entrance to stomach).
      (b) Rugae (folds in mucosa).
      (c) Stomach a storage pouch and churn (for chyme).
      (d) Juice contains hydrochloric acid and enzymes.
      (e) Pyloric sphincter—exit from stomach.
    (2) Disorders of stomach and accessory structures.

      (a) Heartburn and vomiting.
      (b) Hyperacidity and hypoacidity.
      (c) Stomach cancer.
      (d) Peptic ulcer (emotional factors a cause).
      (e) Pyloric stenosis
  D Small intestine.
    (1) Divisions—duodenum, jejunum, ileum.
    (2) Digestive juices and sources.
      (a) Intestinal juice (own secretion).
      (b) Bile from liver through common bile duct (no enzymes).
      (c) Pancreatic juice from pancreas by way of pancreatic duct.
    (3) Digestion—review table of enzymes.
    (4) Absorption—through villi.
      (a) Most food materials absorbed in blood capillaries.
      (b) Some fats absorbed in lacteals (lymphatic).
  E Large intestine.
    (1) Has no enzymes, water absorption occurs through walls.
    (2) Ileocecal valve (sphincter).
    (3) Cecum and appendix.
    (4) Colon (ascending, transverse, descending, and sigmoid parts).
    (5) Rectum and anal canal, surrounded by anal sphincter.
  F Intestinal disorders.
    (1) Enteritis.
    (2) Diarrhea (a symptom).
    (3) Dysentery (bacillary or amebic).
    (4) Spastic and flaccid constipation.
    (5) Cancer of the colon and rectum.
3 Accessory structures.

A Liver and its diseases.
  (1) Liver has many functions.
  (2) Hepatitis may be epidemic.
  (3) Cirrhosis may result in excessive fluid in abdomen.
  (4) Cancer metastasizes to liver.
B Gallbladder and its diseases.
  (1) Gallbladder a storage pouch for bile; discharges bile when needed.
  (2) Cholecystitis—inflammation of gallbladder.
  (3) Cholelithiasis—gallstones.
  (4) Biliary colic is due to spasm of bile duct.
C Pancreas.
  (1) Produces pancreatic juice (3 enzymes).
  (2) Acute pancreatitis—pancreas may digest itself.

  (3) Produces insulin (regulates use of sugar in cells).
4 Peritoneum.
  A Serous membrane lining abdominal wall and covering abdominal organs.
  B Peritoneal structures—mesentery, greater omentum, lesser omentum.
  C Disorders—peritonitis, ascites.
5 Nutrition.
  A Balanced diet necessary for health.
  B Malnutrition—inadequate nutrition.
  C Three basic foods—protective, protein, energy.
  D Most food combinations harmless.
  E A minority of people allergic to some foods.

Questions and Problems

1 Trace the path of an indigestible object from the mouth through all parts of the alimentary canal to the outside and tell what happens on the way.

2 Differentiate between deciduous and permanent teeth as to kinds and numbers of the 2 sets.

3 What is the pharynx? What spaces connect with it?

4 How would you distinguish between "stomach" and "abdomen"?

5 What is peristalsis? Name some structures in which it occurs.

6 Name and describe the purposes of the acid in the stomach juice.

7 Describe the process of absorption.

8 What are the principal enzymes and what is their origin? What does each do?

9 Name several diseases that involve the organs of digestion.

10 Describe what happens in the formation of a peptic ulcer. Where does it occur?

11 What is an important symptom of stomach cancer?

12 What is the mesentery and where is it located? The greater and lesser omenta? What is the principal disease of the peritoneum?

13 List 5 functions of the liver.

14 What constitutes a balanced diet? What are some examples of food fallacies?

15 Is it possible to overdose oneself with vitamins? Explain.

16 What are the most important causes of indigestion?

Chapter 19

The Urinary System and Its Disorders

- A secretion that is an excretion
- Excretions and their mechanisms
- Kidneys, inside and out
- Functions and disorders of the kidneys
- Dialysis and transplants
- Tubes that carry urine to the bladder
- Bladder location and structure
- Function and disease of the bladder
- Excretory tube
- Disorders of the urethra
- Normal urine and what is in it
- Abnormal urine substances and their significance

Glossary

Calyx (pl. calyces) A cup-shaped part.

Cortex Outer layer of an organ.

Dialysis Separation of smaller molecules from larger molecules in a solution by selective diffusion through a semipermeable membrane.

Glomerulus A ball-like cluster of nerve fibers or blood vessels, especially the microscopic tuft of capillaries that is surrounded by the expanded part of each kidney tubule.

Medulla The innermost part of an organ, as seen in the kidneys and adrenal glands; the part of the brain that connects with the spinal cord.

Nephron The microscopic functional unit of kidney tissue, consisting of a glomerulus with its capsule, convoluted tubules, and Henle's loop, plus the collecting tubule.

Pyramid A cone-shaped structure or part.

Reabsorption The process of absorbing again.

Secretion The process of producing a new substance from materials in the blood; the new substance produced by glandular activity, using materials in the blood.

Ureters In the urinary system, the 2 ureters conduct the secretion from the kidneys to the urinary bladder.

Urethra The excretory tube for the bladder.

The urinary system is also called the excretory system, and one of its main functions is to remove certain waste products from the blood and eliminate them from the body.

The terms "elimination" and "excretion" often are used interchangeably. Actually, we usually think of excretion as the function of removing useless substances (*i.e.,* the waste products of cell metabolism) from the blood and lymph. This is accomplished not only by the filtering of these substances from the blood but often by a type of cellular activity, similar to that of gland cells, producing a secretion. On the other hand, elimination indicates the actual emptying of the hollow organs in which these waste products have been temporarily stored. Thus, the kidney is said to excrete, while the urinary bladder eliminates.

Although the focus of this chapter is the urinary system, it is important to remember that body systems work interdependently to maintain the body's constant unchanging balances, namely homeostasis (ho′me-o-sta′sis). Therefore, certain aspects of other systems will be included.

Here it may be of interest to summarize the chief excretory mechanisms of the body, along with some of the substances that they eliminate:

1 The urinary system—water, waste products containing nitrogen, and salts. These are all constituents of the urine.
2 The digestive system—water, some salts, bile, and the residue of digestion. These are all contained in the feces (fe′sez).
3 The respiratory system—carbon dioxide and water. The latter appears as vapor, as breathing on a windowpane will demonstrate.
4 The skin, or integumentary system—water, salts, and very small quantities of nitrogenous wastes. These all appear in perspiration, though evaporation of water from the skin may go on most of the time without our being conscious of it.

Organs of the Urinary System

The main parts of the urinary system, shown in Figure 19-1 are as follows:

1 Two **kidneys**—the glandular organs that are necessary for life. These are the organs that, in addition to other things, extract wastes from the blood.
2 Two **ureters** (u-re′ters)—tubes that conduct the secretion from the kidneys to the urinary bladder.
3 A single **urinary bladder**—the reservoir that receives the urine brought to it by the two ureters.
4 A single **urethra** (u-re′thrah)—the excretory tube for the bladder. Through the urethra, the urine is conducted to the outside of the body and eliminated.

Location of the Kidneys

The two kidneys lie against the muscles of the back in the upper abdomen. They are protected by the lower ribs and the rib (costal) cartilages, since they are up under the dome of the diaphragm. Each kidney is enclosed in a membranous capsule that is made of fibrous connective tissue; it is loosely adherent to the kidney itself. In addition, there is a crescent of fat around the lateral perimeter of the organ. It is called the adipose capsule and is one of the chief supporting structures of the kidney. The peritoneum lies in front of the kidneys so that the kidneys and several other structures are not in the peritoneal cavity. This area is known as the *retroperitoneal* (re′′tro-per′′i-to-ne′al) space, indicating that it is behind the peritoneum. The blood supply of the kidney is illustrated in Figure 19-2.

Structure of the Kidneys

The kidney is a somewhat flattened organ about 10 cm (4 inches) long, 5 cm (2 inches) wide, and 2.5 cm (1 inch) thick. On the inner or medial border there is a notch called the *hilus* (hi′lus), at which region the artery, the vein, and the ureter connect with the kidney. The outer or lateral border is convex (curved outward), giving the entire organ a bean-shaped appearance.

The kidney is divided into three regions: the renal cortex, the renal medulla, and the renal pelvis (Fig. 19-3). The renal *cortex* is the outer portion of the kidney. The renal *medulla* consists of several cone-shaped structures called *pyramids*. The tip of each pyramid points toward the renal pelvis. The renal pelvis is a funnel-shaped basin that forms the upper end of the ureter. Cuplike extensions of the renal pelvis project from the pelvis to surround the tips of the pyramids. These extensions are called *calyces* (kay′li-sez), singular *calyx* (kay′liks). The urine that collects in the pelvis then passes down the ureters to the bladder.

The kidney is a glandular organ; that is, most of the tissue is epithelium with just enough connective tissue to serve as a framework. As is the case with most organs, the most fascinating aspect of the kidney is too small to be seen with the naked eye. This basic unit of the kidney, where the kidney's business is actually done, is called a *nephron* (nef′ron) (Fig. 19-4). The nephron is primarily a tiny coiled tube with a bulb at one end called *Bowman's capsule.* This bulb surrounds a cluster of capillaries called the *glomerulus* (glo-mer′u-lus). A kidney is composed of about a million nephrons;

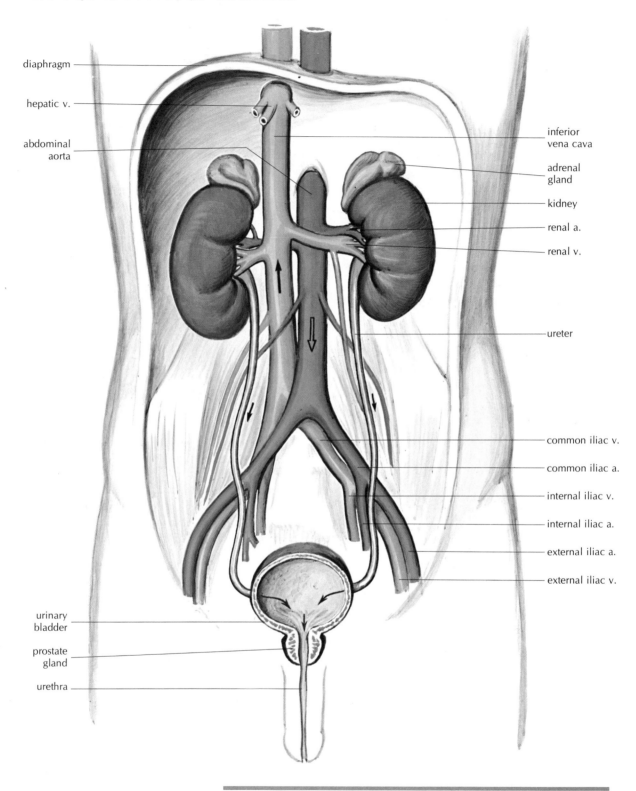

diaphragm

hepatic v.

abdominal
aorta

inferior
vena cava

adrenal
gland

kidney

renal a.

renal v.

ureter

common iliac v.

common iliac a.

internal iliac v.

internal iliac a.

external iliac a.

external iliac v.

urinary
bladder

prostate
gland

urethra

Fig. 19-1 *The urinary system, with blood vessels.*

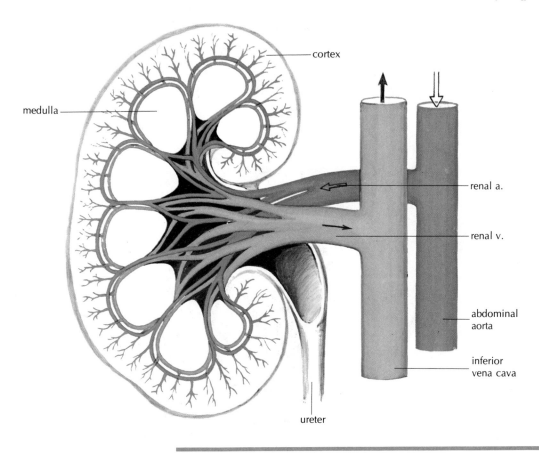

Fig. 19-2 *Blood supply and circulation of kidney.*

if all these coiled tubes were separated, straightened out, and laid end to end, they would span some 120 kilometers (75 miles)!

A small blood vessel, called the *afferent arteriole,* supplies the glomerulus with blood; another small vessel, called the *efferent arteriole,* carries blood from the glomerulus to the capillaries surrounding the coiled tube of the nephron. Since these capillaries surround the tube, they are called the *peritubular capillaries.*

The tubular part of the nephron consists of several portions. The coiled portion leading from Bowman's capsule is called the *proximal convoluted* (kon'vo-lut-ed) *tubule,* and the coiled portion at the other end is called the *distal convoluted tubule.* Between these two coiled portions is the *loop of Henle* (hen'lee).

The distal convoluted tubule curls back toward the glomerulus between the afferent and efferent arterioles. At the point where the distal tubule contacts the arterioles, there are specialized glandular cells that form the *juxtaglomerular* (juks''tah-glo-mer'u-lar) *apparatus* (Fig. 19-5). The function of these specialized cells is discussed later in this chapter.

The glomerulus, Bowman's capsule, and the proximal and distal convoluted tubules of each nephron are within the renal cortex. The loops of Henle extend varying distances into the medulla. The distal end of each tubule empties into a collecting duct which then continues through the medulla toward the renal pelvis.

Renal Physiology
Glomerular Filtration

The process of urine formation begins in the glomerulus and Bowman's capsule. The membranes that form the walls of the glomerular capillaries

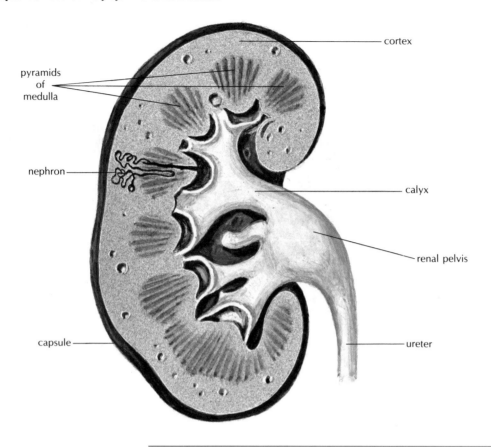

pyramids
of
medulla

nephron

capsule

cortex

calyx

renal pelvis

ureter

Fig. 19-3 *Longitudinal section through the kidney showing its internal structure, including one of more than a million nephrons.*

are sievelike and permit a free flow of water and soluble materials through them. These capillary walls, as is the case with other capillaries, are impermeable (im-per′me-abl) to blood cells and large protein molecules, so these substances remain in the blood (Fig. 19-6).

The afferent arteriole entering the glomerulus allows blood to enter more rapidly than it can leave through the efferent arteriole. Thus, the pressure of the blood in the glomerulus is about three to four times as high as it is in other body capillaries. Consequently, the fluid in the blood is constantly being "squeezed" into Bowman's capsule. This process is known as glomerular filtration, and the fluid that enters Bowman's capsule is called the glomerular filtrate. This filtrate then begins its journey along the tubular system of the nephron. In addition to water and the normal soluble substances in the blood, other substances, such as drugs, may

also be filtered and become part of the glomerular filtrate.

Tubular Reabsorption and Secretion

The process of filtration that occurs in the renal corpuscle is followed by the processes of reabsorption and secretion during the journey of the filtrate through the tubular system. The filtrate is very much like the plasma of the blood in that it contains glucose, amino acids, mineral salts, water, and other needed substances. These are removed by the cells of the proximal convoluted tubule and returned to the tissue fluids and to the blood in the peritubular capillaries by *reabsorption*. As this modified filtrate continues its journey through the loop of Henle and the distal convoluted tubule, more waste materials and often drugs are removed

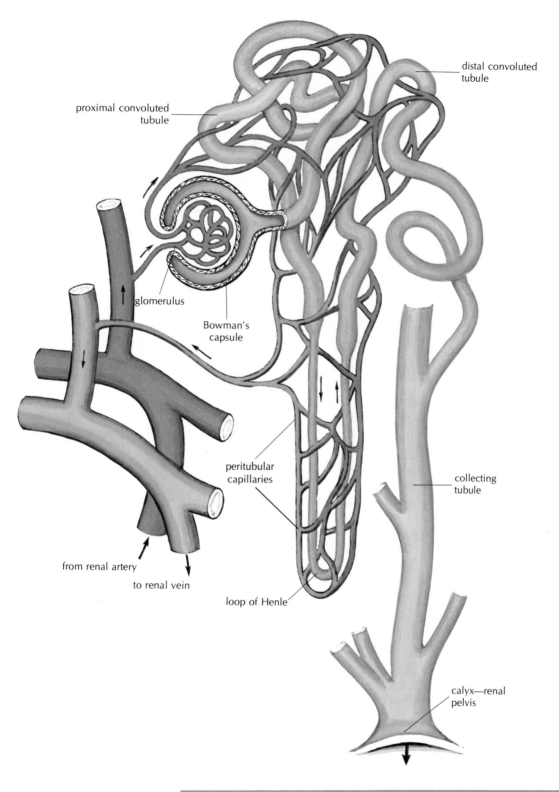

Fig. 19-4 *A simplified nephron.*

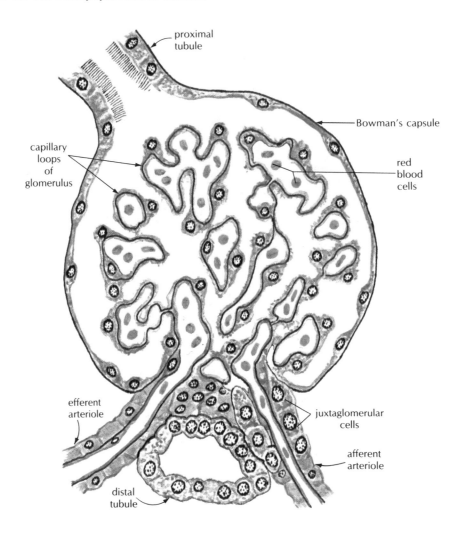

Fig. 19-5 *Structure of juxtaglomerular apparatus. Note how distal tubule contacts the arterioles.*

from the blood by an active process called *secretion.* The original dilute filtrate has now become urine, ready for excretion from the body.

Functions of the Kidneys

1 Excretion of unwanted substances such as **waste products** from cell metabolism and excess salts.
2 Aid in the maintenance of **water balance.**
3 Aid in regulating the **acid–base balance.**
4 Production of hormones, including the hor-

mone **renin** (re′nin), which is important in the regulation of blood pressure.

The use of proteins (in the form of amino acids) by the body cells produces, among other things, waste materials that contain the element nitrogen. Chief among these nitrogen-containing products is *urea* (u-re′ah). The kidneys provide a specialized mechanism for the elimination of these nitrogenous (ni-troj′e-nus) waste products.

A second function of the kidneys involves the maintenance of water balance (Fig. 19-7). Although the amount of water consumed in a day can vary tremendously, the kidneys can adapt to

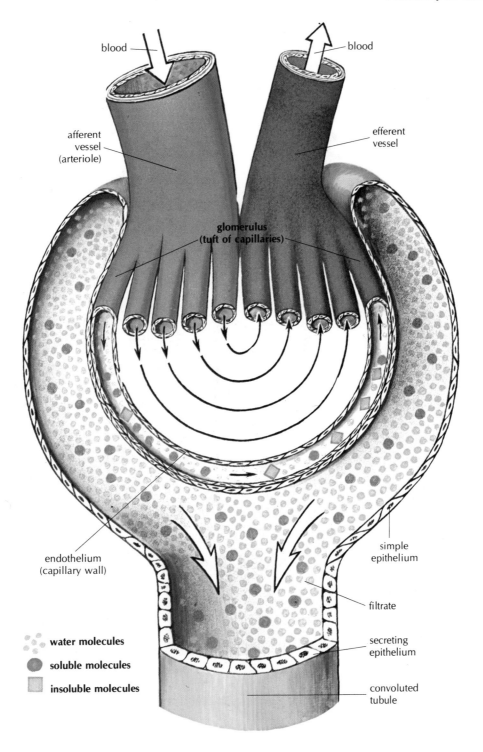

blood

blood

afferent
vessel
(arteriole)

efferent
vessel

**glomerulus
(tuft of capillaries)**

endothelium
(capillary wall)

simple
epithelium

filtrate

secreting
epithelium

convoluted
tubule

water molecules

soluble molecules

insoluble molecules

Fig. 19-6 *Diagram to show the process of filtration in the
formation of urine. The higher pressure inside the small capillaries
of the glomerulus forces the dissolved substances (except the
plasma proteins) and much water into the space inside Bowman's
capsule. The smaller caliber of the efferent vessel as compared
with the larger afferent vessel causes this higher pressure.*

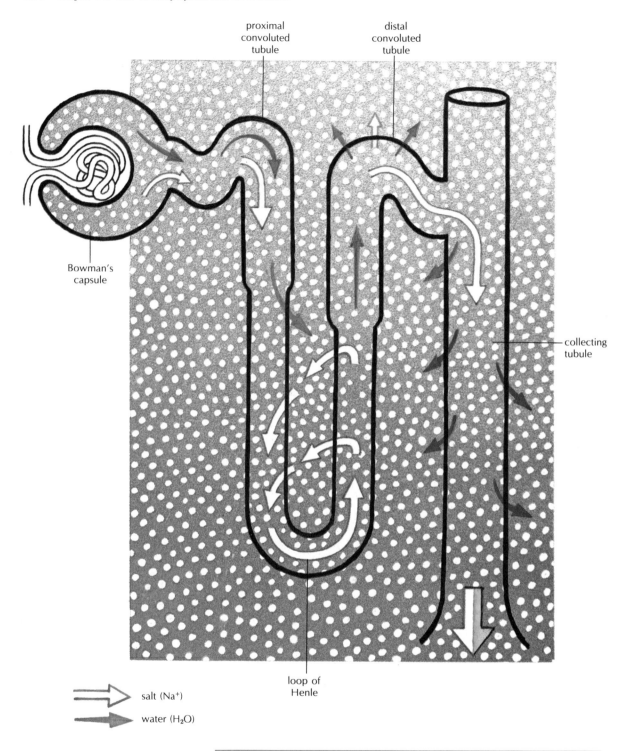

proximal convoluted tubule

distal convoluted tubule

Bowman's capsule

collecting tubule

loop of Henle

salt (Na+)

water (H₂O)

Fig. 19-7   *The loop of Henle, where the proportions of waste and water in urine are regulated according to the body's constantly changing needs. The concentration of urine is determined by means of intricate exchanges of water and salt.*

these variations so that the volume of body water remains remarkably stable from day to day. Water is constantly lost in many ways; from the skin, from the respiratory system during exhalation, and from the intestinal tract. Normally, the amount of water taken in or produced (intake) is approximately equal to the amount lost (output).

A third function of the kidneys is to aid in regulating the acid–base balance of the body fluids. Acids are constantly being produced by cell metabolism and, in addition certain foods can cause acids or bases to be formed in the body. Bases in the form of antacids, such as baking soda, may also be ingested. However, if the body is to function normally, a certain critical proportion of acids and bases must be maintained at all times (see Chaps. 4 and 13).

The fourth function of the kidneys involves the production of hormones, which is accomplished by the juxtaglomerular apparatus. If the blood pressure is low, the cells of the juxtaglomerular apparatus release renin into the blood. There it acts as an enzyme to activate a protein that causes blood vessels to constrict, and thus raise the blood pressure. When the kidneys do not get enough oxygen, they release another hormone-like substance that acts as an enzyme to produce erythropoietin (e-rith''ro-poi'e-tin). Erythropoietin serves to stimulate the red bone marrow and thus prevents anemia.

Kidney Disorders

Kidney disorders may be acute or chronic. Acute conditions usually arise suddenly and, most frequently, are the result of infection with inflammation of the nephrons. These diseases commonly run a course of a few weeks followed by complete recovery. Chronic conditions arise slowly and often are progressive with gradual loss of kidney function.

Acute glomerulonephritis (glo-mer''u-lo-ne-fri'tis) is the most common disease of the kidneys. This condition usually occurs in children about 1 to 4 weeks after a streptococcal infection of the throat. Antibodies formed in response to the streptococci attach to the glomerular membrane and injure it. These damaged glomeruli allow protein, especially albumin, to filter into Bowman's capsule

and ultimately appear in the urine (albuminuria). They also allow red blood cells to filter into the urine (hematuria). Usually, the patient recovers without permanent kidney damage. Sometimes, in an adult patient, the disease becomes chronic with a gradual decrease in the number of functioning nephrons, leading to chronic renal failure.

Pyelonephritis (py''el-o-ne-fri'tis) refers to an inflammation of the kidney pelvis and the tissue of the kidney itself. It may be either acute or chronic. In acute pyelonephritis, the inflammation results from a bacterial infection. Bacteria most commonly reach the kidney by ascending along the lining membrane from an infection in the lower part of the urinary tract. More rarely, bacteria can be carried to the kidney by the blood. Acute pyelonephritis is often seen in persons with partial obstruction of urine flow with stagnation (urinary stasis). This may occur during pregnancy in the female or it may be due to an enlarged prostate in the male. Usually, the disease responds to the administration of antibiotics, fluid replacement, rest, and fever control. Chronic pyelonephritis is a more serious disease and is frequently seen in patients with urinary tract blockage. It may be caused by persistent or repeated bacterial infections. There is progressive damage of kidney tissue, eventually leading to chronic renal failure.

Hydronephrosis (hi''dro-ne-fro'sis) refers to the distension of the renal pelvis and calyces caused by an accumulation of fluid due to an obstruction to normal urine flow. The obstruction may occur at any level in the urinary tract. The most common causes of obstruction are, in addition to pregnancy or an enlarged prostate, a kidney stone that formed in the pelvis and dropped into the ureter, a tumor that presses on a ureter, or scars due to inflammation. Removal of the obstruction within a few weeks, before the kidney is damaged, may result in complete recovery. If the obstruction is not removed, the kidney will be permanently damaged.

Acute renal failure may result from a medical or surgical emergency or from toxins that damage the tubules. This condition is characterized by a sudden, serious decrease in kidney function which may be fatal without immediate medical treatment.

Chronic renal failure results from a gradual loss of nephrons. As more and more nephrons are destroyed, the kidneys gradually lose the ability to perform their normal functions. As the disease progresses, nitrogen waste products accumulate to high levels, and this condition is known as *uremia* (u-re′me-ah).

A few of the characteristic signs and symptoms of chronic renal failure are the following:

1 **Dehydration** (de″hi-dra′shun)—excessive loss of body fluid may occur early in renal failure when the kidneys cannot concentrate the urine and large amounts of water are eliminated.
2 **Edema** (e-de′mah)—accumulation of fluid in the tissue spaces may occur late in chronic renal disease when the kidneys cannot eliminate water in adequate amounts.
3 **Hypertension**—may occur as the result of fluid overload and the increased production of renin.
4 **Anemia**—occurs when the kidneys cannot produce the hormone to activate red bone marrow cell production.
5 **Increased amounts of nitrogen waste products in the blood**—if these levels are very high, urea can be changed into ammonia in the stomach and intestine and cause ulcerations and bleeding.

Even without kidney disease, the kidneys lose some of their ability to concentrate urine owing to the aging process. More water is needed to excrete the normal amount of waste products. Older persons find it necessary to drink more water, and they eliminate larger amounts of urine (polyuria) even at night (nocturia).

Tumors of the kidneys usually grow rather slowly, but occasionally rapidly invading types are found. Blood in the urine and dull pain in the kidney region are warnings that should be heeded at once. Immediate surgery may be lifesaving. A *polycystic* (pol-e-sis′tik) kidney is one in which many fluid-containing sacs develop in the active tissue and gradually, by pressure, destroy the functioning parts. This disorder runs in families, and until now treatment has not proved very satisfactory, except for the use of dialysis machines or kidney transplants.

Kidney stones, or *calculi* (kal′ku-li), are made of certain substances such as uric acid and calcium salts which precipitate out of the urine instead of remaining in solution. They usually form in the renal pelvis, although the bladder can be another site of formation. The causes of this precipitation of stone-building materials include infection of the urinary tract and stagnation of the urine. These stones may vary in size from tiny grains resembling bits of gravel up to large masses that fill the kidney pelvis and extend into the calyces. These are described as *staghorn calculi*. There is no way of dissolving these stones, since substances that would be able to do so also would destroy the kidney tissue. Sometimes instruments can be used to crush smaller stones and thus allow them to be expelled with the urine, but more often surgical removal is required.

Dialysis Machines and Kidney Transplants

Dialysis (di-al′e-sis) means "the diffusion of dissolved molecules through a semipermeable membrane." These molecules tend to pass from the area of greater concentration to one of less concentration. In patients who have defective kidney function, the accumulation of urea and other nitrogen waste products can be reduced by passing the patient's blood through a dialysis machine. This is where the principle of "molecules leaving the area of greater concentration" operates to remove the excess products from the blood.

There are two methods of dialysis in use—hemodialysis and peritoneal dialysis—and both are based on the principle of diffusion of dissolved molecules through a semipermeable membrane. In hemodialysis, the membrane is made of cellophane; in peritoneal dialysis, the surface area of the peritoneum acts as the membrane. An amendment to the Social Security Act in 1973 provides federal financial assistance for persons who have chronic renal disease and require dialysis. Recent improvements have made home dialysis possible for many patients. Access to the bloodstream has been made safer and easier, and the size of the equipment has been reduced. Currently, researchers are developing a portable hemodialysis unit that patients can wear when they are away from home or hospital. With improved methods of peritoneal dialysis, chronic as well as acute renal failure can be treated. Permanent catheters can be implanted into the abdomen, and machines have been developed that can administer the dialyzing fluid automatically.

Many hundreds of kidney transplants have been done successfully during the last several years. Kidneys have so much extra functioning tissue that in the normal individual no problem is posed by losing one kidney. Records show that the percentage of transplant successes is greatest when living, closely related donors are used. However, organs from a deceased donor have also proved satisfactory in many cases. The problem of tissue rejection (the rejection syndrome) is discussed in Chapter 23.

The Ureters
Structure and Function of the Ureters

The two ureters are long, slender, muscular tubes that extend from the kidney basin down to and through the lower part of the urinary bladder. Their length naturally varies with the size of the individual and so may be anywhere from 25 cm to 32 cm (10 to 12 inches) long. Nearly 2.5 cm (one inch) of its lower part enters the bladder by passing obliquely through the bladder wall. They are entirely extraperitoneal; that is, behind and, at the lower part, below the peritoneum.

The wall of the ureter includes a lining of epithelial cells, a relatively thick layer of involuntary muscle, and, finally, an outer coat of fibrous connective tissue. The lining is continuous with that of the renal pelvis and the bladder. The muscles of the ureters are capable of the same rhythmic contraction (peristalsis) found in the digestive system. Urine is moved along the ureter from the kidneys to the bladder by peristalsis at frequent intervals. Because of the oblique direction of the last part of each ureter through the lower bladder wall, compression of the ureters by the full bladder prevents backflow of urine.

Disorders of the Ureters

Abnormalities in structure of the ureter include double portions at the kidney pelves and constricted or abnormally narrow parts, called *strictures* (strik'tures). Narrowing of the ureter also may be caused by abnormal pressures from tumors or other masses outside the tube. Obstruction of the ureters may be the result of stones from the kidneys or a kinking of the tube due to a dropping of the kidney, a condition known as *ptosis* (to'sis).

The passage of a small stone along the ureter causes one of the most excruciating pains known. This intense pain is called renal colic and usually requires morphine or an equally powerful drug for relief. The first "barber surgeons" operating without benefit of anesthesia were permitted by their patients to cut through the skin and the muscles of the back to remove stones from the ureters. "Cutting for stone" in this way was relatively successful, in spite of lack of sterile technique, because of the approach through the back and the avoidance of the peritoneal cavity, with the possibility of deadly peritonitis. Modern surgery for a kidney stone, including the use of special instruments threaded through the urinary tract from the outside, may cause little temporary disability and a short convalescence.

The Urinary Bladder
Characteristics of the Bladder

The urinary bladder, when it is empty, is located below the parietal peritoneum and behind the pubic joint. When it is filled, it pushes the peritoneum upward and may extend well into the abdominal cavity proper. The urinary bladder is a temporary reservoir for urine, just as the gallbladder is a storage bag for bile.

The bladder wall has many layers. It is lined with mucous membrane; the lining, like that of stomach, is thrown into the folds called rugae when the receptacle is empty. Beneath the mucosa is a layer of connective tissue. Then follows a three-layered coat of involuntary muscle tissue which is capable of stretching to a great extent. Finally, there is an incomplete coat of peritoneum that covers only the upper portion of the bladder. When the bladder is empty, the muscular wall becomes thick and the entire organ feels firm. As the organ fills, the muscular wall becomes thinner and the organ may increase from a length of 5 cm (2 inches) up to as much as 12.5 cm (5 inches) or even more. A moderately full bladder holds about 470 ml (one pint) of urine.

Near the outlet of the bladder, circular muscle fibers contract to prevent emptying, and form what is known as the *internal sphincter*. In the infant, a center in the lower part of the spinal cord receives impulses from the bladder and sends motor impulses out to the bladder musculature; the organ is emptied in an action that is automatic (*i.e.,* a *reflex* action). However, with training, the child learns to control this reflex.

Disorders Involving the Bladder

A full (distended) bladder lies in an unprotected position in the lower abdomen, and a blow may rupture it, necessitating immediate surgical repair. Infection and tumors may involve the bladder, and blood in the urine is a rather common symptom of these. Inflammation of the bladder is called *cystitis* (sis-ti'tis) and is ten times as frequent in women as in men. This may be due, at least in part, to the very short urethra in the female (compared with that of the male). Usually, bacteria (*e.g.,* colon bacilli) ascend from the outside through the urethra into the bladder. Pain, urgency, and frequency are common symptoms.

Obstruction by an enlarged prostate gland or from a pregnancy may lead to stagnation and cystitis. Reduction of the general resistance to infection, as in diabetes, may lead to cystitis. The danger is that the infection may ascend to other parts of the urinary tract.

The Urethra
Location and Function of the Urethra

The *urethra* is the tube that extends from the bladder to the outside, and is the means by which the bladder is emptied. The urethra differs in men and women, since in men it is also a part of the reproductive system and it is much longer.

The female urethra is a thin-walled tube about 3.75 cm long. It is behind the pubic joint and is embedded in the muscle of the front wall of the vagina. The external opening is called the urethral meatus and is located just in front of the vaginal opening or within the lower part of the front wall of the vagina.

The male urethra is about 20 cm long. Early in its course, it passes through the prostate gland, where the two ducts carrying the male sex cells join it. From here it leads through the *penis* (pe'nis), the male organ of copulation, to the outside. The male urethra, then, serves the dual purpose of conveying the sex cells and draining the bladder, while the female urethra performs only the latter function.

The process of expelling urine through the urethra is called *urination* or *micturition.* It is controlled by the action of circular muscles continuous with those in the walls of the bladder and in the urethra. These form valvelike structures that are aided by external muscles in the pelvic floor.

Disorders of the Urethra

Congenital *anomalies* (ah-nom'ah-lees) (defects) present at birth involve the urethra as well as other parts of the urinary tract. The opening of the urethra to the outside may be too small, or the urethra itself narrowed. Occasionally it happens that there is an abnormal valvelike structure located at the point where the urethra enters the bladder. These valvelike folds of tissue can cause a back pressure of the urine, with serious consequences if they are not removed surgically. There is also a condition in the male in which the urethra opens on the under surface of the penis instead of at the end. This is called *hypospadias* (hi-po-spa'de-as).

Urethritis, in which inflammation of the mucous membrane and the glands of the urethra are involved, is much more common in the male than in the female and is often due to gonorrhea, although many other bacteria also may be responsible for the infection.

"Straddle" injuries to the urethra are common in men. This type of injury occurs when, for example, a man walking along a raised beam slips and lands with the beam between his legs. Such an accident may catch the urethra between the hard surfaces of the beam and the pubic arch, and rupture the urethra. In accidents in which the bones of the pelvis are fractured, rupture of the urethra is fairly common.

The Urine
Normal Constituents

In this chapter we have learned some of the main constituents of urine. Here they are summarized in a more detailed manner in order to complete the picture of the normal situation.

Urine is a yellowish liquid which is about 95%

water. Dissolved in this water are a number of solids and gases. The amount of these dissolved substances is indicated by the *specific gravity*. If urine were pure water, the specific gravity would be 1.000. However, because of the dissolved materials, the specific gravity of urine normally varies from 1.002 for very dilute urine to 1.040 for very concentrated urine. When the kidneys are diseased, they lose the ability to concentrate urine and the specific gravity will not vary as it does when the kidneys function normally.

Some of the dissolved substances normally found in the urine are the following:

1 **Nitrogenous waste products**—these include urea, uric acid and creatinine (kre-at′i-nin).
2 **Mineral salts**—these include sodium chloride (as in common table salt) and different kinds of sulfates and phosphates. They are excreted in appropriate amounts to keep the blood concentration of the mineral salts constant.
3 **Yellow pigment**—derived from certain bile compounds.

Abnormal Constituents

Urine examination is one of the most important parts of an evaluation of a person's physical state.

Among the most significant abnormal substances found in the urine are the following:

1 **Glucose**—usually an important indication of a disease known as *diabetes mellitus* in which the blood sugar is not oxidized ("burned") in the body cells but is excreted in the urine instead. The presence of glucose in the urine is known as *glycosuria* (gli′′ko-su′re-ah).
2 **Albumin**—normally retained in the blood; may indicate a kidney disorder such as nephritis. Albumin in the urine is known as *albuminuria* (al′′bu-mi-nu′re-ah).
3 **Blood**—usually an important indicator of urinary system disease including nephritis. Blood in the urine is known as *hematuria* (hem′′ah-tu-re′ah).
4 **Acetone** (as′e-tone)—produced when fats are incompletely oxidized; often seen in diabetes mellitus and in starvation.
5 **Pus cells** (leukocytes)—evidence of infection; can be seen by microscopic examination of a centrifuged specimen. Pus in the urine is known as *pyuria* (pi-u′re-ah).
6 **Casts**—molds formed in the microscopic kidney tubules, usually is evidence of disease of the nephrons.

Summary

1 Excretion and elimination.
  A Excretion—removal of useless substances from the body structures.
  B Elimination—emptying of organs in which waste products have been stored.
  C Excretory mechanisms—digestive, urinary, respiratory, skin.
2 Urinary system—kidneys, ureters, bladder, urethra.
3 Kidneys
  A Location—retroperitoneal.
  B Structure.
    (1) Three regions—cortex, medulla, pelvis.
    (2) Nephron—microscopic tubular unit; glomerulus, Bowman's capsule and convoluted tubules in cortex, loops of Henle, and collecting tubules in medulla; collecting ducts empty into pelvis, where ureters begin.
  C Physiology—glomerular filtration; tubular absorption and secretion.
  D Functions—excretion; maintenance of water balance; regulation of acid–base balance; production of hormones.
  E Diseases—glomerulonephritis; pyelonephritis; hydronephrosis; acute renal failure; chronic renal failure and uremia; tumors; calculi.
  F Dialysis and kidney transplants.
4 Ureters.
  A Structure and function—muscular tubes that carry urine from kidney to bladder by peristalsis.
  B Disorders—structures; kinking from ptosis of kidney, renal colic.

5 Bladder.
  A Structure and function—muscular sac capable of stretching; reservoir for urine. Has internal sphincter; impulse to empty a controllable reflex.
  B Disorders—injuries; tumors; stagnation and cystitis.
6 Urethra.
  A Structure and function—tube leading from bladder to outside; longer in male than in female; in male is also part of reproductive system.
  B Disorders—congenital anomalies; urethritis; straddle injuries.
7 Urine.
  A Normal constituents—water (95%); nitrogenous wastes; mineral salts; pigment; specific gravity 1.002 to 1.040.
  B Abnormal constituents—glucose; albumin; blood; acetone; pus cells; casts.

Questions and Problems

1 In what way might secretions and excretions be the same and how do these differ from each other?
2 How do the terms "elimination" and "excretion" differ from each other? Name the body systems that have excretory functions.
3 Where are the kidneys located?
4 Describe the external appearance of the kidneys and tell what tissues form most of the kidney structure.
5 Name and describe the microscopic structure that is the basic kidney unit.
6 What structures empty into the kidney pelvis and what drains this space?
7 In what ways does the kidney adjust the body chemistry?
8 What are some of the infections that involve the kidney, and what parts are most often affected?
9 What are calculi and what are some of the causes of this disorder?
10 What is meant by dialysis and how is this principle used for persons with kidney failure? What kinds of membranes are used for peritoneal dialysis, for hemodialysis?
11 What type of donors are best for kidney transplants?
12 Locate and describe the ureters.
13 What is renal colic?
14 Name and describe the layers of the bladder wall.
15 What is inflammation of the bladder called?
16 Describe the female urethra and tell how it differs from the male urethra in structure and function.
17 What is meant by a congenital anomaly and what is an example of such a condition involving the urethra?
18 What are other disorders that affect the urethra?
19 Define and tell the possible significance of 5 abnormal constituents of the urine.

Chapter 20

Glands and Hormones

Glossary

Endocrine Secreting into tissue fluids, blood, and lymph.

Exocrine Secreting into tubes or ducts that carry the secretion away from the gland to another organ or part, or to the surface of the body.

Hormone A chemical substance that is produced by a body organ or cell and that has a regulatory effect on the activity of a target organ.

Pituitary The "master gland," which produces a number of hormones that regulate many body processes.

Classification of Secretions and Glands

A gland as such is any organ that produces a certain secretion; the secretions themselves are substances manufactured from blood constituents by the specialized cells of which the glands are made.

The secretions of the various glands may be divided into two main groups:

1 **External secretions** are carried from the gland cells to a nearby organ or to the body surface. These external secretions are effective in a limited area near their origin. We have already learned something of most of these secretions: digestive juices, the secretions from the sebaceous glands of the skin, tears from the lacrimal glands, and urine (both a secretion and an excretion).

2 **Internal secretions** are carried to all parts of the body by the blood or lymph. These substances often affect tissues a considerable distance from the point of origin. Internal secretions are known as *hormones;* and the hormones, with the glands that produce them, will be the subject of this chapter.

Glands also fall into two categories:

1 **Exocrine** (ek'so-krin) **glands** have tubes (ducts) to carry the secretion from the gland to another organ or part of the body.

2 **Endocrine** (en'do-krin), or **ductless, glands** (Fig. 20-1) have no ducts, and so must depend upon the blood and the lymph to carry their

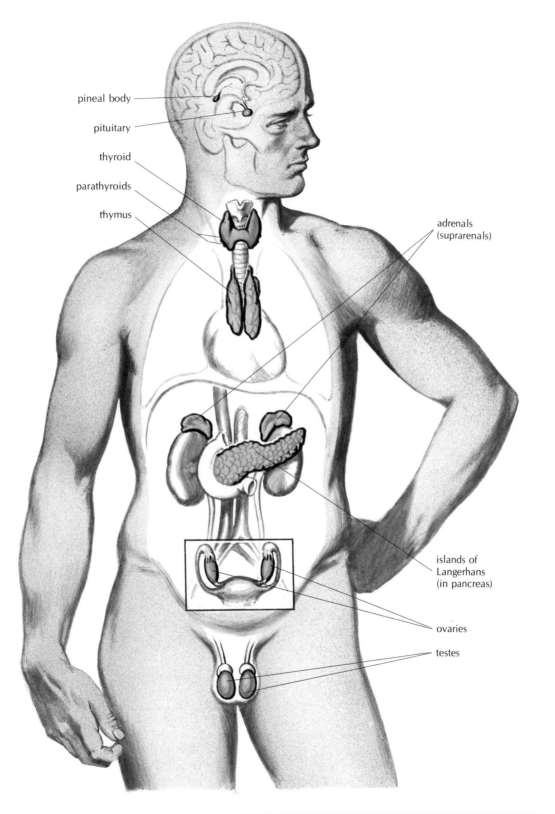

pineal body

pituitary

thyroid

parathyroids

thymus

adrenals
(suprarenals)

islands of
Langerhans
(in pancreas)

ovaries

testes

Fig. 20-1 *Endocrine system, with female sex glands shown in
inset.*

secretions to various body tissues, by way of the capillaries of the glandular tissue.

Sometimes the lymph nodes are spoken of as glands (*i.e.*, the "neck glands," which are actually nodes); but so far as is known the lymph nodes do not produce secretions.

The endocrine glands proper produce only internal secretions (hormones), but some organs contain both exocrine and endocrine gland tissue. For example, the pancreas, the stomach, and the small intestine all produce external secretions (digestive juices) and internal secretions (hormones) (Table 20-1).

Structure of Glands

Exocrine glands vary in complexity from very simple depressions resembling tiny dimples to involved arrangements such as are found in the kidneys. Simple tubelike structures are found in the stomach wall and in the intestinal lining. Complex, treelike groups of ducts are found in the liver, the pancreas and the salivary glands. Most glands are made largely of epithelial tissue with a framework of connective tissue. There may be a tough connective tissue capsule (a fibrous envelope) enclosing the organ, with extensions into the organ which form partitions. Between the partitions are groups of cells, and these units are called *lobes.*

Most endocrine glands, like exocrine glands, are made of epithelial tissue. However, since they have no ducts, they seem to make up for this lack by a most extensive blood vessel network. Operations on endocrine glands such as, for example, on the thyroid, require care in the control of bleeding. The organs believed to have the very richest blood supply of any in the body are the tiny adrenal, or suprarenal, glands which are located near the upper parts of the kidneys.

General Functions of Hormones

Hormones are chemical substances manufactured by the endocrine glands, and their overall function is to regulate the activities of various body organs. In one sense, the action of hormones can be com-

pared with that of the nervous system (in fact, in the chapter covering the nervous system, we saw how the hormone epinephrine acted in conjunction with the autonomic system in an emergency). Hormones sometimes are referred to as "chemical messengers." Some hormones stimulate exocrine tissues to produce their secretions. Another category of hormone stimulates other endocrine glands to action. There are hormones that have a profound effect upon growth, development, and even the personality of the individual. Others regulate the body chemistry: for example, the metabolism of the cells. Still others regulate the contraction of muscle tissues. Finally, there are hormones that control various sex processes. The action of each hormone is specific; that is, each has its particular, specialized job to do and no other.

Endocrine Glands and Their Hormones
The Pituitary, or "Master Gland"

The *pituitary* (pi-tu'i-tar-e) is a small gland about the size of a cherry. It is nearly surrounded by bone except for its area of connection with the brain. The pituitary is located in a saddlelike depression just behind the point of optic nerve crossing, in the midline. It has two important parts called the *anterior* and the *posterior lobes,* each of which produces several different hormones.

The Anterior Lobe

This lobe produces a large number of hormones. Many of them stimulate other glands, and it is for this reason that the pituitary is known as the master gland. Its main hormones are described below:

1 **Growth hormone** or **somatotropic** (so'' mah-to-trop'ik) **hormone** stimulates growth of bones, muscles, and other organs. Varying amounts of this hormone are produced throughout life. A person born with a deficiency of this hormone will remain a small, though well proportioned, individual unless treated with adequate hormones.

2 **Thyroid-stimulating** or **thyrotropic** (thi''ro-trop'ik) **hormone** stimulates the thyroid gland.

Table 20-1 *The endocrine glands and their hormones.*

Gland	Hormone	Principal Functions
Anterior pituitary	ACTH (adrenocorticotropin)	Stimulates adrenal cortex to produce cortical hormones; aids in protecting body in stress situations (injury, pain)
	TSH (thyroid-stimulating hormone)	Stimulates thyroid gland to produce thyroid hormones
	FSH (follicle-stimulating hormone)	Stimulates growth and hormone activity of ovarian follicles; stimulates growth of testes; promotes development of sperm
	GH (human growth hormone)	Promotes growth of all body tissues
	LH (luteinizing hormone)	Causes development of corpus luteum at site of ruptured ovarian follicle in female; stimulates secretion of testosterone in male
	Lactogenic hormone (prolactin)	Stimulates secretion of milk by mammary glands
Posterior pituitary	ADH (antidiuretic hormone; vasopressin)	Promotes reabsorption of water in kidney tubules; stimulates smooth muscle tissue of blood vessels
	Oxytocin	Causes contraction of muscle of pregnant uterus; causes ejection of milk from mammary glands
Adrenal cortex	Cortisol (95% of glucocorticoids)	Aids in metabolism of carbohydrates, proteins, and fats; active during stress
	Aldosterone (95% of mineralocorticoids)	Aids in regulating electrolytes
	Sex hormones	May influence secondary sexual characteristics in male
Adrenal medulla	Epinephrine and norepinephrine	Increases blood pressure and heart rate; activates cells influenced by the sympathetic nervous system plus many not affected by sympathetics
Pancreatic islets	Insulin	Aids transport of glucose into cells; required for cellular metabolism of foods, especially glucose; decreases blood sugar levels
	Glucagon	Stimulates the liver to release glucose, thereby increasing blood sugar levels
Parathyroids	Parathormone	Regulates exchange of calcium between blood and bones; increases calcium level in blood
Thyroid gland	Thyroid hormone (thyroxine and triiodothyronine)	Increases metabolic rate, influencing both physical and mental activities; required for normal growth
	Calcitonin	Decreases calcium level in blood
Ovarian follicle	Estrogens (*e.g.,* estradiol)	Stimulate growth of primary sexual organs (uterus, tubes, etc.) and development of secondary sexual organs such as breasts, plus changes in pelvis to ovoid broader shape
Corpus luteum (in ovaries)	Progesterone	Stimulates development of secretory parts of mammary glands; prepares uterine lining for implantation of fertilized ovum; aids in maintaining pregnancy
Testes	Testosterone	Stimulates growth and development of sexual organs (testes, penis, others) plus development of secondary sexual characteristics such as hair growth on body and face and deepening of voice; stimulates maturation of sperm cells

(continued)

Table 20-1 *The endocrine glands and their hormones.* (*continued*)

Gland	Hormone	Principal Functions
Placenta	Chorionic gonadotropin	Causes continued growth and secretory activity of corpus luteum (of ovary)
	Estrogens	Stimulate growth of mother's reproductive organs; cause relaxation of pelvic ligaments (to make childbirth easier)
	Progesterone	Aids in maintaining nutrition of embryo (due to effects on uterine lining cells)
	Placental lactogen	Promotes growth of maternal breasts
Gastric mucosa	Gastrin	Stimulates secretion of HCL and some enzymes
Intestinal mucosa	Secretin	Activates the pancreas to produce an alkaline watery pancreatic juice (to neutralize HCl)
	Cholecystokinin	Stimulates secretion of pancreatic enzymes: causes contraction and emptying of gallbladder

3 **Adrenocorticotropic** (ad-re″no-kor′te-ko-trop′ik) **hormone** (ACTH) stimulates the cortex of the adrenal glands.

4 **Gonadotropic** (gon″ah-do-trop′ik) **hormones** regulate the growth, development and functioning of the reproductive systems in both the male and the female.

5 **Prolactin** (pro-lak′tin) or **lactogenic** (lak″to-jen′ik) **hormone** stimulates the production of milk in the female.

The Posterior Lobe

This lobe of the pituitary gland stores and releases two hormones. These are produced in the hypothalamus and then trickle down nerve fibers to the posterior lobe. The hormones are described here.

1 **Antidiuretic** (an″ti-di″u-ret′ik) **hormone** (ADH) promotes the reabsorption of water from the kidney tubules and thus decreases the excretion of water. Large amounts of this hormone cause contraction of the smooth muscle of blood vessels and raise blood pressure. Inadequate amounts of ADH cause excessive loss of water and result in a disorder called diabetes insipidus. This type of diabetes should not be confused with diabetes mellitus, which is due to inadequate amounts of insulin.

2 **Oxytocin** (ox″se-tō′sin) causes contraction of the muscle of the uterus and also causes milk ejection from the breasts. Under certain circumstances, commercial preparations of this hormone are administered during or after childbirth to cause the uterus to contract.

Tumors of the Pituitary

The effects of pituitary tumors depend upon what types of cells the new or excess tissue contains. Some of these tumors contain an excessive number of the cells that produce growth hormone. If this occurs in childhood, the person will grow to an abnormally tall stature, a condition called *gigantism* (ji-gan′tizm). Although these people are large, they are usually very weak. If the growth-producing cells become overactive in the adult, a disorder known as *acromegaly* (ak″ro-meg′ah-le) develops. In acromegaly the bones of the face, the hands, and the feet widen. The fingers resemble a spatula, and the face takes on a grotesque appearance: the nose widens, the lower jaw protrudes, and the forehead bones may bulge. Often these pituitary tumors involve the optic nerves and cause blindness.

Tumors or disease may destroy the secreting tissues of the gland so that signs of underactivity develop. Such a patient often becomes obese and sluggish, and may exhibit signs of underactivity of other endocrine glands such as the ovaries, the testes or the thyroid. Evidences of tumor formation in the pituitary gland may be obtained by x-ray examinations of the skull. The saddle-like space for the pituitary body is distorted by the pressure of the tumor.

The Thyroid Gland

The largest of the endocrine glands is the *thyroid,* which is located in the neck. It has two oval parts called the lateral lobes, one on either side of the voice box. A narrow band called the *isthmus* (is'mus) connects these two lobes. The entire gland is enclosed by a connective tissue capsule. This gland produces hormones, the principal one known as *thyroxin* (thi-rok'sin). A hormone called *calcitonin* (kal''si-tō'nin), produced in the thyroid but active in calcium metabolism, will be discussed in connection with the parathyroid gland. The principal function of thyroid hormones is to regulate metabolism for the production of heat and energy in the body tissues. In order that these hormones may be manufactured, there must be an adequate supply of iodine in the blood. The iodine content may be maintained by eating vegetables grown in iodine-containing soils, or by eating seafoods. In some parts of the United States, as well as in certain regions of Italy and Switzerland, the soil is so deficient in iodine that serious defects may result in the inhabitants of these districts. The use of iodized salt may prevent difficulties.

One result of a deficiency of iodine in the blood is the formation of a *goiter,* which is a swelling of the neck due to an enlarged thyroid. As will be seen, there are other causes of goiter as well; but in this first-mentioned case, known as *simple goiter,* the thyroid becomes enlarged as the size and number of glandular cells increase in an attempt to produce enough thyroid hormones.

Another form of goiter is *adenomatous* (ad-e-no'mah-tus), or *nodular, goiter;* and, as the name would indicate, this type of goiter has an accompanying tumor formation which comes about through the overgrowth of the cells of the thyroid tissue. In nodular goiter, the tumor formation may be single or multiple; the former condition appears more likely to become malignant.

For various reasons the thyroid gland may become either underactive or overactive. Underactivity of the thyroid is known as *hypothyroidism* (hi-po-thi'roi-dizm) and shows up as two characteristic states:

1   **Cretinism** (kre'tin-izm), a condition in which there is a serious lack of thyroid activity from the beginning of the individual's life. A blood test of newborns for thyroid hormone is now mandatory in most states. Sometimes this condition is due to the complete absence of thyroid tissue. The infant becomes dwarfed and mentally deficient because of failure of physical growth and mental development. Only if continuous thyroid replacement is begun early is there any hope of altering the outlook. This disorder is fortunately rather rare in the United States, though endemic in certain regions where iodine is lacking.

2   **Myxedema** (mik''se-de'mah), the result of atrophy of the thyroid in the adult. The patient becomes sluggish both mentally and physically. The skin and the hair become dry, and there develops a peculiar swelling of the tissues of the face. Since thyroid extract or the hormone itself may be administered by mouth, the victim of myxedema can be restored to health very easily, though treatment must be maintained throughout the remainder of his life.

Hyperthyroidism is the opposite of hypothyroidism: overactivity of the thyroid gland. The development of a simple goiter might suggest hyperthyroidism, but there is a difference. In a simple goiter the thyroid is usually normal, but enlarges because it has more work to do, just as the heart will enlarge if something causes its work load to increase. Hyperthyroidism, however, is abnormal activity of the thyroid without an accompanying need of it by any other part of the body. A common form of hyperthyroidism is *exophthalmic* (ek-sof-thal'mik) *goiter,* or *Graves' disease,* in which there is a goiter, bulging of the eyes, a strained appearance of the face, intense nervousness, weight loss, a rapid pulse, sweating, and a tremor. Metabolism is stepped up to a terrific rate; it would seem that the victim had a fire raging within him. In many cases, the administration of drugs or surgical removal of a part of the thyroid gland will remedy the condition. An exaggerated form of hyperthyroidism with a sudden onset is called a *thyroid storm.* Untreated, it is usually fatal, but with appropriate care the majority of these persons can be saved.

Tests for Thyroid Function

The most frequently used tests for thyroid function are blood tests in which the uptake of radioactive iodine added to the blood sample is measured.

These tests are named after the type of radioactive iodine used. If these up-take tests are abnormal, the person may have further testing in which radioactive iodine is taken orally and the radioactivity of the thyroid gland measured.

Tests that are used less frequently for determining the activity of the thyroid gland include the basal metabolism test and the protein bound iodine test:

1 The **basal metabolism test** measures the amount of oxygen a person uses while at rest.
2 The **protein-bound iodine** test measures the amount of iodine that is combined with protein in a sample of the person's blood.

The Parathyroid Glands

Behind the thyroid gland, and embedded in its capsule, are four tiny epithelial bodies called the parathyroid glands. The secretion of these glands is called *parathormone* (par''ah-thor'mōn). Parathormone is one of three hormones that regulate calcium metabolism. The other two are *calcitonin* and *hydroxycholecalciferol* (hi-drok''se-ko''le-kal-sif'e-rol). Parathormone promotes the release of calcium from storage areas in bone tissue, thus increasing the amount of calcium circulating in the bloodstream. Calcitonin, which is produced in the thyroid gland, acts to lower the amount of calcium circulating in the blood. Hydroxycholecaliferol is produced from vitamin D after first being modified by the liver and then the kidney. It regulates the absorption of calcium by the intestine.

If these glands are removed, there will follow a series of muscle contractions involving particularly the hand and the face muscles. These spasms are due to a low concentration of blood calcium, and the condition is called *tetany* (tet'ah-ne), which must *not* be confused with the infection called tetanus (lockjaw). On the other hand, if there is an excess production of the secretion of these glands, as may happen in tumors of the parathyroids, calcium (normally stored in the bones for use by the tissues as needed) is removed from its storage place and is poured into the bloodstream, whence it finally is excreted by the kidneys. These persons will have stone formation in the kidneys and easily fractured bones.

The Adrenal Glands and Their Hormones

The *adrenals,* or *suprarenals,* are two small glands, each one situated above a kidney. An adrenal gland has two separate parts each of which acts as a gland. The inner area is called the *medulla,* while the outer portion is the *cortex.*

The Hormones from the Medulla

The principal hormone produced by the medulla is one which we already have learned something about: *epinephrine,* also called *adrenaline* (ad-ren'al-in). Another hormone, *norepinephrine* (nor''ep-i-nef'rin), is closely related chemically and is similar but not identical in its actions. These are referred to as the "fight and flight" hormones because of their effects during emergency situations. Some of these effects are as follows:

1 Stimulation of the sympathetic nerves which supply the involuntary muscle in the walls of the arterioles, causing these muscles to contract and the blood pressure to rise accordingly.
2 Conversion of the glycogen of the liver into sugar, which is poured into the blood and brought to the voluntary muscles, permitting them to do an extraordinary amount of work.
3 Increase of the heartbeat rate.
4 Dilation of the bronchioles, through relaxation of the smooth muscle of their walls.

The Hormones from the Adrenal Cortex

There are three main groups of hormones secreted by the adrenal cortex. Each of these groups of hormones performs certain specific functions.

1 The **glucocorticoids** (gloo''ko-kor'ti-koids) maintain the carbohydrate reserve of the body by controlling the conversion of amino acids into sugar instead of protein. These hormones are produced in larger amounts in times of stress and so aid the body in responding to unfavorable conditions. These hormones have the ability to suppress the inflammatory response, and are often administered as medication for this purpose. A major hormone of this group is cortisol.
2 The **mineralocorticoids** (min''er-al-o-kor'ti-koids) are important in the regulation of elec-

trolyte balance by controlling the reabsorption of sodium and the secretion of potassium by the kidney tubules. The major hormone of this group is aldosterone.

3 The **sex hormones** are normally secreted in small amounts so that their effects in the body are slight.

It should be mentioned once again that production of these hormones by the adrenal cortex is stimulated by ACTH from the "master gland" (pituitary) which is in turn stimulated by impulses from the hypothalamus. Not only are endocrine glands interrelated so they affect each other, but recent research indicates complex nervous and hormone connections.

The adrenal cortex is essential to life because it is largely by means of this part of the adrenal glands that the body succeeds in adapting itself to the constant changes in the environment. Hypofunction of the adrenal cortex gives rise to a condition known as *Addison's disease.* This disease is characterized chiefly by atrophy (loss of muscle tissue), weakness, skin pigmentation, and disturbances in salt and water balance. Hyperfunction of the adrenal cortex results in a condition known as *Cushing's syndrome.* The symptoms include obesity with a round face, thin skin that bruises easily, muscle weakness, bone loss, and elevated blood sugar. Use of steroid drugs may also produce these symptoms.

Adrenal gland tumors give rise to a wide range of symptoms, resulting from an excess or a deficiency of the hormones secreted.

The Pancreas, Insulin, and Diabetes

Scattered throughout the *pancreas* are small groups of specialized cells called *islets* (i'lets), which are also known as the *islands of Langerhans* (lahng'er-hanz). They function independently, and are *not* connected with the ducts with which the exocrine part of the pancreas is so well supplied. The most important hormone secreted by these islets is *insulin.*

Insulin is active in the transport of glucose across the cell membrane. Once inside the cell the glucose can be used for energy metabolism. In the presence of insulin, excessive amounts of carbohydrates enter fat cells, to be converted and stored as fat. Insulin also increases the transport of amino acids into the cells and improves their use in the manufacture of proteins. When insulin is lacking, there is not enough glucose for cell metabolism, and this causes abnormal breakdown of proteins and fats.

If for some reason the pancreatic islets fail to produce enough insulin, sugar is not oxidized ("burned") in the tissues for transformation into energy; instead, the sugar is simply excreted along with the urine. This condition is called *diabetes mellitus* (di-ah-be'teez mel-li'tus). In order that the diabetic patient may lead a normal life, proper utilization of the body's fuel must be restored and maintained. In mild cases of diabetes this can be achieved by a modification of diet, sometimes with the addition of oral medications to increase the output of insulin by the pancreas. In severe cases, however, the patient must also receive insulin from an outside source, in periodic doses. Insulin must be given by injection because it is destroyed by the action of digestive juices. This poses the problem of daily injections for the diabetic patient. As a rule it is considered desirable for the patient to learn to give the injections to himself. He should learn to adjust his diet, his exercise, and his other activities in order to maintain the proper balance between the intake of insulin and sugar needs. He should also carry a special identification card to let people know that he is a diabetic taking insulin, and that a dazed condition might indicate a need for some sugar.

Experimental work involving a mechanical pump that provides a round-the-clock supply of insulin, is now in progress. The insulin is placed in a device which then injects it into the subcutaneous tissues of the abdomen. The consistent blood sugar level thus achieved results in more nearly normal metabolism.

Long-term complications of diabetes are many. Resistance to infection is lessened. The arteries, including those of the retina, the kidneys, and the heart, may be seriously damaged. The peripheral nerves are affected also, with accompanying pain and loss of sensation.

The Sex Glands

The sex glands, including the ovaries of the female and the testes of the male, are important endocrine structures. The hormones produced by these organs play an important part in the development of the sexual characteristics, usually first appearing in the early teens, and in the maintenance of the reproductive apparatus once full development has been attained. The hormone produced by the male sex glands is called *testosterone* (tes-tos'ter-on). It is responsible for the functioning of certain reproductive organs. Those structures directly concerned with reproduction are considered *primary* sexual characteristics. Testosterone is also responsible for such *secondary* sexual characteristics as the deep voice and the growth of facial hair.

In the female, the hormones which most nearly parallel testosterone in their actions are the *estrogens* (es'tro-jens). Estrogens contribute to the development of the female *secondary* sexual characteristics, as well as stimulating the development of the mammary glands, the onset of menstruation, and the development and functioning of the reproductive organs.

There is one other hormone produced by the female sex glands, and it is called *progesterone* (pro-jes'ter-ōn). This hormone assists in the normal development of pregnancy. All of the sex hormones are discussed in more detail in Chapter 21.

Other Hormone-Producing Structures

The kidney (juxtaglomerular apparatus) produces: a hormone (renin) that acts on the vascular system; a hormone (hydroxychole-calciferol) active in calcium metabolism; and other hormones including erythropoietin that stimulate red blood cell production.

The *placenta* (plah-sen'tah) produces several hormones during pregnancy (see Chap. 21). These cause changes in the uterine lining, and later in pregnancy they help to prepare the breasts for lactation. The tests for pregnancy are based on the presence of placental secretions.

The *thymus* produces hormones that stimulate production of the small lymphocytes which function in the body's defense against infection. The thymus secretes a substance that has been given the name thymosin (also called thymic hormone). Thymosin promotes the growth of peripheral lymphoid tissue. The thymus is most active during prenatal life and in infancy.

The *pineal* (pin'-e-al) body, a small, flattened, cone-shaped structure located between the two parts of the thalamus, produces a hormone melatonin (mel-ah-tō'nin), in a number of animals and possibly also in humans. Melatonin, or some other hormone from the pineal, is thought to regulate the release of certain substances from the hypothalamus that may in turn regulate the secretion of gonadotropins from the pituitary. The human pineal body may be invaded by tumor tissue which can either increase the production of pineal hormone or can destroy the gland. Symptoms of these conditions indicate the possible role of the pineal body in gonadal activity.

The *hypothalamus,* located immediately above the pituitary gland, produces substances called neurohormones. These are carried through special blood vessel pathways directly from the hypothalamus to the anterior pituitary where they regulate the secretory activity of that gland.

Hormone-like substances called *prostaglandins* (pros-tah-glan'dins) are the object of active study. They have been found widely distributed in cells throughout the body. Organs that have been named as manufacturers of prostaglandins include the seminal vesicles (male reproductive system), the thymus, the brain, and the kidney medulla. A bewildering array of functions has been ascribed to them. Some cause constriction of blood vessels, of bronchial tubes, and of the intestine; others cause dilation of these same structures. Some of the prostaglandins have been used to induce labor or abortion and have been recommended as possible contraceptive agents. Much has been written about these substances and extensive research continues.

Hormones and Treatment

Many hormones may be extracted from animal tissues for use as medication. However, some hormone and hormone-like substances are available in synthetic form, meaning that they are manufactured in commercial laboratories.

A few examples of the use of natural and synthetic hormones in treatment are noted here:

1   Insulin is used in the treatment of diabetes mellitus.

2 Adrenal cortex hormones, primarily the gluco-corticoids, are used for the relief of inflammation in such diseases as rheumatoid arthritis, lupus erythematosus, and nephritis; for immunosuppression after organ transplants; and for the relief of the stress symptoms of shock.

3 Epinephrine (adrenalin) has many uses, some of which are stimulation of the heart muscle when rapid response is required; treatment of asthmatic attacks by relaxing the muscles of the small bronchial tubes; and treatment of the acute allergic reaction called anaphylaxis (an″ah-fi-lak′sis).

4 Thyroid extracts, either mixtures or purified derivatives of thyroid hormones, are used in the treatment of hypothyroid conditions (cretinism and myxedema) and as replacement therapy following surgical removal of the thyroid gland.

5 Oxytocin is used to contract the uterine muscle.

6 Androgens (an′dro-jens), including testosterone and androsterone, are used in severe chronic illness to promote healing. They may be used to stimulate red blood cell production in chronic kidney failure.

7 Oral contraceptives (birth control pills; "the Pill") contain estrogen or progesterone. They are highly effective in preventing pregnancy. Occasionally, they give rise to unpleasant side-effects, such as nausea. More rarely, they may cause serious complications such as thrombophlebitis, embolism and hypertension. However, these complications may also occur during and following pregnancy.

Summary

1 Secretions.
   A External—carried from gland to nearby organ or body surface.
   B Internal—carried to all parts of body by blood or lymph. Called hormones.
2 Glands—mostly epithelial, connective tissue framework, fibrous capsule; divided into lobes.
   A Exocrine—have ducts to carry secretions.
   B Endocrine—ductless; secretions reach blood by way of capillaries.
3 Hormones—"chemical messengers" regulating activities of various body systems.
4 Pituitary gland.
   A Location and structure—in skull below brain; anterior and posterior lobes.
   B Hormones—ACTH; TSH; FSH; GH; LH; ADH; etc.
   C Effects of tumors—gigantism; acromegaly; obesity; and underactivity of other endocrine glands.
5 Thyroid gland.
   A Location—in neck.
   B Hormones—thyroxine; triiodothyronine.
   C Disorders—simple goiter (lack of iodine); hypothyroidism (cretinism, myxedema); hyperthyroidism (Graves' disease).
6 Parathyroid glands.
   A Location—4 bodies behind thyroid gland.
   B Hormone—parathormone.
   C Disorders—tetany; loss of calcium from bone.
7 Adrenal (or suprarenal glands).
   A Location and structure—2 glands lying above kidneys; each has medulla and cortex.
   B Hormones—cortisol; aldosterone.
   C Disorders—hypofunction of cortex (Addison's); hyperfunction of cortex (Cushing's syndrome).
8 Pancreas.
   A Hormone secreting cells—islets of Langerhans.
   B Hormones—insulin; glucagon.
   C Disorder—diabetes mellitus; insufficient production of insulin.
9 Sex glands. Ovaries and testes; hormones—testosterone, estrogens, progesterone.
10 Kidneys, thymus, placenta, pineal body, hypothalamus.
11 Prostaglandins—wide variety of functions; continuing research.
12 Hormones and treatments—natural and synthetic hormones used to treat hypoactivity of several endocrine glands.

Questions and Problems

1 What is a gland? What is the usual glandular structure? What are the 2 types of glands?

2 What is a secretion? Name the 2 types of secretions.

3 Name some general functions of hormones.

4 Where is the thyroid gland located? What is its hormone and what does it do?

5 What is the cause of simple goiter?

6 Describe the effects of hypothyroidism and hyperthyroidism.

7 Name and describe briefly 3 tests for thyroid function.

8 What is the main purpose of the parathyroid hormone? What are the effects of removal of these glands—Of excess secretion?

9 Name the 2 divisions of the pituitary and describe the effects of the various hormones of each.

10 Name 4 effects of pituitary tumors.

11 What are the main purposes of insulin in the body? Name and describe the condition characterized by insufficient production of insulin.

12 Name the 2 divisions of the adrenal glands and the effects of the hormones of each.

13 What are the results of hypofunction of the adrenal cortex?

14 What are the results of hyperfunction of the adrenal cortex? What common therapy produces similar symptoms?

15 Name the male and female sex hormones and briefly describe what each does.

16 What is the present status in research on the thymus and the pineal body?

17 What are some of the various functions that have been ascribed to prostaglandins?

Chapter 21

Reproduction

Glossary

- Specialized reproductive cells
- Male reproductive system and its disorders
- Female reproductive system and its disorders
- Pregnancy, normal and abnormal
- The menopause

Gamete A reproductive cell; an ovum or a spermatozoon; the sexual form of the malarial parasite found in the stomach of the mosquito.

Gonad An ovary or a testis; a sex gland.

Ovary The female gonad.

Ovulation The discharge of a mature egg cell (ovum) from the follicle of the ovary.

Semen The thick whitish secretion from the male reproductive organs; a combination of male germ cells (spermatozoa) and secretions from the several glands of the reproductive system.

Testis The male gonad.

Zygote The fertilized ovum; the cell formed by the union of the spermatozoon and the egg cell.

This chapter deals with what is certainly one of the most interesting and mysterious attributes of living matter: the ability to reproduce. The lowest forms of life, the one-celled organisms, usually need no partner in order to reproduce; they simply divide by themselves. This form of reproduction is known as *asexual* (nonsexual) reproduction.

In most animals, however, reproduction is *sexual,* meaning that there is a differentiation in the individuals: they are male or female, and both have their own specialized cells designed specifically for the perpetuation of the species. These specialized sex cells are known as *spermatozoa* (sper''mah-to-zo'ah) in the male and *ova* (o'vah) in the female. The sex cells may also be called *germ cells* or *gametes* (gam'etes). Despite the differentiation of the reproductive apparatus in man and woman, the organs of both sexes may be divided into two groups: primary and accessory.

1 The primary organs are the **gonads** (go'nads), or sex glands; they produce the germ cells and also manufacture hormones. The male gonads are the *testes,* and the female gonads are the *ovaries.*

2 The **accessory organs** include a series of ducts that provide for the transport of germ cells as well as various exocrine glands.

The Male Reproductive System
The Testes

The male gonads (testes) are normally located outside the body proper in a sac called the *scrotum* (skro′tum), suspended between the thighs. The testes are egg-shaped organs measuring about 3.7 cm to 5 cm (1.5 to 2 inches) in length and approximately 2.5 cm (one inch) in each of the other two dimensions. The bulk of the specialized tissue of the testes consists of tiny coiled tubules. Cells in the walls of these tubules produce spermatozoa. Between the tubules are specialized cells that secrete the male sex hormone, testosterone.

The hormone *testosterone* (tes-tos′te-rōn) secreted by the testes is absorbed directly into the bloodstream. This hormone acts in two ways. The first is the maintenance of the reproductive structures including development of the spermatozoa. A second function involves the development of the secondary sexual characteristics such as body structure and hair distribution.

The Duct System

The tubes that carry the spermatozoa begin with the tubules inside the testis itself. From these tubes the spermatozoa are collected by a greatly coiled tube, 6 meters (20 feet) long called the *epididymis* (ep″i-did′i-mis), which is located inside the scrotal sac (Fig. 21-1). While they are temporarily stored in the epididymis, the spermatozoa mature and become motile, that is, able to move or "swim" by themselves. The epididymis finally extends upward, and then this straighter part becomes the *vas deferens* (def′er-enz), also called the *ductus deferens*. The vas deferens continues through a small canal in the abdominal wall and then curves behind the urinary bladder. There each vas deferens joins with the duct of the *seminal vesicle* (ves′e-kal) of its own side to form the *ejaculatory* (e-jak′u-lah-to-re) *duct*. The two ejaculatory ducts enter the body of the prostate gland where they empty into the urethra.

The *spermatic cord* is composed of a combination of the vas deferens, blood vessels, lymphatics, and nerves all wrapped in connective tissue. This structure extends upward from the testis on each side and passes through the abdominal wall.

The Seminal Vesicles

The seminal vesicles are tortuous muscular tubes with small outpouchings. They are about 7.5 cm (3 inches) long and are attached to the connective tissue at the back of the urinary bladder. The glandular lining produces a thick yellow secretion that contains large quantities of simple sugar and other substances that provide nourishment for the spermatozoa. The seminal fluid forms a large part of the volume of the *semen*, a mixture of spermatozoa and secretions, that is expelled from the body.

The Prostate Gland

The prostate gland lies immediately below the urinary bladder where it surrounds the first part of the urethra. Ducts from the prostate enter the ejaculatory duct. At this point, the ejaculatory duct contains a mixture of sex cells and seminal fluid. The thin, alkaline prostatic secretion is added to the semen where it serves to enhance the motility of the spermatozoa. The prostate gland is also supplied with muscular tissue, which, upon signal from the nervous system, contracts to aid in the expulsion of the semen from the body.

Mucus-Producing Glands

The largest of the mucus-producing glands in the male reproductive system are a pair of pea-sized organs located in the pelvic floor just below the prostate gland. They are called *Cowper's* or *bulbourethral* (bul″bo-u-re′thral) *glands*. Their ducts extend about 2.5 cm from each side and empty into the urethra before it extends within the penis. Other very small glands secrete mucus into the urethra as it passes through the penis. The mucus from all these glands serve mainly to lubricate the urethra.

The Urethra and the Penis

The male urethra, as we saw earlier, serves the dual purpose of conveying urine from the bladder and carrying the reproductive cells and their accompanying secretions to the outside. The ejection of semen into the receiving canal (vagina) of the female is made possible by the *erection*, or stiffening and enlargement, of the penis, through which the longest part of the urethra extends. The penis is made of a spongelike tissue containing many blood

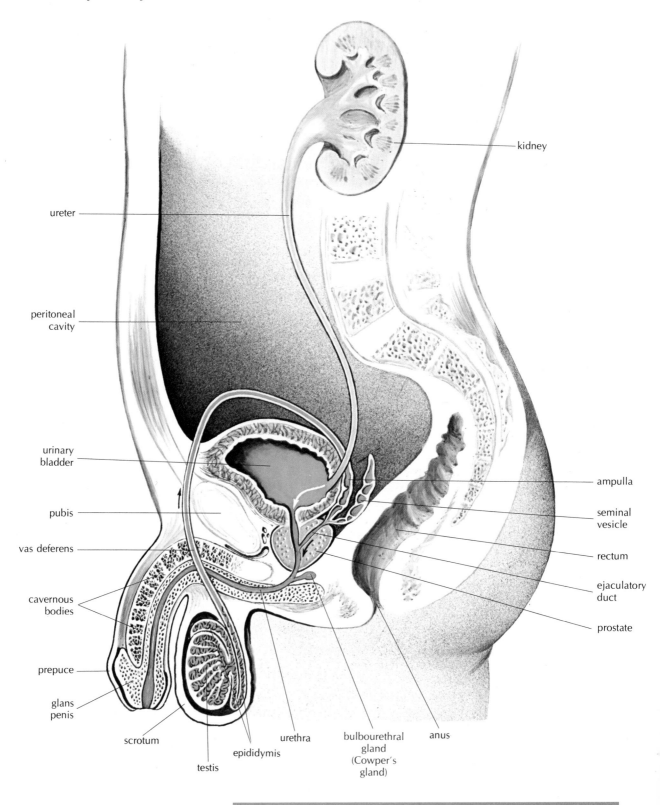

Fig. 21-1 *Male genitourinary system. The black arrows indicate the course of spermatozoa through the duct system; the single white arrow indicates the course of urine.*

spaces that are relatively empty when the organ is flaccid but fill with blood and distend when the penis is erect. The penis and the scrotum are referred to as the external genitalia of the male.

Reflex centers in the spinal cord order the contraction of the smooth muscle tissue in the prostate gland, followed by the contraction of skeletal muscle in the pelvic floor. This provides the force needed for *ejaculation* (e-jak′u-la-shun), the expulsion of semen through the urethra to the outside.

The Spermatozoa

The spermatozoa themselves are tiny detached cells. The fact that at least 200 million spermatozoa are contained in the average ejaculation may give some idea of their size. Spermatozoa are continuously manufactured in the testes. At any given time, live sperm are found throughout the entire duct system. The individual sperm cell is egg-shaped and has a tail which enables it to make its way through the various passages until it reaches the ovum of the female. It is interesting to note that out of the millions of spermatozoa in an ejaculation, only one of these actually fertilizes the ovum. The remainder of the spermatozoa perish within a short time.

Disorders of the Male Reproductive System

Sterility

Sterility means inability to reproduce. The proportion of sterile marriages due to defects involving the male has been estimated variously from one third to one half. The tubules of the testes are very sensitive to x-rays, to infections, to toxins, and to malnutrition, all of which bring about degenerative changes in the tubules. Such damage may cause a decrease in the numbers of spermatozoa produced, leading to a condition called *oligospermia* (ol′′i-go-sper′me-ah). Adequate numbers of spermatozoa are required to disperse the coating around the ovum in order that one sperm can fertilize it. Absence of or an inadequate number of male sex cells is an important cause of sterility.

Intentional sterilization of the male may be accomplished by an operation called a *vasectomy* (vahsek′to-me). In this procedure a portion of the vas deferens on each side is removed and the cut end closed to keep the spermatozoa from reaching the urethra. These tiny cells are absorbed without in-

jury, and the individual retains the ability to produce hormones as well as to perform the sex act.

Cryptorchidism

Cryptorchidism (krip-tor′ki-dizm) means "hidden testes," and is a disorder characterized by failure of the testes to descend to the scrotum. During embryonic life the gonads of both male and female develop from tissue near the kidney. In both sexes the gonads descend to a region considerably lower than the areas of origin. The female gonad descends only as far as the pelvic part of the abdomen, while the testis continues down through the abdominal wall and into the scrotum. This complete descent of the testis is necessary if it is to function normally; in order to produce spermatozoa, the testes must be kept at the temperature of the scrotum, which is lower than that of the abdominal cavity. Undescended testes also are particularly subject to tumor formation. Most testes that are undescended at birth descend spontaneously by age one. Surgical correction is the usual remedy in the remaining cases.

Hernia

Hernia (her′ne-ah), or rupture, refers to the abnormal protrusion of an organ, or part of an organ, through the wall of the cavity in which it is normally contained. Hernias most often occur where there is a weak area in the abdominal wall as, for example, the inguinal canal. This region in the lower abdomen is the place where the testis pushes its way through the muscles and connective tissues of the abdominal wall, carrying with it the blood vessels and other structures that will form the spermatic cord. In the normal adult this area is fairly well reinforced with connective tissue, and there is no direct connection between the abdominal cavity and the scrotal sac. However, this area, as well as some other regions in which openings permit the passage of various structures to and from the abdominal cavity, constitute weak places at which a hernia may occur.

Infections

Infections of various kinds may involve the male reproductive organs, but by far the most common is *gonorrhea*. This disease manifests itself by a discharge from the urethra, which may be accompanied by burning and pain, especially during urination. The infection may travel along the mucous membrane into the prostate gland and into the epididymis; and if both sides are affected and enough scar tissue is formed to destroy the tubules, sterility may be the result. An unpleasant and persistent infection called genital herpes now is the second most common venereal disease (see Table 3 of the Appendix).

Other infectious agents that sometimes invade the reproductive organs include the tubercle bacillus and various staphylococci. The testes may be involved in mumps with a resulting *orchitis* (or-ki'tis), inflammation of the testes.

Tumors

Tumor formation may involve the male reproductive organs, most commonly the prostate, and is quite common in elderly men. Such growths may be benign or malignant. Both cause such pressure on the urethra that urination becomes difficult, and back pressure often causes destruction of kidney tissue, as well as permitting stagnation of urine in the bladder with a resulting tendency to infection. Removal of the prostate or parts of it should be done early in order to prevent serious damage to the urinary system.

Cancer of the prostate is a common disorder in men over fifty. It is frequently detected as a nodule during rectal examination. Surgical treatment may include the removal of the prostate, seminal vesicles and bladder neck. Additional therapy involves radiation of the pelvic lymph glands. Unfortunately, this cancer frequently spreads to the bones with a fatal outcome.

Phimosis

Phimosis (fi-mo'sis) refers to a tightness of the foreskin (prepuce) so that it cannot be drawn back. This may be remedied through circumcision by which part or all of the foreskin is removed. This operation is often done on very young male infants as a routine measure, either for hygienic reasons or because of religious principles.

The Female Reproductive System
The Ovaries, or Female Gonads

In the female the counterparts of the testes are the two *ovaries,* and it is here that the female sex cells, or *ova,* are formed. The ovaries are small, somewhat flattened oval bodies located in the pelvic portion of the abdomen. They are attached at the back of membranous structures, made of two layers of peritoneum, called the broad ligaments (Fig. 21-2).

The outer layer of each ovary is made of a single layer of epithelium. Beneath this layer the ova are produced. The ova begin a complicated process of maturation or "ripening," which takes place in small sacs called *ovarian* (o-va're-an) *follicles* (fal'e-kls). The cells of the ovarian follicle walls secrete estrogens. When an ovum has ripened, the ovarian follicle ruptures, and the ovum is discharged from the surface of the ovary, making its way to the tube known as the *oviduct* (o'vi-dukt), one of which exists for each ovary. The rupture of a follicle allowing the escape of the egg cell is called *ovulation* (ov''u-la'shun).

Although the ovaries contain vast numbers of ova, usually only one ovum is released at a time. Once the ovum has been expelled, the follicle is transformed into a solid glandular mass called the *corpus luteum* (lu'te-um), which means "yellow body." This structure secretes both estrogens and progesterone. Normally, the corpus luteum shrinks and is replaced by scar tissue. When a pregnancy occurs, this structure remains active. Often as a result of normal ovulation the corpus luteum will persist and form a small ovarian cyst (fluid-filled sac). This condition will usually resolve without treatment.

The Oviducts

The egg-carrying tubes of the female reproductive system are also known as *uterine* (u'ter-in) *tubes* or *fallopian* (fah-lo'pe-an) *tubes.* They are small muscular structures, nearly 12.5 cm long, extending from a point near the ovaries to the uterus (womb). There is no direct connection between the ovaries and these tubes. The ova are swept into the oviducts by a current in the peritoneal fluid produced by the small fringelike extensions called *fimbriae* (fim'bre-e) from the edges of the abdominal openings of the tubes.

Unlike the spermatozoon, the ovum cannot move by itself. Its progress through the oviduct toward the uterus is dependent upon the sweeping action of the cilia, part of the lining of the tubes as well as by the peristalsis of the tubes. It takes

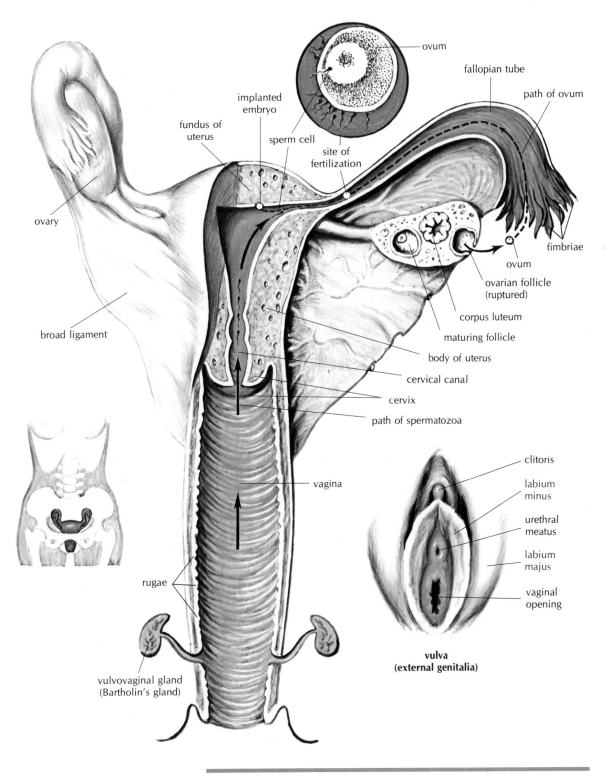

Fig. 21-2   Female reproductive system.

about 5 days for the ovum to reach the uterus from the ovary. During this time the lining of the tube nourishes the ovum.

The Uterus

The organ to which the fallopian tubes lead is the *uterus* (u'ter-us), and it is within this structure that the fetus grows until it is ready to be born.

The uterus is a pear-shaped, muscular organ about 7.5 cm long, 5 cm wide, and 2.5 cm deep. The upper portion rests on the upper surface of the urinary bladder; the lower portion is embedded in the pelvic floor between the bladder and the rectum. The upper portion is the larger and is called the body, or *corpus;* the lower, smaller part is the *cervix* (ser'viks), or neck. The small rounded part above the level of the tubal entrances is known as the *fundus* (fun'dus). The cavity inside the uterus is shaped somewhat like a capital T, but is capable of changing shape and dilating as the embryo (later called the fetus) develops. The cervix leads to the *vagina* (vah-ji'nah), the lower part of the birth canal, which opens to the outside of the body.

The lining of the uterus is a specialized epithelium known as *endometrium* (en-do-me'tre-um), and it is this layer that is involved in menstruation.

The Menstrual Cycle

The menstrual cycle is controlled by the pituitary and by ovarian hormones. The length of this cycle may vary between 22 and 45 days in normal women (Fig. 21-3).

During each cycle, under the influence of follicle stimulating hormone produced by the pituitary, a follicle develops in the ovary. This follicle produces increasing amounts of estrogens as the ovum matures. The estrogens are carried in the bloodstream to the uterus where they start the preparation of the endometrium for a possible pregnancy. This preparation includes thickening of the endometrium and elongation of the glands that produce the uterine secretion. Secretion of follicle-stimulating hormone decreases as the secretion of estrogens increase.

There is a sharp increase in luteinizing (loo''te-in-i'zing) hormone from the pituitary which immediately precedes ovulation. Leuteinizing hormone transforms the ruptured follicle into the corpus luteum, which produces estrogens and progesterone.

Under the influence of these hormones the endometrium continues to thicken, the glands and blood vessels increasing in size. During this time the ovum makes its journey to the uterus by way of the oviduct. If the ovum is not fertilized while passing through the uterine tube, it disintegrates soon after reaching the uterus.

Fourteen days after ovulation, the quantity of hormones secreted by the corpus luteum decreases. Without the hormones to support growth, the endometrium degenerates. Small hemorrhages appear in this lining, producing the bleeding known as *menstrual flow*. Bits of endometrium break away and accompany the flow of blood. The average duration of this discharge is 2 to 6 days.

Before the flow ceases, the endometrium begins to repair itself through the growth of new cells. Within the ovaries a new ovum is ripening, and the cycle begins anew.

The Vagina

The vagina is a muscular tube about 7.5 cm long connecting the uterine cavity with the outside. It receives the cervix, which dips into the upper vagina in such a way that a circular recess is formed, giving rise to areas known as *fornices* (for'ne-sez). The deepest of these spaces is behind the cervix and is called the *posterior fornix* (for'niks) (Fig. 21-4). This recess in the posterior vagina is separated from the lowest part of the peritoneal cavity by a rather thin layer of tissue, so that abscesses or tumor cells in the peritoneal cavity can sometimes be detected by vaginal examination.

The lining of the vagina is a wrinkled mucous membrane something like that found in the stomach. The folds (rugae) permit enlargement so that childbirth will not tear the lining (as a rule). In addition to being a part of the birth canal, the vagina is the organ that receives the penis during sexual intercourse. At or near the vaginal (vaj'i-nal) canal opening to the outside there sometimes may be found a more or less definite fold of membrane called the *hymen.*

The Greater Vestibular Glands

Just above and to each side of the vaginal opening are the mucus-producing *greater vestibular* (ves-tib'u-lar) or *Bartholin's glands*. These glands open

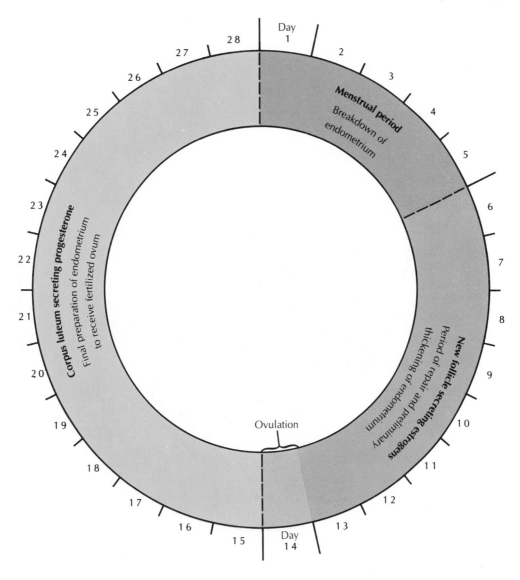

Fig. 21-3 Summary of events in an average 28-day menstrual cycle.

into an area near the vaginal opening known as the *vestibule*. They may become infected, then painfully swollen, and, finally, abscessed. A surgical incision to promote drainage may be required.

The Vulva and the Perineum

The external parts of the female reproductive system form the *vulva* (vul'vah). These include two pairs of lips, or *labia* (la'be-ah), the *clitoris* (kli'to-ris), which is a small organ of great sensitivity,

and related structures. Although the entire pelvic floor is properly called the *perineum* in both the male and the female, those who care for the pregnant woman usually refer to the limited area between the vaginal opening and the anus as the perineum. To prevent the pelvic floor tissues from being torn during childbirth as often happens, the physician may cut the perineum just before the infant is born and then repair this clean cut immediately after childbirth. Such an operation is called an *episiotomy* (e-piz''e-ot'o-me).

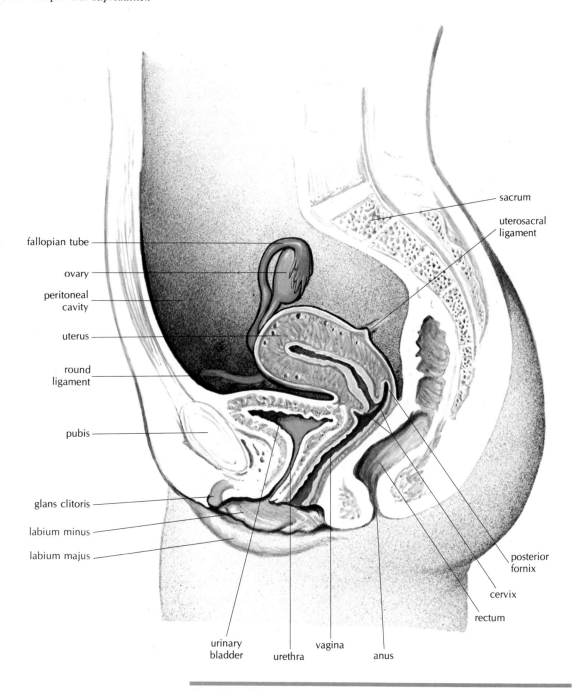

Fig. 21-4 *Female reproductive system, as seen in sagittal section.*

Disorders of the Female Reproductive System
Leukorrhea

A nonbloody vaginal discharge, usually whitish in color, is called leukorrhea (loo''ko-re'ah). In many cases, it is merely the colorless mucus produced by the cervical glands; these glands produce more mucus during ovulation. Leukorrhea is not a disease, but it can be a sign of irritation or infection involving the cervix or vagina. A common causative organism is a protozoan called *Trichomonas* (trik''o-mo'nas) *vaginalis*. There may be other causes, and a microscopic examination of the discharge should be done in order to make a diagnosis. Tight, nonabsorbent clothing makes this condition worse.

Menstrual Disorders

Absence of the menstrual flow is known as *amenorrhea* (ah-men''o-re'ah). This condition can be symptomatic of such a disorder as insufficient hormone secretion, or of a congenital abnormality of the reproductive organs. Very often, psychological factors play a part in stoppage of the menstrual flow. For example, a change in the pattern of living such as a shift in working hours can cause a woman to miss a period. Any significant change in the general state of health can cause this also. The most common cause of amenorrhea (except, of course, for the menopause) is pregnancy.

Dysmenorrhea (dis''men-o-re'ah) means painful or difficult menstruation. It may be due to immaturity of the uterus in young women. Dysmenorrhea is frequently associated with cycles in which ovulation has occurred. Often the pain can be relieved by drugs that block prostaglandins, since some prostaglandins are known to cause painful uterine contractions. In many cases, women have been completely relieved of menstrual cramps by the first pregnancy. Apparently, the cervical openings are thus enlarged adequately. Artificially dilating the cervical openings may alleviate dysmenorrhea for several months. Often such health measures as sufficient rest, a well-balanced diet, and appropriate exercises will remedy dysmenorrhea. During the attack, the application of heat over the abdomen usually relieves the pain, just as it may ease other types of muscular cramps.

Premenstrual tension is a condition in which nervousness, irritability, and depression precede the menstrual period. It is thought to be due to fluid retention in various tissues, including the brain. Sometimes a low-salt diet and appropriate medication for the 2 weeks before the menses prevent this disorder. This treatment also may avert dysmenorrhea.

Abnormal uterine bleeding includes excessive menstrual flow, too-frequent menstruation, and nonmenstrual bleeding. Any of these may cause serious anemias and deserve careful medical attention. Nonmenstrual bleeding may be an indication of a tumor, possibly cancer.

Benign Tumors

Fibroids, which are more correctly called myomas (see Chap. 2), are common tumors of the uterus. Studies indicate that about 50% of women who reach the age of 50 have one or more of these growths in the walls of the uterus. Very often they are small, and usually they remain benign and produce no symptoms. They develop between puberty and the menopause and ordinarily stop growing after a woman has reached the age of 50. In some cases, these growths interfere with pregnancy and if the patient is under 40, the surgeon may simply shell out the tumor and leave the uterus fairly intact. Normal pregnancy has developed after such surgery.

Fibroids may become so large that pressure on adjacent structures causes grave disorders. In some cases invasion of blood vessels near the uterine cavity causes serious hemorrhages. For these and other reasons, it may be necessary to remove the entire uterus or the larger part of it. Surgical removal of the uterus is called a *hysterectomy* (his''te-rek'to-me).

Malignant Tumors

Cancer of the breast is the most common malignant disease in women. The tumor is usually a painless, movable mass that is first noticed by the woman—and all too frequently ignored. However, in recent years, there has been increasing emphasis on the importance of regular self-examination of the breasts. Any lump, no matter how small, should be reported to a physician immediately. For years the surgical treatment of this disease has been a *radical mastectomy* (mas-tek'to-me) a procedure that involves total removal of the affected breast together with removal of the axillary lymph nodes and muscles on the chest wall. Underway are long-range studies to evaluate the effectiveness of simple versus radical mastectomy, with or without radiation therapy. Breast cancer frequently has more than one primary tumor and may spread by way of the bloodstream to the lungs, bones, or other parts of the body.

The second most common cancer of the female reproductive organs is cancer of the endometrium (the lining of the uterus). This type of cancer usually affects women during or after the menopause. It is seen more frequently in women who have had few pregnancies, abnormal bleeding, or cycles in which ovulation did not occur. Symptoms include an abnormal discharge or irregular bleeding. The usual treatment methods include surgery and radiation.

Cancer of the cervix is the third most common cancer of the female reproductive system. It is most frequent in women from 30 to 50 years of age. Appropriate screening allows the discovery and treatment of many early cases. Although no specific cause has been identified, statistics indicate that the incidence of cervical cancer is strongly affected by various risk factors, such as first sexual intercourse at an early age, having many sexual partners, and genital herpes infection. The decline in the death rate from this type of cancer is directly related to the use of the *Papanicolaou* (pap''ah-nik''o-la'oo) *test,* also known as the *Pap test* or *Pap smear.* The Pap smear is a microscopic examination of cells obtained from scrapings of the cervix and swabs of the cervical canal. All women should be encouraged to have these tests every year, although certain low-risk groups may have them less frequently.

Infections

The common venereal diseases that involve the male reproductive system also attack the female genital organs (Fig. 21-5). The most common (as in the male) are gonorrhea and genital herpes. Syphilis also occurs in women, and the fetus of an untreated syphilitic mother may be stillborn; an infant born alive may have highly infectious lesions of the palms or the soles as well as other manifestations of the disease.

Salpingitis (sal-pin-ji'tis) means "inflammation of a tube." However, the term is used most often to refer to disease of the uterine tubes. In most cases, infection of the uterine tubes is caused by gonorrhea, but other bacteria can bring it about. Salpingitis may cause sterility by obstructing the tubes, thus preventing passage of the ovum.

Sterility

In the female, sterility is much more difficult to diagnose and evaluate than it is in the male. Whereas a microscopic examination of properly collected seminal fluid may be all that is required to determine the presence of abnormal or too-few spermatozoa, no such simple study can be made in the case of the female. Sterility may be relative or absolute, as is also true in the male. Causes of

female sterility include infections, endocrine disorders, psychogenic factors, and abnormalities in the structure and function of the reproductive organs themselves. In all cases, the male partner should be investigated first, since the procedures for determining sterility in the male are much simpler, less costly, and, in any case, essential for the evaluation.

Pregnancy
First Stages of Pregnancy

When semen is deposited in the vagina, the many spermatozoa immediately wriggle about in all directions. They travel into the uterus and the oviducts. Some dissolve the coating surrounding the ovum, so that when a spermatozoon encounters an ovum, it can penetrate the last barrier, namely the cell membrane of the ovum. The result of the union of these two sex cells is a single cell which can now divide and grow into a new individual; this new cell is called a *zygote* (zi'gote). The zygote begins the process of dividing into two cells and then four cells, and soon a ball of cells is formed. During this time, the ball of cells is traveling toward the uterine cavity, pushed along by the cilia and by the peristalsis of the tube.

After reaching the uterus, the little ball of cells burrows into the greatly thickened uterine lining, where it is soon completely covered and implanted. Following implantation, the ball of cells is called an *embryo* (em'bre-o). Soon the cords of villi (embryonic cells) project outward from the ball-like mass, invading the uterine wall and the maternal blood vessels. This eventually leads to the formation of the *placenta* (plah-sen'tah), a flat, circular organ that consists of a spongy network of blood-filled lakes. The embryo is connected to the developing placenta by a stalk of tissue that eventually becomes the *umbilical* (um-bil'e-kal) *cord.* The placenta serves as the organ of nutrition, respiration, and excretion for the developing individual. Another function of the placenta is endocrine in nature. Beginning soon after implantation, some of the embryonic cells produce a hormone called *chorionic gonadotropin* (ko''re-on'ik gon''ah-do-tro'pin). This hormone stimulates the corpus luteum of the ovary, prolonging its life span (to 11 or 12 weeks) and causing it to secrete increasing amounts of progesterone and estrogens. Progester-

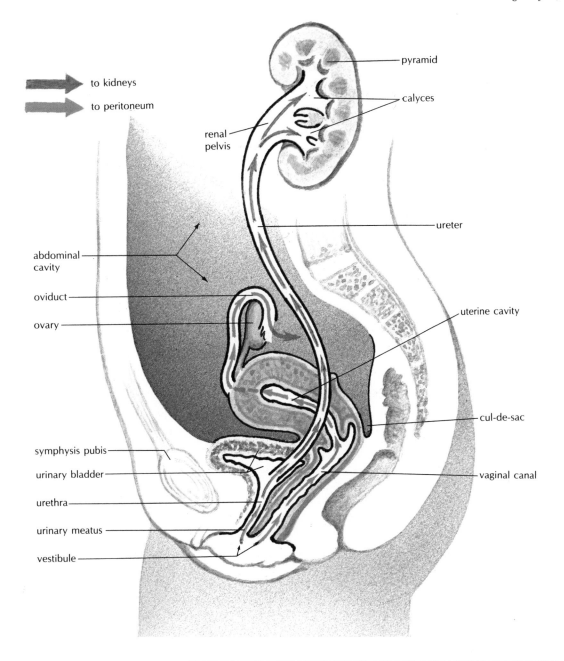

to kidneys

to peritoneum

pyramid

calyces

renal pelvis

ureter

abdominal cavity

oviduct

ovary

uterine cavity

cul-de-sac

symphysis pubis

urinary bladder

vaginal canal

urethra

urinary meatus

vestibule

Fig. 21-5 *Pathway of infection from outside to peritoneum and into urinary system.*

one is essential for the maintenance of pregnancy. It promotes endometrial secretions to nourish the embryo, and it decreases the ability of the uterine muscle to contract, thus preventing the embryo from being expelled from the body. During pregnancy, progesterone also helps to prepare the breasts for the secretion of milk. Estrogens promote enlargement of the uterus and breasts. By the 11th or 12th week of pregnancy, the corpus luteum is no longer needed; by this time, the placenta itself can secrete adequate amounts of progesterone and estrogens.

Development of the Embryo

Embryology (em''bre-ol'o-je) is the study of the development of the embryo (em'bre-o). Embryonic life begins with the fertilization of the ovum. The cellular mass consists of cells that have not yet begun to assume any specialized function. The embryo develops from a very small part of the original ball of unspecialized cells. The placenta and the sac that surrounds the embryo as well as the *umbilical* (um-bil'i-kal) *cord* also originate largely from some of the primitive cells of this ball. Among the first organs to develop in the embryo are the heart and the brain. By the end of the first month, the embryo is about 0.62 cm long with four small swellings at the sides called *limb buds,* which will develop into the four extremities. At this time, the heart produces a prominent bulge at the front of the embryo. By the end of the second month, the embryo takes on an appearance that is recognizably human. The developing individual is called an embryo until the third month (Fig. 21-6).

The growing embryo is sustained by the *placenta.* The maternal side of this organ consists of blood in sinuses into which the villi of the fetus project. The barrier between the two sides of this organ allow for the necessary exchange of substances such as oxygen and waste products. The embryo is connected to the placenta by a stalk of tissue that becomes the umbilical cord. The cord contains two arteries and one vein (Fig. 21-7). As mentioned previously, the placenta serves as the organ of nutrition, respiration, and excretion for the embryo (later called the fetus). The placenta also secretes several hormones, the primary ones being estrogens, progesterone, and placental lactogen. As the pregnancy progresses, these hormones prepare the breasts for lactation, cause changes that prepare the body for delivery such as relaxation of ligaments, and promote the storage of nutrients required for lactation.

The Fetus

From the beginning of the third month until birth, the developing individual is referred to as a *fetus* (fe'tus). During this period, there is continued growth and maturation of the organ systems. By the end of the fourth month, the fetus is almost 15 cm long with sufficient development of the external genitalia to reveal its sex. By the seventh month, the fetus is usually about 35 cm long and weighs about 1.1 kg. At the end of pregnancy, the normal length of the fetus is 45 cm to 56 cm, and the weight varies from 2.7 kg to 4.5 kg.

After the ball of cells became attached to the wall of the uterus, auxiliary organs designed to serve the fetus began developing also. These include the placenta and the umbilical cord, as well as the *amniotic* (am-ne-ot'ik) *sac* (Fig. 21-8). This sac is filled with a clear liquid known as *amniotic fluid* that serves as a protective cushion for the fetus. The amniotic sac, which ruptures at birth, is popularly called the bag of waters. The skin of the fetus is protected by a layer of cheeselike material called *vernix* (ver'niks) *caseosa* (ka'se-o-sa).

The Mother

The total period of pregnancy, from fertilization of the ovum to birth, is about 280 days. During this period, the mother must supply all the food and oxygen for the fetus, and eliminate its waste materials as well. To support the additional demands of the growing fetus, the mother's metabolism changes markedly with increased demands on several organ systems:

1   The heart pumps more blood to supply the needs of the uterus and its contents.
2   The lungs provide more oxygen to supply the fetus by increasing the rate and depth of respiration.
3   The kidneys excrete nitrogenous wastes from the fetus as well as from the mother's body.
4   Nutritional needs are increased to provide for the growth of the maternal organs (uterus and breasts) and growth of the fetus, as well as preparation for labor and for the secretion of milk.

Nausea and vomiting are common discomforts in early pregnancy. The specific cause is not known, but these symptoms may occur because of the great changes in hormone levels. The nausea and vomiting usually last for only a few weeks. Frequency of urination and constipation are often present during the early stages of pregnancy and then usually disappear as the pregnancy progresses. These symptoms may reappear late in pregnancy as the

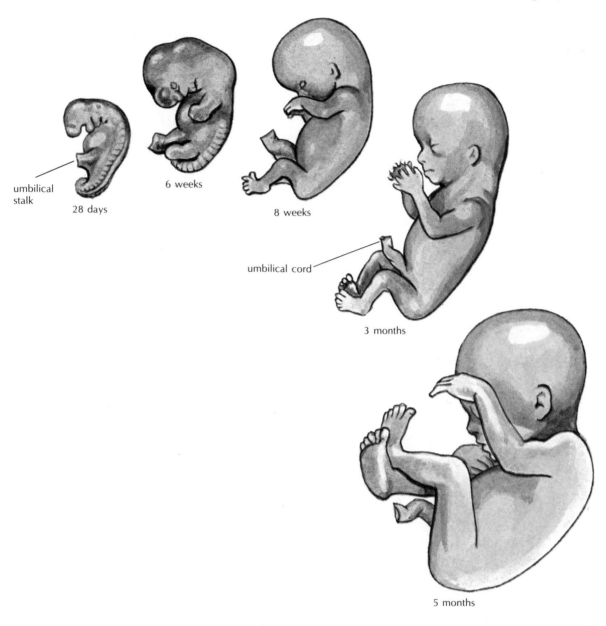

umbilical
stalk

28 days

6 weeks

8 weeks

umbilical cord

3 months

5 months

Fig. 21-6 *Development of embryo into fetus.*

head of the fetus drops from the abdominal region down into the pelvis, pressing on the rectum and the urinary bladder.

Childbirth

The mechanisms that trigger the beginning of uterine contractions are still unknown. However, it is recognized that the uterine muscle becomes increasingly sensitive to oxytocin (from the pituitary gland) late in pregnancy. Once labor is started, stimuli from the cervix and vagina produce reflex secretion of this hormone which, in turn, increases the uterine contractions.

The process by which the fetus is expelled from the uterus is known as *labor* and *delivery;* it also

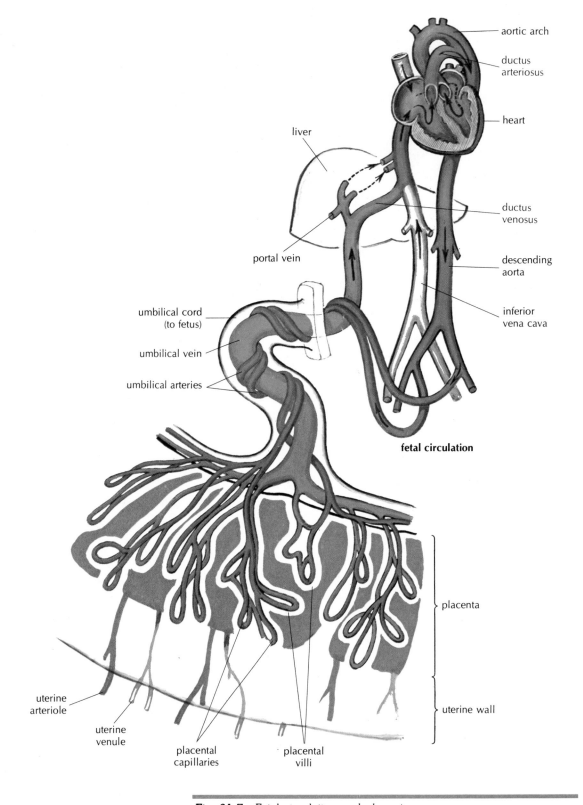

aortic arch

ductus arteriosus

heart

liver

ductus venosus

portal vein

descending aorta

inferior vena cava

umbilical cord (to fetus)

umbilical vein

umbilical arteries

fetal circulation

placenta

uterine wall

uterine arteriole

uterine venule

placental capillaries

placental villi

Fig. 21-7 *Fetal circulation and placenta.*

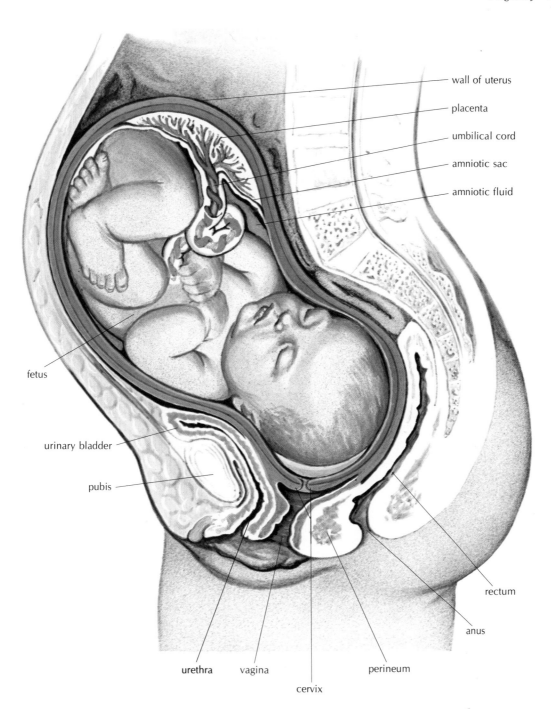

wall of uterus

placenta

umbilical cord

amniotic sac

amniotic fluid

fetus

urinary bladder

pubis

rectum

anus

urethra

vagina

cervix

perineum

Fig. 21-8 *Midsagittal section of pregnant uterus.*

may be called confinement, or *parturition* (par'tu-rish'un). It is divided into four stages:

1 The **first stage** begins with the onset of regular contractions of the uterus. With each contrac-

tion, the cervix becomes thinner and the opening larger. Rupture of the amniotic sac may occur at any time with a gush of fluid from the vagina.

2 The **second stage** begins when the cervix is

completely dilated and ends with the delivery of the baby. This stage involves the passage of the fetus, usually head first, through the cervical canal and the vagina to the outside.

3 The **third stage** begins after the child is born and ends with the expulsion of the *afterbirth*. The afterbirth includes the placenta, the membranes of the amniotic sac, and the umbilical cord, except for a small portion remaining attached to the baby's *umbilicus*.

4 The **fourth stage** begins with the expulsion of the afterbirth and constitutes a period in which bleeding is controlled. The contraction of the uterine muscle acts to close off the blood vessels leading to the placental site.

The Mammary Glands and Lactation

The *mammary glands,* or the breasts of the female, are accessories of the reproductive system. They are designed to provide nourishment for the baby after its birth; and the secretion of milk at this period is known as *lactation* (lak-ta′shun).

The mammary glands are constructed in much the same manner as the sweat glands. Each of these glands is divided into a number of lobes composed of glandular tissue and fat, and each lobe, in turn, is subdivided. The secretions from the lobes are conveyed through *lactiferous* (lak-tif′er-us) *ducts,* all of which converge at the nipple (Fig. 21-9).

The mammary glands begin developing during puberty, but they do not become functional until the end of a pregnancy. A lactogenic hormone called *prolactin,* produced by the anterior lobe of the pituitary, stimulates the secretory cells of the mammary glands. The first of the mammary gland secretions is a thin liquid called *colostrum* (ko-los′trum). It is nutritious but has a somewhat different composition from milk. Within a few days, milk is secreted, and it will continue for several months if frequently removed by the suckling baby or by pumping the breast.

The digestive tract of the newborn baby is not ready for the usual mixed diet of an adult. Mother's milk is more desirable for the young infant than milk from other animals for several reasons. Some of these are as follows:

1 Infections that may be transmitted by foods exposed to the outside air are avoided by nursing the infant.

2 Antibodies may be unaffected by the less potent digestive juices found in the infant. Thus, these antibodies may help to protect the baby against pathogens.

3 The particular proportion of the various nutrients and other substances in human milk is believed to be especially well suited to the human infant. While substitutes are made to imitate as nearly as possible the qualities of human milk, it is not likely that every detail of the content of human milk is well enough known to make an exact replica possible. Nutrients are present in more desirable amounts if the mother's diet is well balanced.

4 The psychological and emotional satisfactions of nursing the child are of infinite value to both the mother and the infant.

Multiple Births

Statistics indicate that twins occur in about 1 in every 80 to 90 births, varying somewhat in different countries. Triplets occur much less frequently, usually once in several thousand births, while quadruplets occur very rarely indeed, and the birth of quintuplets represents an historical event unless the woman has been taking fertility drugs.

Twins originate in two different ways, and on this basis are divided into two groups:

1 **Fraternal** twins are formed as a result of the fertilization of two different ova by two spermatozoa. Two completely different individuals, as different from each other as other brothers and sisters, except in age, are produced. Each fetus has its own placenta and surrounding sac.

2 **Identical** twins develop from a single zygote formed from a single ovum fertilized by a single spermatozoon. Obviously, they are always the same sex and carry the same inherited traits. Sometime during the early stages of development the embryonic cells separate into two units. Usually there is a single placenta, although there must be a separate umbilical cord for each individual.

Other multiple births may be fraternal, identical, or combinations of these. The tendency to multiple births seems to be hereditary.

Fertility drugs have increased the number of multiple births. These drugs stimulate the ovary either directly or indirectly (by way of the pitui-

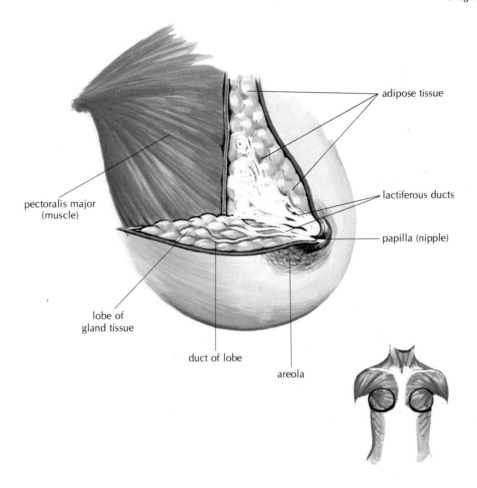

Fig. 21-9 *Section of breast.*

tary). The usual prematurity of multiple births causes a very high death rate. Newer drugs that will cause less drastic stimulation are being investigated, with the hope that single births and more living children will be the end result.

Disorders of Pregnancy

Ectopic Pregnancy

A pregnancy that develops in a location outside the uterine cavity is said to be an *ectopic* (ek-top'ik) pregnancy, "ectopic" meaning "out of normal place." The most common type is the *tubal* ectopic pregnancy, in which the growth of the embryo takes place in the uterine tube. However, this structure, which is not designed by nature for pregnancy, is not able to expand to contain the growing pregnancy and soon ruptures. The ruptured tube causes internal hemorrhage, and prompt surgical removal of the affected tube is required to save the mother's life.

Placenta Previa

Placenta previa (pre'via) is an abnormal condition in which the placenta is attached at or near the internal opening of the cervix. Whereas the placenta is usually attached to the upper part of the uterus, in placenta previa it becomes attached to the lower segment of the organ. The normal softening and dilation of the cervix that occur in later pregnancy will separate part of the placenta from its attachment. The result will be painless bleeding as well as interference with the fetal oxygen supply. Sometimes placenta previa necessitates *cesarean* (se-zar're-an) *section,* which is delivery of the fetus by way of an incision made in the abdominal wall and the wall of the uterus.

A valuable diagnostic tool that avoids the use

of undesirable x-ray is a form of vibrational energy called ultrasound (see Chap. 12). By this method, soft tissues can be visualized and such abnormalities as ectopic pregnancies and placenta previa can be accurately delineated. The relatively inexpensive ultrasound equipment has been found useful in detecting abnormalities of the fetus as well as tumors and other disorders of the reproductive system.

Lactation Disturbances

Disturbances in lactation may be due to a variety of reasons, including the following:

1 Malnutrition or anemia, which may prevent lactation entirely.
2 Emotional disturbances, which may affect lactation (as they may other glandular activities).
3 Abnormalities of parts of the mammary glands or injuries to these organs, which may cause interference with their functioning.
4 **Mastitis** (mas-ti′tis), which means inflammation of the breast, and which would make nursing the child inadvisable.

Toxemia of Pregnancy

Toxemia of pregnancy is a serious, often life-threatening disorder that can develop in the latter part of the pregnancy. The causes of this disorder are unknown. However, it is most common in women whose nutritional state is poor and who have received little or no health care during pregnancy. Symptoms include hypertension, protein in the urine, general edema, and sudden weight gain. If untreated, convulsions, kidney failure, and finally death of both mother and infant can occur.

Live Births and Fetal Deaths

The duration, or average term, of a human pregnancy is 9 calendar months, 10 lunar months, or 40 weeks. However, a pregnancy may end before that time.

The term *live birth* is used if the baby breathes or shows any evidence of life such as heartbeat, pulsation of the umbilical cord, or movement of voluntary muscles.

An *immature* or *premature* infant is one born before the organ systems are mature. Infants born

before the 37th week of gestation or weighing less than 2500 grams are considered preterm.

Loss of the fetus is classified according to the duration of the pregnancy:

I The term **abortion** refers to loss of the embryo or fetus before the 20th week or weight of about 500 grams. This loss can be either spontaneous or induced.
  1 **Spontaneous abortions** occur naturally with no interference. The most common causes are related to an abnormality of the embryo or fetus. Other causes include abnormality of the mother's reproductive organs, infections, or chronic disorders such as kidney disease or hypertension. *Miscarriage* is the lay term for spontaneous abortions.
  2 **Induced abortions** occur as a result of artificial or mechanical interruption. This classification includes *criminal abortions,* which are performed illegally and which are the cause of many tragic and unnecessary deaths each year. *Therapeutic abortions* are abortions performed by physicians as a form of treatment for a variety of reasons. With more liberal use of this type of abortion, there has been a dramatic decline in deaths related to illegal abortions, particularly among poor people.
II The term **fetal death** refers to the loss of the fetus after the 20th week of pregnancy. The fetus is considered *viable,* that is, able to live outside the uterus, after this point in the pregnancy. *Stillbirth* refers to the delivery of an infant that is lifeless.

Immaturity is a leading cause of death in the newborn. A fetus expelled before the 28th week or a weight of 1000 grams has less than a 50% chance of survival. Those born at a point closer to the full 40 weeks stand a much better chance of survival. Greater numbers of immature infants are being saved owing to the advances in neonatal intensive care.

The Menopause

The *menopause* (men′o-pawz), often called *change of life,* is that period at which menstruation ceases altogether. It ordinarily occurs between the ages of 45 and 55 and is caused by normal decline in ovarian function. The ovary becomes chiefly scar tissue and no longer produces ova or appreciable amounts of estrogens. Eventually, the uterus, the oviducts, the vagina, and the vulva all gradually become somewhat atrophied.

Although the menopause is an entirely normal condition, its onset sometimes brings about effects that are temporarily disturbing. The decrease in estrogens can cause such nervous symptoms as irritability, "hot flashes," and dizzy spells.

Summary

1 Reproduction.
  A Asexual in some of simplest forms of life.
  B Sexual in most higher forms. Specialized cells—ova in female, spermatozoa in male.
  C Common to both male and female; gonads, passageways for sex cells, accessory organs.
2 Male reproductive system.
  A Testes produce spermatozoa and hormone.
  B Ducts to carry sperm toward outside.
  C Seminal vesicles, prostate gland, and bulbourethral glands produce lubricating and alkalinizing secretions.
  D Penis contains urethra, of erectile tissue, distal end has prepuce (foreskin).
  E Disorders—sterility, infections, tumors.
3 Female reproductive system.
  A Ovaries produce ova and hormones.
  B Oviducts convey ova and provide place for fertilization.
  C Uterus has fundus, body, and cervix; involved in menstrual cycle and pregnancy.
  D Vagina receives spermatozoa, part of birth canal.

  E External genitalia—vulva including clitoris and labia; perineum (pelvic floor).
  F Disorders—leukorrhea, dysmenorrhea, tumors of uterus and breast (most common), infections, sterility.
4 Pregnancy.
  A Ovulation, fertilization, implantation.
  B Embryo—heart and brain develop early.
  C Fetus—surrounded by amniotic fluid, umbilical cord connects placenta and fetus.
  D Mother—supplies nutrition and oxygen and eliminates waste products for fetus and for herself; burden for lungs, heart, kidneys.
  E Labor and delivery—stages.
  F Mammary glands—lobes and ducts; lactation and advantages of breast feeding.
  G Multiple births—fraternal and identical.
  H Disorders—ectopic pregnancy, placenta previa, toxemia.
  I Fetal deaths—causes, immaturity.
5 Menopause—normal cessation of production of ova and hormones; sometimes temporary discomforts.

Questions and Problems

1 In what fundamental respect does reproduction in some single-celled animals such as the ameba differ from that in most animals?
2 Name the sex cells of both the male and the female.
3 Name all the parts of the male reproductive system and describe the function of each.
4 What is cryptorchidism? Why does this condition cause sterility?
5 Name and describe a disorder of the male reproductive system that is common in elderly men.
6 Name the principal parts of the female reproductive system and describe the function of each.

7 Describe the process of ovulation.
8 Beginning with the first day of the menstrual flow, describe the events of one complete cycle, including the role of the various hormones.
9 Distinguish between dysmenorrhea and amenorrhea.
10 What is a Pap test? Why is it important?
11 What is the most common malignant disease in women? For early detection, what should a woman do at regular intervals?
12 What are the two most common cancers of the uterus?
13 What are some causes of sterility in both the male and the female?

14 Distinguish between the following: zygote, embryo, fetus.

15 Name two auxiliary organs that are designed to serve the fetus. What is their origin and what are their functions?

16 Describe some of the changes that take place in the mother's body during pregnancy.

17 What is the major event of each of the 3 stages of labor and delivery?

18 List some of the advantages associated with breast-feeding the baby.

19 Define ectopic pregnancy; placenta previa; abortion (2 categories); premature, or preterm, infant.

20 What is the menopause? What causes this event? What are some of the changes that take place in the body?

Chapter 22

Heredity and Hereditary Diseases

- Mendel's discoveries
- Congenital vs. hereditary
- Chromosomes contain genes
- Functions of genes
- Genetic disorders
- Pedigrees and karyotypes
- Genetic counseling

Glossary

Congenital Present at and usually before birth.

Hereditary Characteristics transmitted from parents to offspring.

Meiosis A special method of cell division occurring during the development of sex cells (ova and sperm) in which the number of chromosomes is reduced, so that there are only half as many in the mature gamete as there are in other body cells of the species.

Mutation A variation in an inheritable characteristic, a permanent transmissible change in which the offspring differ from the parents.

Pedigree A diagram or chart of a person's ancestors.

Often, we are struck by the resemblance of a baby to one or both of its parents, yet rarely do we stop to consider *how* various traits are transmitted from parents to offspring. This subject—heredity—has fascinated mankind for thousands of years; the Old Testament contains numerous references to heredity (though, of course, the word was unknown in biblical times). However, it was not until the nineteenth century that methodical investigation into heredity was begun. At that time an Austrian monk, Gregor Mendel, discovered through his experiments with garden peas that there was a precise pattern in the appearance of differences occurring among parents and their progeny. Mendel's most important contribution to the understanding of heredity was the demonstration that there are independent units of hereditary influence. Later, these independent units were given the name "genes." Mendel demonstrated further that the traits—hence the genes that denote the traits—could be either dominant or recessive. Available evidence indicates that heritable characteristics include the following:

1 Color of skin, eyes, and hair.
2 Blood type.
3 Body build and body dimensions.
4 Life span.
5 Skull shape.
6 Form of forehead, nose, and jaws, and arrangement of teeth.
7 Texture and shape of hair.

8 Handedness.
9 Certain diseases.
10 Susceptibility to contract certain diseases.

Study of the last two of these, with which we shall be chiefly concerned, will help us to understand the workings of heredity and its functional unit—the gene.

Congenital vs. Hereditary

Before we discuss hereditary diseases we need to distinguish them from other congenital diseases. To illustrate, let us assume that two infants are born within seconds in adjoining delivery rooms of the same hospital. It is noted that one infant has a clubfoot, a condition called *talipes;* (tal′i-pes) the second infant has a rudimentary extra finger attached to the fifth finger of each hand, a condition called *polydactyly* (pol-y-dac′tyl-y). Are both conditions hereditary? Both congenital? Is either hereditary? We can answer these questions by defining the key terms, congenital and hereditary. Congenital means existing from the time of birth; hereditary means genetically transmitted or transmissible. Thus, one condition may be both congenital and hereditary; another, congenital yet not hereditary. On the other hand, a hereditary condition will usually be congenital, since many disorders are evident at birth or soon thereafter. However, certain inherited disorders such as adult polycystic kidney and Huntington's chorea, a nervous disorder, do not manifest themselves until about midlife (40 to 50 years of age). In the case of our earlier examples, the clubfoot is congenital, but not hereditary, having resulted from severe distortion of the developing extremities during intrauterine growth; the extra fingers are hereditary, a familial trait that appears in another relative, a grandparent, perhaps, or a parent, and in this case is also evident at the time of birth.

Now let us take a look at the mechanism that underlies Mendel's findings.

Chromosomes and Genes

As described in Chapter 2, the nucleus of each cell contains chromosomes composed of deoxyribonucleic acid (DNA), on a protein framework. Each chromosome contains thousands of genes, and each gene carries a specific trait. Another way to state this fact is, "Each gene is coded for a specific trait." The three types of traits so carried are physical, biochemical, and physiologic, and they thus influence an individual's physical appearance, physiologic makeup, and susceptibility or tendency to contract certain diseases, as well as the activities of all the cells in his body.

The human ovum and the human sperm each contain 23 chromosomes; except for the pair of chromosomes that contain the sex determinants, each chromosome in the sperm is similar in size and shape to one in the ovum. Thus, when the sperm unites with the ovum, the fertilized ovum contains 23 pairs of chromosomes, or a total of 46.

During cell division (mitosis, see Chap. 2), the chromosomes duplicate themselves, so that each new cell thus produced contains the same number and kind of chromosomes as the original (a process usually termed replication). The ovum and the sperm are formed by a process of cell division called *meiosis* (mi-o′sis) such that each sperm or ovum receives only one member of each chromosome pair. One pair of chromosomes—the sex chromosomes, which determine the sex of offspring—is very different from the other 22 pairs; the female pair has two similar members called X chromosomes, whereas the two members in the male chromosome differ from each other and are called the X and the Y chromosomes. Each male egg cell contains either an X or a Y chromosome; if the sperm has a Y chromosome the infant will be male; if an X, it will be female (Fig. 22-1). Then, as the fertilized ovum grows, by the process of cell division (mitosis, see Chap. 2), the chromosomes duplicate themselves so that each new cell thus produced contains the same number and kind of chromosomes as the original.

Mechanism of Gene Function
Manufacture of Enzymes

The primary action of each gene is to control the manufacture of a specific protein. Remember that DNA—the genetic material—controls the forma-

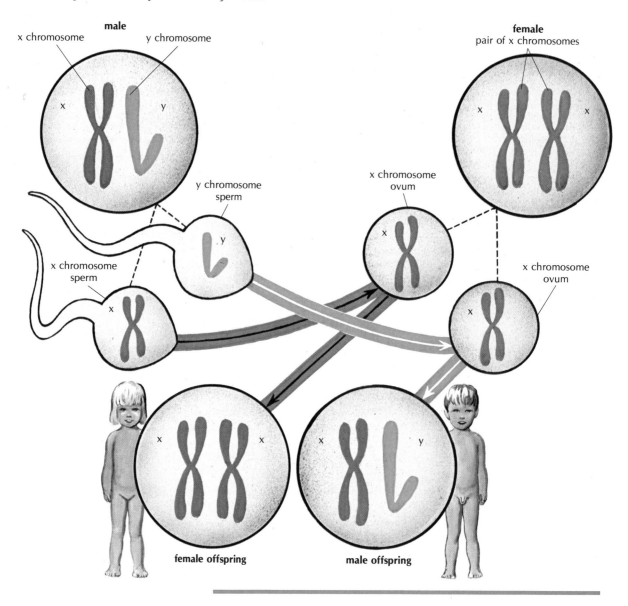

Fig. 22-1 *Male X chromosome unites with female X chromosome—child is female; male Y chromosome unites with female X chromosome—child is male.*

tion of RNA (ribonucleic acid, see Chap. 4), which in turn spreads throughout the cell and controls the manufacture of both *structural* proteins—the main components of skin, muscle, and so on;—other proteins, such as hemoglobin; and *enzymes*—the proteins that promote all of the chemical reactions that take place in the cells. The genes are reproduced several hours before mitosis occurs, and are replicated only once. Some traits are determined through the collaboration of many genes

located at various positions along the chromosome; some, by a single gene. Genes are said to be *dominant* or *recessive:* a dominant gene is one that expresses its effect in the daughter cell regardless of whether the gene at the same site on the matching chromosome is the same as or different from the dominant gene. The effect of a recessive gene will not be evident unless the gene at that site in the matching chromosome in the pair is also recessive.

Gene Mutation

As a rule, chromosomes replicate exactly during cell division. Occasionally, for reasons not yet clearly understood, there is a change in the number of chromosomes, or chromosomal breakage, in which there is loss of or rearrangement of gene fragments, resulting in genetic mutation.

A mutation is any change in a chromosome or a gene occurring spontaneously, and is, obviously, inheritable. If the mutation occurs in an ovum or a sperm involved in reproduction, the altered trait will be expressed in the offpsring. The vast majority of harmful mutations never are expressed because the affected fetus dies and is spontaneously aborted; and most mutations are so inconsequential that they have no visible influence. Beneficial mutations tend to be spread throughout a population.

Genetic Diseases

Advances in genetic research have made it possible to identify the causes of many disorders and—what is more to the point—to develop methods of genetic screening. Persons who are "at risk" for having a child with a genetic disorder, and fetuses and newborn in whom the presence of an abnormality may be suspected can have chromosome studies done to identify genetic abnormalities.

Any disorders that involve the genes may be said to be genetic, but in some cases they are not hereditary. Nonhereditary genetic disorders may begin during the maturation of the sex cells or even during the development of the embryo. The best-known example of a genetic disorder that is not inherited is *Down's syndrome.* In most cases this abnormality results from the presence of an extra chromosome per cell. It is usually recognizable at birth. The afflicted child has distinctive facial features. The face is round, with close-set eyes that slant upward at their lateral extremities. The head is small and grows at an unusually slow rate. The nose is flat; the tongue is large and protruding. The muscles and joints are lax. Intellectually, the child will not achieve a "normal" level of functioning. However, the amount of skill he can gain depends on the severity of his disease and his family and school environments. It is important to recognize that this disorder is not inherited. Usually,

both parents are normal as are the child's siblings. However, the birth of one child with Down's syndrome does increase the likelihood that an additional child may be similarly affected.

Various toxins may damage the genes but the disorders they produce are not hereditary. Environmental agents, such as mercury and some chemicals used in industry (for example, certain phenols and PCB), as well as some drugs, notably LSD, are known to disrupt genetic organization.

A familial disease is a genetic disease that is hereditary, that is, it is passed on from parent to child by way of the spermatozoa and ova. In the case of a dominant trait, one parent carries the abnormal gene that gives rise to the disorder, as is the case in Huntington's chorea. The disturbance appears in the parent and any of the offspring who receive the defective gene. If the trait is a recessive one, as is the case in the majority of inheritable disorders, the defective genes must come from both parents. Among important inheritable diseases that are carried as recessive traits are diabetes mellitus, cystic fibrosis, and sickle cell anemia.

Earlier, it was stated that genes control the production of specific enzymes. In the case of *PKU, phenylketonuria* (fen′′il-ke′′to-nu′re-ah), the lack of a certain enzyme prevents the proper metabolism of *phenylalanine* (fen′′il-al′ah-nin), one of the common amino acids. The phenylalanine accumulates in the infant's blood; if the condition remains untreated, it leads to mental retardation before the age of 2 years. PKU screening is done routinely on newborn infants.

Sickle cell disease is described in Chapter 13, where it is stated that the disease is found almost exclusively in members of the black race. By contrast, *cystic fibrosis* is most common in members of the Caucasian race; in fact, it is possibly the most frequently inherited disease in white persons. It is characterized by excessively viscid (thickened) secretions of the linings of the bronchi, the intestine, and the ducts of the pancreas. Owing to the latter, the flow of pancreatic juice to the small intestine is prevented. Obstruction and blockage of these vital organs follows, associated with frequent respiratory infections, with uncontrollable intestinal losses, particularly of fats (and the vitamins these fats carry), as well as massive salt loss. Treatment includes oral administration of pancreatic enzymes and special pulmonary exercises. Once a fatal disease in children and adolescents, now, with appropriate care, life expectancies are extending into the third decade.

Another group of heritable muscle disorders is known collectively as the *progressive muscular atrophies*. Atrophy means wasting due to decrease in size of a normally developed part. The absence of normal muscle movement in the infant proceeds within a few months to extreme weakness of the respiratory muscles, until ultimately the infant is unable to breathe adequately. Most afflicted babies die within several months. The name "floppy baby syndrome," as the disease is commonly called, provides a vivid description of its effects.

Albinism is an inherited disorder that is carried by recessive genes. It is of particular interest because of the easily recognizable appearance it lends to the affected person. The skin and hair color are strikingly white, and do not darken with age. The skin is abnormally sensitive to sunlight and may appear wrinkled. Albinos are especially susceptible to skin cancer and to some severe visual disturbances.

Treatment and Prevention of Genetic Diseases

The list of genetic diseases is so lengthy that many pages of this book would be needed to simply enumerate them. Moreover, the list continues to grow as sophisticated research techniques and advances in biology make it clear that verious diseases whose cause formerly was not understood are now known to be genetic—some actually hereditary, while others are not. Can we identify which are inherited genetic disorders and which are due to environmental factors? Can we prevent the occurrence of any of them?

Genetic Counseling

Strange as it may seem, it is possible to prevent genetic disorders, even those that are inherited, to some extent at least, as well as to effectively treat some of them. The most effective method of preventing genetic disease is through genetic counseling, a specialized field of health care. Genetic counseling centers use a team approach of medical, nursing, laboratory, and social service professionals to advise and care for the clients.

The Family History

An accurate and complete family history of both of the prospective parents is necessary. It includes information about relatives regarding age, onset of a specific disease, health status, and cause of death. The families' ethnic origins may be relevant, since some genetic diseases have a definite relationship to certain ethnic groups. Hospital and physician records are studied, as are photographs of family members. The age of the prospective parents is a factor, as is parental or ancestral relationship (for example, marriage between first cousins). The complete, detailed family history, or tree, is called a *pedigree*.

Karyotype

Abnormalities in the number of chromosomes can be detected by analysis of the *karyotype* (kar'eotype) (karyon means nucleus), the chromosomal elements typical of a cell, identified and arranged according to a definite classification. A karyotype is produced by growing certain cells in a special medium, and arresting the cell division at the stage called metaphase. The chromosomes, visible under the microscope, are photographed, cut out, and arranged in groups according to their size and form. Abnormalities in number and structure of chromosomes—called chromosomal errors—can thereby be detected.

A technique that enables the geneticist to prepare a karyotype of an unborn fetus is *amniocentesis* (am''ne-o-sen-te'sis). During this procedure, a small amount of amniotic fluid, which surrounds the fetus and is often referred to as the "waters," is withdrawn. Cells in the amniotic fluid are removed, grown (cultured), and separated for study. A karyotype is prepared, and the chromosomes are examined.

Counseling the Prospective Parents

The counselor, armed with all the available pertinent facts, as well as with his special knowledge of the recurrence risk rate, is now equipped to inform the prospective parents of their possibility of having genetically abnormal offspring. The couple may then elect to have no children; to have an adoptive family; to undergo sterilization; to terminate the pregnancy; or to accept the risk.

Progress in Medical Treatment

The mental and physical ravages of many genetic diseases are largely preventable provided the disease is diagnosed and treated very early in the individual's life. Some of these diseases respond very well to dietary control. One such disease, which goes by the interesting name "maple syrup urine disease," responds to very large doses of thiamine along with control of the intake of certain amino acids. The disastrous effects of Wilson's disease, in which abnormal accumulations of copper in the tissues cause tremor, rigidity, uncontrollable stagger, and finally extensive liver damage, can be prevented by a combination of dietary and drug therapy. Phenylketonuria is perhaps the best-known example of dietary management of inherited disease. If undiagnosed and untreated, 98% of patients will be severely mentally retarded by 10 years of age; whereas if the condition is diagnosed and treated before the baby reaches the age of 6 months and treatment is maintained for several years, mental deficiency will be prevented. A simple test, which is now mandatory in many states, is performed immediately after birth to determine whether phenylketonuria is a potential problem.

The rate of population growth slows down nationwide as couples tend to have smaller families, and concern about the health and well-being of each newborn infant increases. Hence, we can anticipate greatly improved methods of screening, diagnosis and treatment of genetic diseases.

Summary

1 Heredity and genetics.
  A Genetics is a branch of biology dealing with heredity and its laws.
  B Mendel discovered that
    (1) Inherited factors may be dominant or recessive.
    (2) Dominant and recessive traits appear according to a particular pattern.
  C Hereditary characteristics.
    (1) Physical features.
    (2) Blood type.
    (3) Body build and dimensions.
    (4) Susceptibility to some diseases.
    (5) Inheritance of some diseases.
2 Hereditary and congenital diseases.
  A Congenital—existing from the time of birth; may or may not be hereditary.
  B Hereditary—transmitted through familial lines.
  C Genetic—Abnormality of genes; may or may not be hereditary.
3 Chromosomes and genes.
  A Germ cell nucleus contains chromosomes composed of DNA; genes are bits of DNA molecule.
  B Thousands of genes strung along each chromosome; each gene carries specific trait.
  C Ovum and sperm each contain 23 chromosomes
    (1) 22 chromosomes in sperm similar to 22 chromosomes in ovum.
    (2) 1 pair—sex chromosomes—different in male and female.
      (a) Female pair contains two X chromosomes.
      (b) Male pair contains one X and one Y chromosome.
      (c) If ovum fertilized by male X chromosome, fetus will be female; if by male Y chromosome, fetus will be male.
  D Mutations—spontaneous changes in genetic material.
    (1) Most mutations have no visible effect.
    (2) Most harmful mutations cause fetal death.
4 Gene function.
  A Genes control formation of all body cells.
    (1) Structural proteins—skin, muscle.
    (2) Enzymes—chemical reactions.
  B Gene types.
    (1) Dominant—may hide presence of recessive factor.
    (2) Recessive—reveals itself if both parents transfer it to offspring.
5 Genetic diseases.
  A Prenatal diagnosis by amniocentesis.
  B Some recognizable at birth.

C Some testable at birth.

D Some not apparent until adolescence.

6 Treatment and prevention of genetic disorders.

    A Genetic counseling provides information to prospective parents about probable genetic makeup of offspring.

        (1) Counselor's special knowledge of heredity.

        (2) Pedigree.

        (3) Karyotype.

    B Some genetic disorders treatable by careful control of diet, medication, or by combination of both; some correctable by surgical means.

Questions and Problems

1 Is hair color and texture a hereditary trait? Why?

2 A baby is born with syphilis. Is this congenital or hereditary? Why?

3 What types of traits are coded by the genes?

4 In what way does a recessive gene differ from a dominant one?

5 What purpose does a pedigree serve?

6 What is a karyotype and what is its purpose?

7 What is Down's syndrome and what is found in the karyotype of this disorder?

8 What is PKU and how should this disease be treated?

9 What are some evidences of albinism and what are the risks in this disorder?

10 What heritable disorder is more common among black persons and how does it manifest itself?

11 What is the most common heritable disease among white persons and what are some of its symptoms?

Chapter *23*

Immunity, Vaccines, and Serums

- Conditions for infection
- Defenses of the body
- What immunity means
- Antigens and antibodies
- Immunity, inborn and acquired
- Vaccines and booster shots
- Serums and borrowed antibodies
- Allergy
- Transplants and the rejection syndrome

Glossary

Immunity Protection against a particular disease; absence of susceptibility to the harmful effects of foreign agents.

Infection Invasion and multiplication of microorganisms in tissues.

Inflammation A protective response to injury or destruction of tissue.

Resistance Natural ability of an organism to remain unaffected by harmful agents in the environment.

Specificity Pertaining to or characterizing a species; special or distinctive.

Toxin A poison.

Vaccine A substance used to cause antibody formation. Usually, a suspension of attenuated or killed pathogens given by inoculation in order to prevent a specific disease.

Virulence The power of an organism to overcome the defenses of its host.

The Occurrence of Infection

This chapter deals primarily with the various defenses which the body brings to bear against invading disease organisms, cancer cells, or other substances that are foreign or harmful to it. Included is discussion of the series of chemical processes producing *immunity.*

It should be repeated that although the body is constantly being exposed to pathogenic invasion, a large number of conditions determine whether or not an infection will actually occur. Many pathogens have a decided preference for certain body tissues. For example, some viruses will attack only nerve tissue, as is the case with the poliomyelitis pathogen. Even though it may be inhaled or swallowed in large numbers and therefore may be in direct contact with the mucous membrane, no apparent disorder of these respiratory or digestive system linings occurs. On the other hand, such pathogens as the influenza and cold viruses do attack these mucous membranes.

The respiratory tract is a common *portal of entry* for many pathogens. Other important avenues of entry include the digestive system and the tubes that open into the urinary and the reproductive systems. Any break in the skin or in a mucous membrane allows organisms such as staphylococci easy access to the deeper tissues and nearly always leads to infection, while the unbroken skin or membrane usually is not affected at all. The portal of entry, then, is an important condition influencing the occurrence of infection.

The *virulence* (vir′u-lens), or the power of an organism to overcome the defenses of its host, must also be considered. Virulence has two aspects: one may be thought of as "aggressiveness," or invasive power; the other is the ability of the organism to produce *toxins,* which damage the body. The virulence of different organisms varies, and the virulence of a specific organism also can change. In other words, an organism can be more dangerous at some times than at others. As a rule, organisms that come from an already infected host are more "vicious" than the same type of organism grown under laboratory conditions.

The number of pathogens that invade the body also has much to do with whether or not an infection develops. Even if the virulence of a particular organism happens to be low at the moment, if a large number of them enter the body, infection has a better chance of occurring than if the number is small.

Finally, there are the defenses of the body itself, considered in sum as its *resistance.* There are certain protective devices common to all living things, effective against any harmful agent. These devices might be classified as the body's *nonspecific resistance.* Then there are devices that act against a certain specific agent and no other. These defenses are referred to as *specific resistance,* or *immunity.*

The Body's Defenses Against Disease

The devices that protect the body against disease are usually considered as successive "lines of defense," beginning with the relatively simple first, or outer, line and proceeding through the progressively more complicated lines until the ultimate defense mechanism—immunity—is reached.

The first line of defense against invaders is the combination of the skin and mucous membranes, which serve as mechanical barriers as long as they remain intact, by virtue of their thickness alone. Certain other properties of the skin and the mucous membranes help to discourage parasites; for example, their acid secretion. Also the cilia of some mucous membranes serve to keep their surfaces swept clean.

Included in this first line are other defenses of a mechanical or chemical nature. Certain reflexes aid in the removal of pathogens. Sneezing and coughing, for instance, are reflexes that tend to remove foreign matter, including microorganisms, from the upper respiratory tract. In the digestive tract, the acid stomach juice destroys many organisms. Vomiting and diarrhea are ways in which toxins (poisons) and bacteria may be expelled.

The second great line of defense is the process of *inflammation,* which is the body's effort to get rid of anything that irritates it (or, if this proves impossible, to minimize the harmful effects of the irritant). Inflammation can occur as a result of any irritant, not only bacteria. Friction, fire, chemicals, x-rays, and cuts or blows all can be classed as irritants. If the irritant is due to pathogenic invasion, the resulting inflammation is termed an *infection.* With the entrance of pathogens and their subsequent multiplication, a whole series of defensive processes begins. This is called an *inflammatory reaction,* and accompanying it are the four classic symptoms: heat, redness, swelling, and pain. What takes place in the course of an inflammatory reaction is briefly this. When the parasite enters the tissues, the small blood vessels dilate, admitting more blood into the area. This is the basis of the heat, redness, and swelling.

With the increased blood flow come a vast number of leukocytes. Now a new phenomenon occurs: the walls of the tiny blood vessels become "coarsened" in their texture (as a piece of cloth will do when stretched), the blood flow slows down, and the leukocytes move through these altered walls and into the tissue, where they can get at the irritant directly. Blood vessel dilation and changes in the walls of the capillaries, allowing leukocytes and more fluid to leak from them, is due to the release of *histamine* (his′tah-mēn), a substance found in all tissues. When this response occurs in a local area, it is useful in preventing the spread of the foreign agent. The mixture of leukocytes and the fluid from the blood plasma is the *inflammatory exudate.* The pressure of this material on the nerve endings, as well as that of the increased amount of blood in the vessels, causes the pain of inflammation.

The leukocytes now proceed to surround, engulf and digest the invaders. As was mentioned in Chapters 13 and 16, this process is called *phagocytosis* (fag''o-si-to'sis) (see Fig. 13-2). The bacteria fight back. They discharge their toxins and destroy large numbers of white blood cells so that eventually the area becomes filled with dead leukocytes. The mixture of exudate, living and dead white blood cells, and pathogens plus destroyed tissue cells is *pus.*

Meanwhile, the regional lymph nodes become enlarged and tender, a sign that they are performing their own protective function in working overtime to produce phagocytic cells which "clean" the lymph drained from the inflamed area; at the same time, the lymph nodes are manufacturing lymphocytes at an accelerated rate. These cells figure in the production of *antibodies,* to be discussed shortly.

Finally, we arrive at the ultimate defense against disease, immunity, to which most of this chapter is devoted.

The Processes of Immunity

Immunity can be defined as the power of an individual to resist or overcome the effects of a particular disease or other harmful agent. Sometimes the words "immunity" and "resistance" are used interchangeably; but it is more accurate to think of immunity as a process that nullifies the effect of the invading bacteria *before* they have had a chance to set up an infection. Also, it is useful to consider immunity as a selective process; that is, a person may be immune to measles but not to diphtheria, or vice versa. This selective characteristic has a name: *specificity* (spes-i-fis'i-te).

The chemical processes that produce immunity can be described briefly as follows. Every pathogenic microorganism that enters the body carries within itself a substance called an *antigen* (an'te-jen). When the antigen is introduced into the body, it causes certain body cells to produce protein compounds called *antibodies.* These antibodies destroy the toxins or the pathogens, or else act on them in a way that will make the microorganisms more susceptible to the action of the white blood cells

or other phagocytes. Antigens vary in their chemical structure, and a specific antigen will stimulate the body to produce only a specific antibody in response to it. The antibody, then, will react only with the kind of antigen that caused its production, and with no other. This is the reason for the selective nature of immunity; so that immunity to one disease does not necessarily cause a person to be immune to another. Indeed, it is possible to have immunity to one disease and *susceptibility,* its opposite, to a different disease.

Reaction to foreign substances is mediated by two different types of lymphocytes found in lymphoid tissue and in the circulating blood (see Fig. 13-7). These lymphocytes differ in their development and method of response. Both types of lymphocytes arise, originally, from bone marrow. Some of the immature stem cells from the bone marrow migrate to the thymus and become T cells, which constitute about 90% of the lymphocytes in the circulating blood. These thymus-derived cells produce an immunity that is said to be cell-mediated.

1 T cells attack the pathogen or foreign cell directly.
2 On continued exposure to the invader (antigen), the T cells become "sensitized" and then attach directly to the invader.
3 Once attached, T cells release substances that stimulate other lymphocytes and macrophages, large phagocytic cells, to assist in the destruction of the foreign cell.
4 This part of the immune system is responsible for defense against cancer cells, certain viruses, and some bacteria, and for the rejection of tissue transplanted from another person.

The B-lymphocytes do not migrate to the thymus but rather to the lymphoid tissues associated with the small bowel, to the tonsils, to the appendix, and into the blood. After exposure to an antigen, the B-lymphocytes manufacture great quantities of antibodies, which circulate in the blood and are active in a number of ways.

1 They dissolve cell membranes, acting with complement (a combination of enzymes) to coat bacterial cells and increase the effectiveness of the antibodies.

2 The antibodies produced by B-lymphocytes cause antigens to stick or clump together.

3 They cause the release of chemicals that attract white blood cells to the site of irritation.

4 Certain antibodies become attached to basophils, a type of leukocyte. When an antigen contacts this antibody, the basophil ruptures and releases histamine.

Kinds of Immunity

There are two main categories of immunity: *inborn* (or inherited) *immunity* and *acquired immunity.* This second type may be acquired by *natural* or *artificial* means. In addition, an acquired immunity may be either *active* or *passive.* Let us investigate each category in turn.

Inborn Immunity

Although certain diseases found in animals may be transmitted to humans, many infections such as chicken cholera, hog cholera, distemper in dogs, and various other animal diseases do not affect human beings. On the other hand, the constitutional differences that make human beings immune to these disorders also make them susceptible to others that do not affect the lower animals. Such infections as measles, scarlet fever, diphtheria, and influenza do not seem to affect the animals contacted by human beings during the time they are experiencing illness. Both humans and animals have what is called a *species immunity* to many of each other's diseases.

Another form of inborn immunity is termed *racial immunity.* Indications seem to be that some racial groups have a greater inborn immunity to certain diseases than other racial groups. For instance, in our own country, Blacks are apparently more immune to poliomyelitis, malaria, and yellow fever than are members of the white race. Of course, it is often difficult to tell how much of this variation in resistance to infection is due to environment and how much is due to actual inborn traits of the particular racial group.

Some members of a given group have a more highly developed *individual immunity* than other members. Newspapers and magazines sometimes feature the advice of an elderly person who is asked to give his secret for living to a ripe old age, and his answer may be that he practiced temperance and lived a carefully regulated life with the right amount of rest, exercise, and work. The next oldster interviewed may boast of his use of alcoholic beverages, his constant smoking, his lack of exercise, and other kinds of reputedly unhygienic behavior. Could it be that the latter person has lived through the onslaughts of toxins and disease organisms, resisting infection and maintaining health in spite of his environment rather than because of it, thanks to the resistance factors and immunity to disease that he inherited?

Acquired Immunity

The difference between an inborn immunity and an acquired immunity is that in the latter case the immunity is not due to inheritance factors. An immunity can be *naturally acquired* before birth through the transmission of antibodies from the mother to the fetus by way of the placenta. An immunity also may be naturally acquired by contracting the disease itself.

On the other hand, an immunity can be *artificially acquired* by the administration of a vaccine or an immune serum.

An acquired immunity also can be classed as *active* or *passive.* The difference is that in an actively acquired immunity the antibodies are made "on the premises"—in the person's own tissues. In a passively acquired immunity, the antibodies come from some outside source. Let us look more closely at typical active and passive situations.

Active Immunity

In actively acquired immunity, the person's tissues and cells *actively* manufacture antibodies by themselves which then act against the infecting agent or its toxins. Each time a person is invaded by the organisms of a disease, his cells may manufacture antibodies that give him immunity against this particular infection for years, and in some cases for life. Sometimes, a small number of relatively nonvirulent organisms may cause so little disturbance that the host is not conscious of the invasion. His tissues nevertheless may produce antibodies which give an active immunity of a natural type.

Now suppose that for one reason or other a person fails to be exposed to repeated small doses of a particular organism. Having no antibodies, he would be defenseless against a heavy onslaught of that particular pathogen, and the result might be disastrous. Therefore, artificial measures are taken to cause the person's tissues to actively manufacture antibodies. One could inject the virulent pathogen into the tissues, but obviously this would be dangerous. What is done, then, is to take some of the pathogen (or toxin), treat it to reduce its virulence (that is, *attenuate* it), and then inject it. In this way the tissues are made to produce antibodies without causing a serious illness. This process is known as *vaccination* or *inoculation,* and the solution containing the pathogen (with reduced virulence) is a *vaccine.* By means of vaccination an active immunity of the artificially acquired type is accomplished.

Passive Immunity

In a passively acquired immunity, it was noted, the antibodies are borrowed, not made by the person's own tissues. We already have seen an example of this in the case of the fetus, which receives antibodies from the mother's blood by way of the placenta. The result of this borrowing (or rather, donation) of antibodies is that at birth the infant has much more resistance to contagious diseases than he does when he is several months old. The antibodies borrowed from the mother do not last as long as those actively produced by the child himself, but they serve to "tide him over" during the period when his constitution might not otherwise withstand exposure to various infections. Nursing the infant may lengthen this period owing to the presence of specific antibodies in breast milk. These are the only known examples of naturally acquired passive immunity.

If a person receives a large dose of virulent organisms with no established immunity to them, he stands in great danger, since it takes several weeks to produce a naturally acquired active immunity, and even longer to produce an artificial active immunity through the administration of a vaccine. In order to prevent catastrophe, then, the victim must receive a counteracting dose of borrowed antibodies in a hurry. This is accomplished through the administration of a *serum,* the nature and origin of which will subsequently be explained. The serum gives a short-lived but effective protection against the invaders, and its action is an example of an artificially acquired passive immunity.

Vaccines and Serums
Vaccines

The purpose of a vaccine, we learned, is to provide an artificially acquired active immunity to a specific disease. A vaccine is a preparation made of the actual cause of the disease—the organism or its toxin—treated in such a way that it will not cause the disease when injected but nevertheless will stimulate antibody formation. Ordinarily, the administration of a vaccine is a preventive measure, designed to provide protection in anticipation of an invasion by a certain disease organism.

Sometimes the terms "vaccine" and "antigen" are confused, understandably, since both are concerned with antibody formation. Think of it this way: all vaccines are antigens, but not all antigens are vaccines. Actually, the word "antigen" includes a much broader area of biologic activity. Antigens include many protein substances, such as the Rh factor in blood, the A and B proteins which are in part responsible for the four blood groups, such toxins as snake venom, and many other materials. The Rh factor from an Rh positive baby, entering the blood stream of the Rh negative mother, causes in some cases the production of antibodies against itself. This Rh factor is an antigen, but we would not think of it as a vaccine. Vaccines, then, are merely one small group of a large number of antigenic substances, and should be thought of only as agents given to prevent disease.

Examples of Vaccines

To nearly everyone the word "vaccination" has meant inoculation against smallpox. According to the World Health Organization, smallpox is virtually an extinct disease. Mandatory vaccination has been discontinued because the side-effects of the vaccine are thought to be more hazardous than the probability of contracting the disease. The appearance of a few isolated cases may lead to some rethinking about the need for vaccination for smallpox.

Because of the seriousness of whooping cough in the young infant, early inoculation with whooping cough or *pertussis* (per-tus'is) vaccine, made from heat-killed whooping cough bacteria, is recommended. This vaccine usually is given in conjunction with diphtheria toxoid and tetanus toxoid, all in one mixture. A *toxoid* is a form of vaccine containing the weakened toxin of the disease organism instead of the organism proper. This combination, usually referred to as DPT, may be given as early as the second month, and should be followed by additional injections during the first year of life and again at the time the child enters a nursery, a school, or any other environment in which he might be exposed to one of these contagions.

Vaccines are now available for nearly all of the common contagious diseases with the exception of the common cold and chicken pox. The decrease in cases of smallpox and typhoid fever is so great that immunizations for these no longer are recommended in the United States.

A great deal of intensive research in viruses has lead to the development of vaccines for an increasing number of virus diseases. Spectacular results in preventing poliomyelitis have been obtained by the use of a variety of vaccines. The first of these was the Salk vaccine. Now the more convenient oral vaccines, such as the Sabin, are used most. A number of vaccines have been developed for influenza, which is caused by several different strains of virus. The measles (rubeola), mumps, and rubella (German measles) vaccine, MMR, is proving to be effective. The use of a rubella vaccine should lower the number of birth defects because, although the disease itself is very mild, it has serious effects on the developing fetus (see Appendix, Table 3).

An exception to the usual rule of a vaccine being given before the invasion of the disease organism is the rabies vaccine. Rabies is a virus disease transmitted by the bite of such animals as dogs, cats, wolves, coyotes, foxes, and bats. There is no actual cure for rabies; it is fatal in nearly 100% of cases. However, the disease develops so slowly following the transmission of the organism that the "treatment" consists of the administration of a vaccine, since there is time enough to develop an active immunity. Anyone bitten by an animal suspected of having rabies should begin this *Pasteur treatment* at once. The most desirable method of controlling rabies is to immunize all dogs.

A final word about the long-term efficacy of vaccines: in many cases an active immunity acquired by artificial (or even natural) means does not last a lifetime. Repeated inoculations, called booster shots, administered at relatively short intervals, help in maintaining a high level of immunity. The number of such booster injections recommended varies with the disease and with the environment or range of exposure of the individual.

Serums

A serum that is given for the purpose of producing an immunity should properly be called an *immune serum,* but in this discussion it will be referred to simply as a serum for the sake of convenience.

There are a number of differences between vaccines and serums. When a vaccine is given, it results in antibody formation by the body tissues. In the administration of a serum, the antibodies are supplied "ready made." The administration of a serum produces immediate immunity, but this passive immunity does not last as long as that actively produced by the body tissues.

There is a basic difference, too, in the content of vaccines and serums. Whereas the principal element of a vaccine is a weakened form of the disease organism or its toxin, a serum contains neither of these. In an earlier chapter we saw that serum as such consists of blood plasma minus the fibrinogen content. An immune serum is this basic serum with the addition of antibodies.

A serum prepared for immune purposes is often derived from animals, mainly horses. It has been found that the tissues of the horse produce large quantities of antibodies in response to the injection of organisms or their toxins. After repeated injections, the horse is bled, using careful sterile technique; and because of the size of the animal it is possible to remove large quantities without injury. The blood is allowed to clot, the serum is removed, and it is packaged in sterile glass vials or other appropriate containers. It is then sent to the hospital, clinic, or doctor's office for use. In most cases the use of a serum is in the nature of an emergency; that is, there is no time to wait until an active immunity has developed. Injecting humans with serum derived from animals is not without its problems. The foreign proteins in animal serums may cause a sensitivity reaction so that *serum sickness,* often a serious disorder, can occur (see Chap. 13).

Examples of Serums

Some immune serums contain antibodies that are known as *antitoxins;* that is, they neutralize the toxins but have no effect upon the toxic organisms themselves. Certain antibodies act directly on the pathogens, engulfing and destroying them, or preventing their continued reproduction. Some serums are obtained from animals, others from human sources. The following are some immune serums:

1   Diphtheria serum (from horses) contains large amounts of antitoxin.
2   Tetanus immune globulin is effective in preventing lockjaw (tetanus), which is often a complication of neglected wounds. Because tetanus immune globulin is of human origin there is less chance of untoward reactions than in the case of serums obtained from horses.
3   Measles immune globulin, from human serum, is used for susceptible infants or debilitated children who have been exposed to measles. Active immunization with the live vaccine should be done eight to ten weeks after the immune serum has been given.
4   Immune serum globulin, from pooled normal human plasma, may be effective in the prevention of infectious hepatitis.
5   The immune globulin Rh_0 (D), a concentrated antibody, is given to prevent the formation of active antibodies against the Rh factor in an Rh negative mother, following the birth of an Rh positive infant (or even in a miscarriage of a presumably Rh positive fetus) (see Chap. 13). It is also given when Rh transfusion incompatabilities occur.
6   Anti-snake bite serum or *antivenin* (an-te-ven′in) is used to combat the effects of bites of certain poisonous snakes.
7   Botulism antitoxin, from horses, is a serum that offers the best hope for botulism victims, and then only if given early.

Allergy

This is as appropriate a place as any to discuss the subject of *allergy,* since it has been touched upon several times without benefit of adequate explanation; moreover, allergy involves antigens and antibodies, and its chemical processes are much like those of immunity.

Allergy (a broader term for it is hypersensitiveness) can be defined informally as the tendency of some individuals to react unfavorably to the presence of certain substances that are normally harmless to most people.

These substances are called *allergens* and, like any antigen, are often of a protein nature. Examples of typical allergens are pollens, house dust, horse dander (dander is the term for the minute scales that are found on hairs and feathers), and certain food proteins. When the tissues of a susceptible person are repeatedly exposed to an allergen—for example, the nasal mucosa to pollens—these tissues become *sensitized;* that is, antibodies are produced in them. When the next invasion of the allergen occurs, there is an antigen–antibody reaction. Now, normally this type of reaction takes place in the blood without harm, as it does in immunity. In allergy, however, the antigen–antibody reaction takes place within the cells of the sensitized tissues, with results that are disagreeable and sometimes dangerous. In the case of the nasal mucosa that has become sensitized to pollen, the allergic manifestation is *hay fever,* with symptoms much like those of the common cold.

An important allergic manifestation that may occur in connection with serums is serum sickness as mentioned previously. Some people are allergic to the proteins in serum derived from the horse or some other animal, and show such symptoms as fever, vomiting, joint pain, enlargement of the regional lymph nodes, and hives or *urticaria* (ur-ti-ka′re-ah). This type of allergic reaction can be severe, but is rarely fatal.

Many drugs can bring about the allergic state, particularly aspirin, barbiturates, and the antibiotics (especially penicillin). In some cases of allergy, it is possible to desensitize a person by means of repeated injections of the offending allergen at short intervals. This form of protection, unfortunately, does not last long.

The antigen–antibody reaction in sensitive individuals may cause the release of excessive amounts of histamine. The histamine causes dilation and leaking from capillaries as well as contraction of involuntary muscles (*e.g.,* in the bronchi). Sometimes a group of drugs called antihistamines are effective in treating certain cases of allergy.

An interesting sidelight on some allergic disorders is that they are strongly associated with emotional disturbances. Asthma and *migraine* (mi′-grane), or sick headache, are two good examples of this type. In such disorders the interaction of body and mind still is not fully understood.

Autoimmunization

Autoimmunization (aw''to-im''u-ni-za'shun) refers to an abnormal reactivity to one's own tissues. The body's immune system reacts to its own cells as if they were foreign substances. Normally, the tolerance of the immune system to the body's tissues develops early in life. One theory is that the loss of this immune tolerance may be a cause of such disorders as rheumatic heart disease, glomerulonephritis, rheumatoid arthritis, and lupus erythematosus.

Transplants and the Rejection Syndrome

The hope that organs and tissues could be obtained from animals or other human beings to replace injured or incompetent parts of the body has long been under discussion. Much experimental work with *transplantation* (grafting) of organs and tissues in animals has preceded transplant operations in the human. Replacement by grafting of bone marrow, lymphoid tissue, skin, eye corneas, parathyroid glands, ovaries, kidneys, lungs, heart, liver, and uterus are among those that have been attempted. The natural tendency for every organism to reject foreign substances, especially tissues from another person or any other animal, has been the most formidable obstruction to complete success. This normal quality, an antigen-antibody reaction, has been called the *rejection syndrome.*

In all cases of transplanting or grafting, the tissues of the donor, the person donating the part, should be typed in much the same way that blood is typed whenever a transfusion is given. Blood types are much fewer in number than tissue substances; thus the process of obtaining matching blood is much less involved than is the process of trying to match tissues. Tissue typings are being done in a number of laboratories, and an effort is being made to obtain donors whose tissues contain relatively few antigens that might cause transplant rejection.

Because it has been impossible to completely match all the antigens of a donor with those of the recipient (the person receiving the part), drugs that suppress the action of antibodies against the transplanted organ are given to the recipients. The goal is to avoid suppressing the action of antibodies against organisms that might cause infection and, at the same time, prevent rejection of the transplant. Much of the reaction against the foreign material in transplants is believed to be generated by the thymus-derived T-lymphocytes. Drugs are being used to suppress the action of these cells without damaging the antibodies produced by the B-lymphocytes. The B cells produce humoral antibodies—those that circulate in the blood and lymph—and they are thought to be most important in preventing infections.

Summary

1 Influences on the occurrence of infection.
  A Portal of entry of pathogen.
  B Virulence of pathogen.
  C Number of pathogens.
  D Resistance of the body.
2 Defenses against disease.
  A Skin and mucous membranes.
  B Reflex actions.
  C Inflammation (phagocytosis).
  D Immunity (antibodies).
3 Immune process.
  A Pathogen contains antigens which stimulate antibody formation.
  B Antibodies destroy pathogens or neutralize toxins.
  C Immunity process is specific.
  D Mediated by lymphocytes.
4 Kinds of immunity.
  A Inborn (inherited)—species, racial, individual.
  B Acquired.
    (1) Naturally acquired—active or passive.
    (2) Artificially acquired—active or passive.
5 Acquired immunity.
  A Naturally acquired.
    (1) Active (by contracting disease).

(2) Passive (by transmission of antibodies through placenta).

B Artificially acquired.

   (1) Active (by administration of vaccine).

   (2) Passive (by administration of serum).

6 Vaccines and serums.

A Vaccines—cause tissues to produce antibodies; contain organism or toxoid. Examples—MMR, DPT, Sabin (for polio), rabies. Booster inoculations supplement vaccines, maintain immunity. Effects of vaccines long-lasting.

B Serums—provide antibodies directly; derived from blood serum of humans or horses and other animals. Examples—diphtheria, antivenin, botulism, Gamma globulins (human) given for measles, tetanus, hepatitis. Human serum administration avoids aller-

gic reactions to animal proteins. Effects of serums are of short duration.

7 Allergy.

A Some individuals are susceptible to allergens (usually foreign protein).

B Allergens cause antigen–antibody reaction in tissues, with accompanying irritation or other symptoms.

C Desensitization sometimes done. Antihistamines sometimes useful in treatment.

D Some allergies associated with nervous disturbances

8 Autoimmunization.

9 Transplants and the rejection syndrome.

A Normal antigen–antibody reaction.

B Suppress undesirable antibodies without injury to those needed to resist infection.

Questions and Problems

1 Name 4 conditions that determine whether or not an infection will occur in the body.

2 What are the body's "lines of defense" against disease?

3 Describe the process of inflammation.

4 Define immunity and describe its basic process.

5 Give 3 examples of inborn immunity.

6 What is the basic difference between inborn and acquired immunity?

7 Outline the various categories of acquired immunity and give an example of each.

8 What is a vaccine? A toxoid? Give examples of each. What is a booster shot?

9 What is a serum? Give examples. Define an antitoxin.

10 Name 2 origins of serums. Why is one sometimes used in preference to another?

11 Define allergy. How is its process like that of immunity, and how do they differ?

12 What is an allergen? Name some examples.

13 Name and describe some typical allergic disorders. Why would the diagnosis of some of these be especially difficult?

14 What does autoimmunization mean? Name 4 disorders.

15 What is meant by the rejection syndrome and what is being done to offset it?

Medical
Terminology

Medical terminology, the special language of the health occupations, is based upon an understanding of a relatively few basic elements. These elements—combining forms, roots, prefixes, and suffixes—form the foundation of almost all medical terms. A useful way to familiarize yourself with each term is to learn to pronounce it correctly and say it aloud several times. Soon it will become an integral part of your vocabulary.

The foundation of a word is the "word root." Examples of word roots are *abdomin-*, referring to the belly region; and *aden-*, pertaining to a gland. A word root is often followed by a vowel to facilitate pronunciation, as in *abdomino-* and *adeno-*. We then refer to it as a "combining form." The hyphen appended to a combining form indicates that it is not a complete word, and if the hyphen precedes the combining form, then it commonly appears as the terminal element or the word ending, as in *-algia*, meaning "a painful condition."

A "prefix" is a part of a word that precedes the word root and changes its meaning. For example, the prefix *mal-* in *malunion* means "an abnormal" union. A "suffix" or word ending is a part that follows the word root and adds to or changes its meaning. The suffix *-rrhea* means "profuse flow" or "discharge," as in *diarrhea*, a condition in which there is excessive discharge of liquid stools.

Many medical words are "compound" words; that is, they are made up of more than one root or combining form. Examples of such compound words are *erythrocyte* (red blood cell) and *hydrocele* (a fluid-containing sac), and many more difficult words, such as *sternoclavicular* (indicating relationship to both the sternum and the clavicle).

A general knowledge of language structure and spelling rules is also helpful in mastering medical terminology. For example, adjectives include words that end in *-al*, as in *sternal* (the noun is sternum), and words that end in *-ous*, as in *mucous* (the noun is mucus).

The following list includes some of the most commonly used word roots, combining forms, prefixes, and suffixes, and examples of their use.

a-, an- absent, deficient, lack of: *atrophy, anemia, anuria.*

ab- away from: *abduction, aboral.*

abdomin-, abdomino- the belly or abdominal area: *abdominalgia, abdominocentesis, abdominoscopy.*

acou- hearing, sound: *acoustic.*

acr-, acro- extreme ends of a part, especially of the extremities: *acral, acromegaly, acromion.*

actin-, actini-, actino- a relationship to raylike structures or, more commonly, to light or roentgen (x-) rays, or some other type of radiation: *actiniform, actinodermatitis.*

ad- (sometimes converted to ac-, af-, ag-, ap-, as-, at-) toward, added to, near: *adrenal, accretion, agglomerated.*

aden-, adeno- gland: *adenectomy, adenitis, adenocarcinoma.*

-agogue inducing, leading, stimulating: *cholagogue, galactagogue.*

alge-, algo-, algesi-, pain: *algetic, algophobia, algesia, analgesic.*

-algia pain, painful condition: *myalgia, neuralgia.*

amb-, ambi-, ambo- both, on two sides: *ambidexterity, ambivalent, amboceptor.*

ambly- dimness, dullness: *amblyopia.*

ant-, anti- against; to prevent, suppress, or destroy: *antarthritic, antibiotic, anticoagulant.*

ante- before, ahead of: *antenatal, antepartum.*

antero- a position ahead of or in front of (*i.e.,* anterior to) another part: *anterolateral, anteroventral.*

arthr-, arthro- joint or articulation: *arthral, arthrolysis, arthrostomy.*

-asis see -sis.

audio- sound, hearing: *audiogenic, audiometry, audiovisual.*

aut-, auto- self: *autistic, autodigestion, autoimmune.*

bi- two, twice: *bifurcate, bisexual.*

bio- life, a living organism: *biopsy, antibiotic.*

blast-, blasto-, -blast an early stage, an immature cell or a bud: *blastula, blastophore, erythroblast.*

blenn-, blenno- mucus: *blennuria, blennogenic, blennorrhea.*

bleph-, blephar-, blepharo- eyelid, eyelash: *blepharism, blepharitis, blepharospasm.*

brachi- arm: *brachial, brachiocephalic, brachiotomy.*

brachy- short: *brachydactylia, brachyesophagus.*

brady- slow: *bradycardia.*

bronch- windpipe or other air tubes: *bronchiectasis, bronchoscope.*

bucc- cheek: *buccally.*

carcin- cancer: *carcinogenic, carcinoma.*

cardi-, cardia-, cardio- heart: *carditis, cardiac, cardiologist.*

-cele swelling; an enlarged space or cavity: *cystocele, meningocele, rectocele.*

centi- relating to 100 (used in naming units of measurements): *centigrade, centimeter.*

cephal-, cephalo- head: *cephalalgia, cephalopelvic.*

cheil-, cheilo-, lips; a brim or an edge: *cheilitis, cheilosis.*

cheir-, cheiro- (also written **chir-, chiro-**) hand: *cheiralgia, cheiromegaly, chiropractic.*

chol-, chole-, cholo- bile, gall: *chologogue, cholecyst, cholecystitis, cholochrome.*

chondr-, chondri-, chondrio- cartilage: *chondric, chondrocyte, chondroma.*

chrono- time: *chronograph, chronology, chronophobia.*

-cid, -cide to cut, kill or destroy: *bactericidal, germicide, suicide.*

circum- around, surrounding: *circumoral, circumorbital, circumrenal.*

colp-, colpo- vagina: *colpectasia, colposcope, colpotomy.*

contra- opposed, against: *contraindication, contrastimulus.*

cost-, costa-, costo- ribs: *costiform, intercostal, costosternal.*

counter- against, opposite to: *counterirritation, countertraction.*

crani-, cranio- skull: *craniectomy, craniotomy.*

cry-, cryo-, crymo- low temperature: *cryalgesia, cryogenic, crymotherapy.*

crypt-, crypto- hidden, concealed: *cryptic, cryptogenic, cryptorchidism.*

cut- skin: *cutization, subcutaneous.*

cysti-, cysto- sac, bladder: *cystitis, cystoscope.*

cyt-, cyto-, -cyte cell: *cytemia, cytolytic, cytoplasm, erythrocyte.*

dacry-, dacryo- lacrimal glands: *dacryagogue, dacryocyst.*

dactyl-, dactylo- digits (usually fingers, but sometimes toes): *dactylitis, dactylology.*

derm-, derma-, dermo-, dermat-, dermato- skin: *dermic, dermatitis, dermatology, dermatosis.*

di-, diplo- twice, double: *diglossia, dimorphism, diplopia.*

dia- through, between, across, apart: *diaphragm, diaphysis.*

dis- apart, away from: *disarticulation, distal.*

dolicho- long: *dolichocephalic, dolichomorphic.*

dorsi-, dorso- back (in the human, this combining form refers to the same region as **postero-**): *dorsiflexion, dorsonuchal.*

-dynia pain, tenderness: *myodynia, neurodynia.*

dys- disordered, difficult, painful: *dysentery, dysphagia, dyspnea.*

-ectasis expansion, dilation, stretching: *angiectasis, bronchiectasis.*

ecto- outside, external: *ectoderm, ectogenous.*

-ectomize, -ectomy surgical removal or destruction by other means: *thyroidectomize, appendectomy.*

-emia blood: *glycemia, hyperemia.*

encephal-, encephalo- brain: *encephalitis, encephalogram.*

end-, endo- within, innermost: *endarterial, endocardium.*

enter-, entero- intestine: *enteritis, enterocolitis, enteroptosis.*

epi- on, upon: *epicardium, epidermis.*

eryth-, erythro- red: *erythema, erythrocyte.*

-esthesia sensation: *anesthesia, paresthesia.*

eu- well, normal, good: *euphoria, eupnea.*

ex-, exo- outside, out of, away from: *exanthem, excretion, exocrine.*

extra- beyond outside of, in addition to: *extracellular, extrasystole, extravasation.*

fasci- fibrous connective tissue layers: *fasciectomy, fasciitis, fascicle.*

-ferent to bear, to carry: *afferent, efferent.*

fibr- fibro- threadlike structures, fibers: *fibrillation, fibroblast, fibrositis.*

galact-, galacta-, galacto- milk: *galactemia, galactagogue, galactocele.*

gastr-, gastro- stomach: *gastritis, gastroenterostomy.*

-gen an agent which produces or originates: *allergen, pathogen.*

-genic produced from, producing: *endogenic, pyogenic.*

genito- organs of reproduction: *genitoplasty, genitourinary.*

geno- a relationship to reproduction or sex: *genodermatology, genotype.*

geny- jaw: *genyantrum, genyplasty.*

-geny manner of origin, development or production: *ontogeny, progeny.*

glio-, -glia a gluey material; specifically, the connective tissue of the brain: *glioma, neuroglia.*

gloss-, glosso- tongue: *glossitis, glossopharyngeal.*

gly-, glyco- sweet, relating to sugar: *glycemia, glycosuria.*

gon- seed; knee: *gonad, gonarthritis.*

-gram a record, that which is recorded: *electrocardiogram, electroencephalogram.*

-graph an instrument for recording: *electrocardiograph, electroencephalograph.*

gyn-, gyne-, gyneco-, gyno- female sex (women): *gynatresia, gynecology, gynecomastia, gynoplasty.*

hem-, hema-, hemato-, hemo- blood: *hematoma, hematuria, hemorrhage.*

hemi- one half: *hemianopia, heminephrectomy, hemiplegia.*

hepat-, hepato- liver: *hepatitis, hepatogenous.*

heter-, hetero- other, different: *heteradenoma, heterocrine, heterogeneous, heterosexual.*

hist-, histio- tissue: *histology, histicyte.*

homeo-, homos- unchanging, the same: *homeostasis, homosexual.*

hydr-, hydro- water: *dehydration, hydrocele, hydrocephalus.*

hyper- above, over, excessive: *hyperesthesia, hyperglycemia, hypertrophy.*

hypo- deficient, below, beneath: *hypochondrium, hypodermic, hypogastrium.*

hyster-, hystero- uterus: *hysterectomy, hysterodynia.*

-iatrics, -trics medical practice specialties: *pediatrics, obstetrics.*

idio- self, one's own, separate, distinct: *idiopathic, idiosyncrasy.*

ilio- flank, ilium (part of os coxae or hip bone): *iliocolotomy, iliotibial.*

im-, in- in, into; lacking: *implantation, inanimate, infiltration.*

inter- between: *intercostal, interstitial.*

intra- within a part or structure: *intracranial, intracellular, intraocular.*

-itis inflammation: *dermatitis, keratitis, neuritis.*

kerat-, kerato- cornea of the eye, certain horny tissues: *keratin, keratitis, keratoplasty.*

lact-, lacto- milk: *lactation, lactogenic.*

leuk-, leuko- (also written as **leuc-, leuco-**) white: *leukocyte* or *leucocyte, leukoplakia.*

lith-, litho- stones (also called calculi): *lithiasis, lithopedion.*

-logy, -ology the study of: *graphology, gynecology.*

lyso-, -lysis flowing, loosening, dissolution (dissolving of): *lysobacteria, hemolysis.*

macro- large, abnormal length: *macroblast, macrocolon.* See also **mega-, megalo-**.

mal- disordered, abnormal: *malnutrition, malocclusion, malunion.*

malac-, malaco-, -malacia softening: *malacoma, malacosarcosis, osteomalacia.*

mast-, masto- breast: *mastectomy, mastitis, mastocarcinoma.*

meg-, mega-, megal-, megalo- unusually or excessively large: *megacolon, megalencephalon, megaloblast.*

men- meno- physiologic uterine bleeding: *menses, menorrhagia.*

mening-, meningo- membranes covering the brain and spinal-cord: *meningitis, meningocele.*

ment-, mento- mind, chin: *menticide, dementia, mentolabial, mentum.*

mes-, mesa-, meso- middle, midline: *mesencephalon, mesaortitis, mesoderm.*

meta- a change, beyond, after, over, near *metabolism, metacarpus, metaplasia.*

micro- very small: *microabscess, microbiology, microcyte.*

my-, myo- muscle: *myenteron, myocardium, myometrium.*

myc-, mycet-, myco- fungi: *mycid, mycete, mycology, mycosis.*

myel-, myelo- marrow (often used in reference to the spinal cord): *myeloid, myeloblast, osteomyelitis, poliomyelitis.*

necr-, necro- death, corpse: *necrectomy, necropsy, necrosis.*

neo- new, strange: *neopathy, neoplasm.*

neph-, nephro- kidney: *nephrectomy, nephritis, nephron.*

neur-, neuro- nerve: *neuralgia, neuroma.*

noct-, nocti- night: *noctambulation, nocturia, noctiphobia.*

nos-, noso- disease: *nosema, nosophilia, nosophobe.*

ocul-, oculo- eye: *oculist, oculomotor, oculomycosis.*

odont-, odonto- teeth: *odontalgia, odontiasis, odontology.*

-oid likeness, resemblance: *lymphoid, myeloid.*

olig-, oligo- few, a deficiency: *oligemia, oligospermia, oliguria.*

-oma tumor, a swelling: *hematoma, sarcoma.*

onych-, onycho- nails: *paronychia, onychoma.*

oo-, ovi-, ovo- ovum, egg: *oocyte, oviduct, ovoplasm* (do not confuse with **oophor-**).

oophor-, oophoro- ovary: *oophorectomy, oophoritis, oophorocystectomy.* See **ovar-**.

ophthalm-, ophthalmo- eye: *ophthalmia, ophthalmologist, ophthalmoscope.*

orth-, ortho- straight, normal: *orthesis, orthodontist.*

oscillo- to swing to and fro: *oscillography, oscilloscope.*

oss-, osseo-, ossi-, oste-, osteo- bone, bone tissue: *ossature, osseous, ossicle, osteitis, osteomyelitis.*

-ostomy creation of a mouth or opening by surgery: *colostomy, gastroenterostomy.*

ot-, oto- ear: *otalgia, otitis, otomycosis.*

-otomy cutting into: *iliocolotomy, phlebotomy.*

ovar-, ovario- ovary: *ovariectomy, ovariorhexis.* See **oophor-.**

para- near, beyond, apart from, beside: *paramedical, parametrium, parathyroid.*

path-, patho-, -pathy disease, abnormal condition: *pathema, pathogen, pathognomonic, pathology, endocrinopathy.*

ped-, pedia- child; foot: *pedialgia, pedophobia, pediatrician.*

-penia lack of: *leukopenia, thrombocytopenia.*

per- through, excessively: *peracidity, percutaneous, perfusion.*

peri- around: *pericardium, perichondrium, periostitis.*

-pexy fixation: *nephropexy, proctopexy.*

phag-, phago- to eat, to ingest: *phage, phagocyte.*

-phagia, -phagy eating, swallowing: *aphagia, dysphagia, aerophagy.*

-phasia speech, ability to talk: *aphasia, dysphasia.*

-phil, -philic to be fond of, to like (have an affinity for): *eosinophilia, hemophilic.*

phleb-, phlebo- vein: *phlebitis, phleboclysis, phlebotomy.*

phob-, -phobia fear, dread, abnormal aversion: *phobic, acrophobia, hydrophobia, photophobia.*

pile-, pili-, pilo- hair, resembling hair: *pileous, piliation, pilonidal.*

-plasty molding, surgical formation: *gastroplasty, kineplasty.*

pleur-, pleuro- side, rib, the serous membrane covering the lung and lining the chest cavity: *pleurisy, pleurotomy.*

-pnea air, breathing: *dyspnea, eupnea.*

pneum-, pneuma-, pneumo-, pneumon-, pneumato- lung, air: *pneumectomy, pneumatics, pneumograph, pneumonia, pneumatocardia.*

pod-, podo- foot: *podiatry, pododynia.*

-poiesis making, forming: *erythropoiesis, hematopoiesis.*

polio- gray: *polioclastic, polioencephalitis, poliomyelitis.*

poly- many: *polyarthritis, polycystic.*

post- behind, after, following: *postnatal, postocular, postpartum.*

pre- before, ahead of: *precancerous, preclinical, prepatellar.*

presby- old age: *presbyophrenia, presbyopia.*

pro- in front of, before: *prodromal, prosencephalon, provitamin.*

proct-, procto- rectum: *proctitis, proctocele, proctologist, proctopexy.*

pseud-, pseudo- false: *pseudoarthrosis, pseudomania.*

psych-, psycho mind: *psychasthenia, psychosomatic, psychotherapy.*

-ptosis downward displacement, falling, prolapse: *enteroptosis, nephroptosis.*

pulmo-, pulmono- lung: *pulmonic, pulmonology, pulmotor.*

py-, pyo- pus: *pyuria, pyogenic, pyorrhea.*

pyel-, pyelo- kidney pelvis: *pyelitis, pyelogram, pyelonephrosis.*

rachi-, rachio- spine: *rachicentesis, rachischisis, rachiocentesis.*

radio- emission of rays or radiation: *radioactive, radiography, radiology.*

ren- kidney: *renal, renopathy.*

retro- backward, located behind: *retrocecal, retroperitoneal.*

rheo- flow of matter, or of a current of electricity: *rheology, rheoscope.*

rhin-, rhino- nose: *rhinitis, rhinophyma.*

-rrhage, -rrhagia excessive flow: *hemorrhage, menorrhagia.*

-rrhaphy suturing of or sewing up of a gap or defect in a part: *enterorrhaphy, perineorrhaphy.*

-rrhea flow, discharge: *diarrhea, gonorrhea, seborrhea.*

salping-, salpingo- tube: *salpingitis, salpingoscopy.*

scler-, sclero- hardness: *scleredema, scleroderma, sclerosis.*

scolio- twisted, crooked: *scoliosis, scoliosometer.*

-scope an instrument used to look into or examine a part: *bronchoscope, cystoscope, endoscope.*

semi- mild, partial, half: *semicanalis, semicoma.*

sep-, septic- poison, rot, decay: *sepsis, septicemia.*

-sis condition or process, usually abnormal: *dermatosis, enteroptosis.*

somat-, somato- body: *somatalgia, somatotype.*

sono- sound: *sonogram, sonography.*

splanchn-, splanchno- internal organs: *splanchnic, splanchnoptosis.*

sta-, stat- stop, stand still, remain at rest: *stasis, static.*

sten-, steno- contracted, narrowed: *stenosis, stenostomia.*

sthen-, stheno-, -sthenia, -sthenic strength: *sthenometry, sthenophotic, asthenia, asthenic.*

sub- under, below, near, almost: *subclavian, subcutaneous, subluxation.*

super- over, above, excessive: *superego, supernatant.*

supra- location above or over: *supranasal, suprarenal.*

sym-, syn- with, together: *symbiosis, symphysis, synapse.*

syring-, syringo- fistula, tube, cavity: *syringectomy, syringomyelia.*

tacho-, tachy- rapid, fast, swift: *tachogram, tachycardia.*

tars-, tarso- eyelid, foot: *tarsitis, tarsoplasty, tarsoptosis.*

-taxia, -taxis order, arrangement: *ataxia, chemotaxis, thermotaxis.*

tens- stretch, pull: *extension, tensor.*

therm-, thermo-, -thermy heat: *thermalgesia, thermocautery, diathermy.*

tox-, toxic-, toxico- poison: *toxemia, toxicology, toxicosis.*

trache- windpipe: *trachea, tracheitis, tracheotomy.*

trans- across, through, beyond: *transorbital, transpiration, transplantation.*

tri- three: *triad, triceps.*

trich-, tricho- hair: *trichiasis, trichocardia, trichosis.*

-trophic, -trophy nutrition (nurture): *atrophic, hypertrophy.*

-tropic turning toward, influencing, changing: *adrenotropic, gonadotropic, thyrotropic.*

ultra- beyond or excessive: *ultramicroscope, ultrasound, ultraviolet.*

uni- one: *unilateral, uniovular.*

-uria urine: *glycosuria, hematuria, pyuria.*

vas-, vaso- vessel, duct: *vascular, vasectomy, vasodilation.*

viscer-, viscero- internal organs: *viscera, visceroptosis.*

xero- dryness: *xeroderma, xerophthalmia, xerosis.*

Suggestions for
Further Study

Anderson L et al: Nutrition in Health and Disease, 17th ed. Philadelphia, JB Lippincott, 1982

Anderson WA and Fuller K: Pathology, 10th ed. St Louis, CV Mosby, 1980

Arey LB: Developmental Anatomy (embryology), 7th ed. Philadelphia, WB Saunders, 1974

Ayala FJ, Kiger JA Jr: Modern Genetics. Menlo Park, CA, Benjamin-Cummings, 1980

Barnhart ML et al: Sickle Cell. Kalamazoo, A Scope Publication, Upjohn, 1974

Beeson PB et al (eds): Cecil's Textbook of Medicine, 15th ed, Vol 1 & 2. Philadelphia, WB Saunders, 1979

Bellanti JA: Immunology: Basic Processes. Philadelphia, WB Saunders, 1979

Bevelander G, Ramsley J: Essentials of Histology, 8th ed. St Louis, CV Mosby, 1979

Boyd W, Sheldon H: Introduction to the Study of Disease, 8th ed. Philadelphia, Lea & Febiger, 1980

Brobeck JR (ed): Best & Taylor's Physiological Basis of Medical Practice, 10th ed. Baltimore, Williams & Wilkins, 1979

Brunner LS, Suddarth DS: Textbook of Medical-Surgical Nursing, 4th ed. Philadelphia, JB Lippincott, 1980

Brunner LS, Suddarth DS: The Lippincott Manual of Nursing Practice, 3rd ed. Philadelphia, JB Lippincott, 1982

Buchanan RE, Gibbons NE (eds): Bergey's Manual of Determinative Bacteriology, 8th ed. Baltimore, Williams & Wilkins, 1974

Burton GW: Microbiology for the Health Sciences. Philadelphia, JB Lippincott, 1979

Carter, S et al: Principles of Cancer Treatments. New York, McGraw-Hill, 1981

Chaffee EE, Lytle IM: Basic Physiology and Anatomy, 4th ed. Philadelphia, JB Lippincott, 1980

Conn HF (ed): Current Therapy. Philadelphia, WB Saunders, 1981

Creasy WA: Cancer, An Introduction. New York, Oxford University Press, 1981

Crouch JE: Functional Human Anatomy, 3rd ed. Philadelphia, Lea & Febiger, 1978

Crouch JE: Essential Human Anatomy. Philadelphia, Lea & Febiger, 1981

DeGroot LJ et al: Endocrinology. New York, Grune & Stratton, 1979

di Fiore M, Schmidt I: Atlas of Human Histology. Philadelphia, Lea & Febiger, 1981

Eckstein G: The Body Has a Head (abridged). New York, Bantam Books, 1980

Flitter H: An Introduction to Physics in Nursing, 7th ed. St Louis, CV Mosby, 1976

Frenay A: Understanding Medical Terminology, 6th ed. St Louis, The Catholic Hospital Assoc, 1977

Fudenberg HH, Stites DP, Caldwell JL et al (eds): Basic & Clinical Immunology, 3rd ed. Los Altos, CA, Lange Medical Publications, 1980

Ganong WF: Review of Medical Physiology, 10th ed. Los Altos, CA, Lang Medical Publications, 1981

Garb S: Laboratory Tests in Common Use, 6th ed. New York, Springer-Verlag, 1976

Gilbert E, Huntington R: An Introduction to Pathology. New York, Oxford University Press, 1978

Goldberger E: A Primer of Water, Electrolyte and Acid–Base Syndromes, 6th ed. Philadelphia, Lea & Febiger, 1980

Goodhard RS, Shils ME: Modern Nutrition in Health and Disease, 6th ed. Philadelphia, Lea & Febiger, 1980

Grammick R: Echocardiography. Journal of the American Medical Association, Vol 229, p 1099, Aug 1974.

Guyton AC: Basic Human Physiology, 2nd ed. Philadelphia, WB Saunders, 1977

Guyton AC: Physiology of the Human Body, 5th ed. Philadelphia, WB Saunders, 1981

Ham AW, Cormack D: Histology, 8th ed. Philadelphia, JB Lippincott, 1979

Hamilton H (ed): Nurses' Reference Library: Diagnostics. Horsham, PA, Intermed Communications, 1981

Hamilton, H (ed): Nurses' Reference Library: Drugs. Horsham, PA, Intermed Communications, 1982

Hole JW Jr: Human Anatomy and Physiology. Dubuque, Wm C. Brown, 1978

Holum JR: Elements of General and Biological Chemistry, 5th ed. New York, John Wiley & Sons, 1979

Jawetz E, Melnick JL, Adelberg EA: Review of Medical Microbiology, 14th ed. Los Altos, CA., Lange Medical Publications, 1980

King EM, Wieck L, Dyer M: Illustrated Manual of Nursing Techniques, 2nd ed. Philadelphia, JB Lippincott, 1981

Kozier B, Erb G: Fundamentals of Nursing: Concepts and Procedures, Reading, MA. Addison-Wesley Publishing Co, 1979

Krause MV, Mahan LK: Food, Nutrition and Diet Therapy, 6th ed. Philadelphia, WB Saunders, 1979

Lin-Fu, JS: Sickle Cell Anemia. Washington, DC, US Department of Health, Education, and Welfare, 1972

Merrell DJ: Ecological Genetics. Minneapolis, University of Minnesota Press, 1981

Metheny NM, Snively WD: Nurses' Handbook of Fluid Balance, 3rd ed. Philadelphia, JB Lippincott, 1979

Nagle JJ: Heredity and Human Affairs, 2nd ed. St Louis, CV Mosby, 1979

Naval Education and Training Program: The Metric System; America Measures Up. Washington, DC, United States Suprintendent of Documents, 1979

Nicksic E: The Plus and Minus of Fluids and Electrolytes. Reston, VA, Reston Publishing Co, 1981

Pansky B: Review of Gross Anatomy, 4th ed. London, Macmillan, 1979

Rodman MJ, Smith DW: Pharmacology and Drug Therapy in Nursing Text, 2nd ed. Philadelphia, JB Lippincott, 1979

Rothwell NV: Understanding Genetics, 2nd ed. New York, Oxford University Press, 1976

Rubens RD, Knight RK: A Short Textbook of Clinical Oncology. Philadelphia, JB Lippincott, 1980

Rubin P (ed): Clinical Oncology, 5th ed. Rochester, American Cancer Society, 1978

Sackheim G, et al: Chemistry for the Health Sciences, 3rd ed. New York, Macmillan, 1977

Schottelius BA, Schottelius DD: Textbook of Physiology, 18th ed. St Louis, CV Mosby, 1978

Smith AL: Microbiology and Pathology, 12th ed. St Louis, CV Mosby, 1980

Smith AL: Principles of Microbiology, 9th ed. St Louis, CV Mosby, 1981

Sobotta J: Atlas of Human Anatomy, 3 vols, 11th text ed. Baltimore, Urban and Schwarzenberg, 1978

Thompson RB: A Short Textbook of Haematology. Philadelphia, JB Lippincott, 1976

Thompson RB: Disorders of the Blood. New York, Churchill-Livingston, 1978

Turek SL: Orthopaedics, 3rd ed. Philadelphia, JB Lippincott, 1977

Vaughan D, Asbury T: General Ophthalmology, 9th ed. Los Altos, CA.; Lange, 1980

Volk WA, Wheeler MF: Basic Microbiology, 4th ed. Philadelphia, JB Lippincott, 1981

Vredevoe DL et al: Concepts of Oncology Nursing, New York, Prentice-Hall, 1981

Wintrobe MM et al: Clinical Hematology, 8th ed. Philadelphia, Lea & Febiger, 1981

Appendix

Typical Disease Conditions and Causative Organisms

Table 1   Bacterial diseases.

Organism	Disease and Description
Cocci	
Neisseria gonorrhoeae (gonococcus)	Gonorrhea. Acute inflammation of mucous membranes of the reproductive and urinary tracts (with possible spread to the peritoneum in the female). Bloodstream infection may cause gonococcal arthritis and endocarditis. Organism also causes ophthalmia neonatorum, an eye inflammation of the newborn.
Neisseria meningitidis (meningococcus)	Epidemic meningitis. Inflammation of the membranes covering brain and spinal cord.
Streptococcus pneumoniae (*Diplococcus pneumoniae*)	Pneumonia. Inflammation of the alveoli, bronchioles, and bronchi. May be prevented by use of polyvalent pneumococcal vaccine.
Staphylococcus aureus and other staphylococci	Boils, carbuncles, impetigo, osteomyelitis, staphylococcal pneumonia, cystitis, pyelonephritis, empyema, septicemia, and food poisoning. Strains resistant to antibiotics a cause of infections originating in the hospital such as wound infections.
Streptococcus pyogenes and *Streptococcus hemolyticus* plus other streptococci	Septicemia; septic sore throat; scarlet fever (an acute infectious disease characterized by red skin rash, sore throat, "strawberry" tongue, high fever, enlargement of lymph nodes); puerperal sepsis; erysipelas (an acute infection of skin, occurring in lymph channels, usually of face); streptococcal pneumonia; rheumatic fever (an inflammation of the joints, usually progressing to heart disease); subacute bacterial endocarditis (an inflammation of the heart valves); acute glomerulonephritis (inflammation of the glomeruli).
Bacilli	
Escherichia coli, Proteus bacilli, and other colon bacilli	Normal inhabitants of the colon, and usually harmless there. Cause of local and systemic infections; diarrhea (especially in children); septicemia and septic shock. *E. coli* is the most common organism in hospital-transmitted infections.
Pseudomonas aeruginosa	Ubiquitous organism is a frequent cause of wound and urinary infections in debilitated hospitalized patients. Often found in solutions that have been standing for long periods.
Mycobacterium tuberculosis (tubercle bacillus)	Tuberculosis. An infectious disease in which the organism causes primary lesions called tubercles. These break down into cheeselike masses of tissue, a process known as caseation. Any body organ can be infected, but in adults the usual site is the lungs; still one of the most widespread diseases in the world, treated with chemotherapy; resistant strains have developed.
Mycobacterium leprae (Hansen's bacillus)	Leprosy. A chronic illness in which hard swellings occur under the skin, particularly of the face, causing a grotesque appearance. In one form of leprosy the nerves are affected, resulting in loss of sensation in the extremities.
Legionella pneumophila	Legionnaires' disease (pneumonia). Seen in localized epidemics, may be transmitted by air conditioning towers and by contaminated soil at excavation sites. Not spread person to person. Characterized by high fever, vomiting, diarrhea, cough, and bradycardia. Mild form of the disease called Pontiac Fever.
Clostridium tetani	Tetanus. Acute, often fatal poisoning caused by introduction of the organism into deep wounds. Characterized by severe muscular spasms. Also called lockjaw.
Clostridium perfringens	Gas gangrene. An acute wound infection. The organisms cause death of tissues accompanied by the generation of gas within them.
Clostridium botulinum	Botulism. A very severe poisoning caused by eating food in which this organism has been allowed to grow and excrete its toxin. Can cause paralysis of the muscles, death from asphyxiation.
Bacillus anthracis	Anthrax. A disease acquired from animals. Characterized by a primary lesion called a pustule. Can develop into a fatal septicemia.
Corynebacterium diphtheriae	Diphtheria. Acute inflammation of the throat with the formation of a leathery membranelike growth (pseudomembrane) which can obstruct air passages and cause death by asphyxiation. Toxin produced by this organism can damage heart, nerves, kidneys, etc. Disease preventable by appropriate vaccination.

Table 1 *Bacterial diseases. (continued)*

Organism	Disease and Description
Bordetella pertussis	Pertussis (whooping cough). Severe infection of the trachea and bronchi. The "whoop" is caused by the effort to recover breath after coughing. All children should be inoculated with appropriate vaccine.
Salmonella typhi (and others)	Salmonellosis occurs as enterocolitis, bacteremia, localized infection or typhoid. Depending on type, presenting symptoms may be fever, diarrhea, abscesses; complications include intestinal perforation and endocarditis. Carried in water, milk, meat, and other food.
Shigella dysenteriae (and others)	A serious bacillary dysentery. An acute intestinal infection with diarrhea (sometimes bloody); may cause dehydration with electrolyte imbalance or septicemia. Transmitted through fecal oral route or other poor sanitation.
Yersinia pestis (formerly called *Pasteurella pestis*)	Plague, the "black death" of the Middle Ages. Transmitted by fleas from infected rodents to humans. Symptoms of the most common form are swollen, infected lymph nodes or buboes, another form may cause pneumonia. All forms may lead to a rapidly fatal septicemia.
Francisella tularensis	Tularemia or deer fly fever. Transmitted by contact with an infected animal or bite of tick or fly. Symptoms are fever, ulceration of the skin, enlarged lymph nodes.
Brucella abortus (and others)	Brucellosis or undulant fever is a disease of animals such as cattle and goats. Transmitted to humans through unpasteurized dairy products or undercooked meat. Acute phase of fever and weight loss; chronic disease with abscess formation and depression.

Note: The following organisms are smaller than other bacteria and vary in shape. They grow within cells as do the viruses but differ in that they are affected by antibiotics.

Chlamydia psittaci	Psittacosis is also called ornithosis and is transmitted by various birds, including parrots, ducks, geese, and turkeys. Primary symptoms are chills, headache, and fever, more severe in older persons. The duration may be from 2 to 3 weeks, often with a long convalescence. Antibiotic drugs are effective remedies.
Chlamydia trachomatis (the same organism causes trachoma)	Lymphogranuloma venereum (LGV) is a venereal disease, characterized by swelling of inguinal lymph nodes, accompanied by signs of general infection. Later scar tissue forms in the genital region, possibly resulting in complete rectal stricture.
Chlamydia trachomatis	Trachoma. A common cause of blindness in underdeveloped areas of the world. An infection of the conjunctiva and cornea; characterized by redness, pain, and lacrimation. Antibiotic therapy effective if begun before there is scarring.
Chlamydia oculogenitalis	Inclusion conjunctivitis, acute eye infection. Carried in genital organs, transmitted during birth or through water in inadequately chlorinated swimming pools.
Rickettsia prowazekii	Epidemic typhus. Transmitted between humans by lice; associated with poor hygiene and war. Main symptoms are headache, hypotension, delirium, and a red rash. Frequently fatal in older persons.
Rickettsia typhi	Endemic or murine typhus. A milder disease transmitted to man from rats by fleas. Symptoms are fever, rash, headache, and cough. Rarely fatal.
Rickettsia rickettsii	Rocky Mountain spotted fever. A tickborne disease occurring throughout the United States. Symptoms are fever, muscle aches, and a rash that may progress to gangrene over bony prominances. Rarely fatal.
Coxiella burnetii	Q fever. An infection transmitted from cattle, sheep, and goats to man by contaminated dust and also carried by arthropods. Symptoms are fever, headache, chills, and pneumonitis. Practically never fatal.
Curved, Wavy or Corkscrew Rods ***Spirilla*** *Vibrio cholerae* (*Vibrio comma*)	Cholera. Acute infection of the intestine characterized by prolonged vomiting and diarrhea, leading to severe dehydration, electrolyte imbalance, and in some cases, death.

(continued)

Table 1   *Bacterial diseases.* (*continued*)

Organism	Disease and Description
Spirochetes	
Treponema vincentii (formerly called *Borelia vincentii* or *Spirillum vincentii*)	Vincent's angina (trench mouth). Infection of the mouth and throat accompanied by formation of a pseudomembrane, and with ulceration.
Borrelia recurrentis (and others)	Relapsing fever. A generalized infection in which attacks of fever alternate with periods of apparent recovery. Organisms spread by lice, ticks, etc.
Leptospira	Leptospirosis is an infection of rodents and certain domestic animals transmitted to man by way of contaminated water or by direct contact. The organisms may penetrate the mucous membranes and broken skin. It causes hepatitis, with or without jaundice, nephritis and meningitis.
Treponema pallidum	Syphilis. An infectious disease transmitted mainly by sexual intercourse. Untreated syphilis is seen in the following three stages. Primary—formation of primary lesion (chancre). Secondary—skin eruptions and infectious patches on mucous membranes. Tertiary—development of generalized lesions (gummas), destruction of tissues resulting in aneurysm, heart disease, degenerative changes in brain, spinal cord and ganglia, meninges.
	Also a cause of intrauterine fetal death or stillbirth.
Treponema pertenue	Yaws. A tropical disease characterized by lesions of the skin, deformities of hands, feet, and face.

Table 2   *Fungous diseases.*

Disease	Description
Candidiasis	An infection that can involve the skin and mucous membranes. May cause diaper rash, infection of the nail beds, infection of the mucous membranes of the mouth, throat, and vagina.
Histoplasmosis	This fungus may cause a variety of disorders ranging from mild respiratory symptoms or enlargement of liver, spleen and lymph nodes to cavities in the lungs with symptoms similar to tuberculosis.
Ringworm (tinea capitis) (tinea corporis) (tinea pedis)	Common fungous infections of the skin, many of which cause blisters and scaling with discoloration of the affected area. All are caused by similar organisms from a group of fungi called dermatophytes. They are easily transmitted from person to person or by contaminated articles.
Actinomycosis	"Lumpy jaw," which occurs in cattle and humans. The organisms cause large masses of tissue to form, and these masses are often accompanied by abscesses. The lungs and liver may be involved.
Blastomycosis	A general term for any infection caused by a yeastlike organism. There may be skin tumors and lesions in the lungs, bones, liver, spleen, and kidneys.
Coccidioidomycosis	Also called San Joaquin Valley fever. It is another systemic fungous disease. Because it often attacks the lungs, it may be mistaken for tuberculosis.

Table 3 *Viral diseases.*

Disease	Description
Chickenpox (varicella)	A usually mild infection, almost completely confined to children, characterized by blister-like skin eruptions.
Shingles (herpes zoster)	The cause of this disease is the virus of chickenpox. Herpes is a very painful eruption of blisters of the skin which follow the course of certain peripheral nerves. These blisters eventually dry up and form scabs that resemble shingles.
Cold sores (herpes simplex)	Cold sores or fever blisters appearing about the mouth and nose of patients with colds or other illness accompanied by fever. This condition should not be confused with herpes zoster.
Measles (rubeola)	Acute respiratory inflammation followed by fever and a generalized skin rash. Patients are prone to develop dangerous complications, such as bronchopneumonia and other secondary infections caused by staphylococci and streptococci.
Yellow fever	An acute infectious tropical disease transmitted by the bite of an infected mosquito. The disease is marked by jaundice, severe gastrointestinal symptoms, stomach hemorrhaging, and nephritis which may be fatal.
Infectious hepatitis	Liver inflammation caused by type A hepatitis virus. The portal of entry and exit is often, but not always, the digestive tract.
Serum hepatitis	Liver disease caused by type B hepatitis virus. It was formerly thought to be transmitted by injection into the tissues or blood as by contaminated needles, surgical instruments, blood specimens. It is now known that this virus may also enter by the oral route. It is a more serious and prolonged illness than is infectious hepatitis.
Poliomyelitis	An acute viral infection which may attack the anterior horns of the spinal cord, resulting in paralysis of certain voluntary muscles. The degree of permanent paralysis depends upon the extent of damage sustained by the motor nerves. Three types of causative viruses are known (Types 1, 2, and 3).
Rabies	An acute, fatal disease transmitted to man through the saliva of an infected animal. Rabies is characterized by violent muscular spasms induced by the slightest sensations. Because the swallowing of water causes spasms of the throat, the disease is also called hydrophobia ("fear of water"). There is a final stage of paralysis ending in death.
Viral encephalitis	"Encephalitis" usually is understood to be any brain inflammation accompanied by degenerative tissue changes, and it can have many causes besides viruses. There are several forms of viral encephalitis (Western and Eastern epidemic, equine, St. Louis, Japanese B, etc.), some of which are known to be transmitted from birds and other animals to man by insects, principally mosquitoes.
Mumps (epidemic parotitis)	Acute inflammation with swelling of the parotid salivary glands. Mumps can have many complications, such as orchitis (an inflammation of the testes), especially in children.
German measles (rubella)	A less severe form of measles, but especially dangerous during the first 3 months of pregnancy because the disease organism can cause heart defects, deafness, mental deficiency, and other permanent damage in the fetus.
Common cold (coryza)	Viral infection of the upper respiratory tract. Victims are highly susceptible to complications such as pneumonia and influenza.
Influenza	An epidemic viral infection, marked by chills, fever, muscular pains, and prostration. The most serious complication is bronchopneumonia caused by *Hemophilus influenzae* (a bacillus) or streptococci.
Genital herpes	An acute inflammatory disease of the genitalia, often recurring. Caused by herpes simplex II virus. A very common venereal disease.

Table 4 *Protozoal diseases.*

Organism	Disease and Description
Amebae	
Entamoeba histolytica	Amebic dysentery. Severe ulceration of the wall of the large intestine caused by amebae. Acute diarrhea may be an important symptom. This organism also may cause liver abscesses.
Ciliates	
Balantidium coli	Gastrointestinal disturbances and ulcers of the colon.
Flagellates	
Giardia lamblia	Gastrointestinal disturbances.
Trichomonas vaginalis	Inflammation and discharge from the vagina of the female. In the male it involves the urethra and causes painful urination.
Trypanosoma	African sleeping sickness. Disease begins with a high fever, followed by invasion of the brain and spinal cord by the organisms. Usually the disease ends with continued drowsiness, coma, and death.
Leishmania donovani (and others)	Kala-azar. A disease in which there is enlargement of the liver and spleen, as well as skin lesions.
Sporozoa	
Plasmodium; varieties include *vivax, falciparum, malariae*	Malaria. Characterized by recurrent attacks of chills followed by high fever. Severe attacks of malaria can be fatal because of kidney failure, cerebral disorders, and other complications.
Toxoplasma gondii	Toxoplasmosis is a common infectious disease transmitted by cats and raw meat. Mild forms cause fever and enlargement of lymph nodes. Infection of a pregnant woman is a cause of fetal stillbirth or congenital damage.

Index

Page numbers followed by *t* indicate tabular material; page numbers in *italics* indicate glossary terms.